MEDICINE IN NORTHUMBRIA

ESSAYS ON THE HISTORY OF MEDICINE IN THE NORTH EAST OF ENGLAND

MEDICINE IN NORTHUMBRIA

ESSAYS ON THE HISTORY OF MEDICINE IN THE NORTH EAST OF ENGLAND

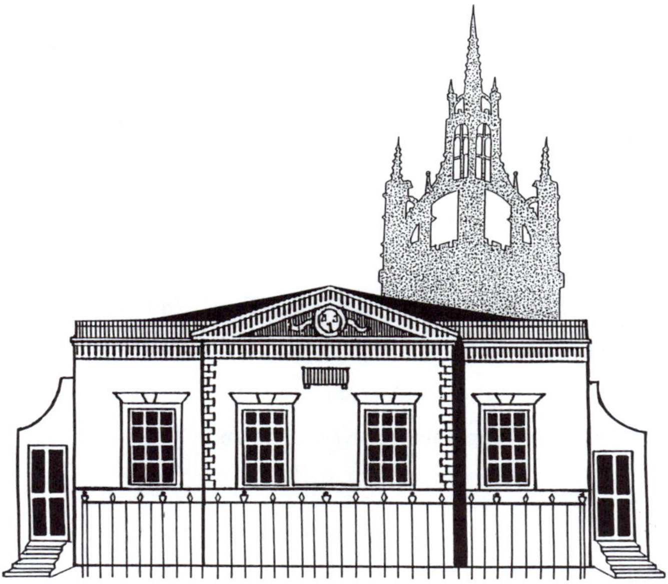

THE PYBUS SOCIETY
FOR THE HISTORY AND BIBLIOGRAPHY OF MEDICINE
Newcastle-upon-Tyne

Imageset by Alpha Word Power for the Pybus Society
1993

First published 1993 by

The Pybus Society for the History and Bibliography of Medicine,
c/o The Children's Department, Newcastle General Hospital,
Westgate Road, Newcastle upon Tyne NE4 6BE.

Edited by

David Gardner-Medwin, Anne Hargreaves and Elizabeth Lazenby

Cover designed by Elizabeth Lazenby

Imageset by Alpha Word Power, Durham

Printed by Athenaeum Press Limited, Newcastle upon Tyne

ISBN: 0 9522097 0 5

Readers may be amused to identify the following people and buildings on the cover: Saxon Leeches, Hewson, Trotter, Heysham, Snow, Johnston, St. Nicholas Church, the Barber Surgeons' Hall, Bell's Court door, the old Infirmary, Dispensary, Lying-in Hospital, House of Recovery, Floating Hospital, High Level Bridge and Tyne Bridge.

CONTENTS

LIST OF FIGURES

LIST OF THE AUTHORS

Lindsay Allason-Jones BA, MLitt, FSA, FSA (Scot), MIFA. Archaeological Museums Officer for the University of Newcastle upon Tyne. Author of a number of books and articles on Roman artefacts from Britain and Europe.

CN Armstrong MD (Dunelm), B Hyg, DPH, FRCP. Consultant Physician to the Royal Victoria Infirmary, Newcastle upon Tyne, 1931-1962; formerly Subdean and Lecturer in Clinical Medicine, University of Newcastle upon Tyne and Director of the Regional Postgraduate Institute of Medicine and Dentistry.

Anthony Ashcroft MD, FRCGP. Retired General Practitioner.

GAG Binnie MRCGP, LRCP&S (Edin), DObstRCOG. General Practitioner in a rural dispensing single-handed practice in Norham, near Berwick on Tweed and Clinical Assistant in Accident and Emergency and Ophthalmology to Berwick Infirmary, 1964-1990. Librarian of the Berwickshire Naturalists' Club.

W Alec Campbell DSc, MLitt, FRSC. Chartered chemist.

E J Carmichael MB BS(Dunelm) FRCGP. Retired Family Doctor.

Gordon Dale MD, BSc (Newcastle), MBBS (Dunelm). Senior Lecturer in Paediatric Biochemistry, University of Newcastle upon Tyne; Consultant Chemical Pathologist, Newcastle General Hospital.

Hewan A Dewar MD (Dunelm), FRCP. Formerly Consultant Physician and Cardiologist to the Royal Victoria Infirmary, Newcastle upon Tyne.

Joan S Emmerson MA (Dunelm). Formerly Medical Librarian at the University of Newcastle upon Tyne. Pybus Fellow 1966-68.

Rex Gardner FRCOG, MA, FSA (Scot). Consultant Obstetrician and Gynaecologist, Sunderland Hospitals (retired).

David Gardner-Medwin MD, FRCP. Consultant Paediatric Neurologist, Newcastle General Hospital. Honorary Secretary of the Pybus Society.

Elspeth M Gould RGN, RSCN, RM, RHV. Senior Health Adviser in the Department of Genito-Urinary Medicine (formerly the Joint Committee's Venereal Diseases Clinic, then known as Ward 34) at Newcastle General Hospital.

Ralph Wales Gould MB BS (Dunelm). Retired General Practitioner.

John R Guy BA, PhD, ARHistS. Vicar of Betws Cedewain, a rural parish in mid-Wales. Author of a number of papers on various aspects of medical history; co-editor of the Proceedings of the 12th Congress of the BSHM - *A Pox on the Provinces!* published by Bath University Press in 1990. Currently working on a biography of the 19th century public health reformer, Thomas Southwood Smith.

Reginald R Hall MS, FRCS. Consultant Urologist, Freeman Hospital, Newcastle upon Tyne and Senior Lecturer in Urology, University of Newcastle Medical School. Special interest in urological oncology.

G E M Hallett LDS, MDS, FDSRCS Eng and Edin, FFDRCS Ire, Hon FDSRCPS Glas, Silver Medal Ville de Paris. Emeritus Professor of Child Dental Health and former Dean of Dentistry, University of Newcastle upon Tyne.

A S Hargreaves BDS, PhD. Clinical Lecturer, University of Newcastle upon Tyne. Chairman of the Lindsay Society for the History of Dentistry.

W P Honeyman BSc, MB, ChB. Retired General Practitioner, has a longstanding interest in the medical history of Carlisle, where he was born and worked. As a trustee for a medical charity fund arising from the Carlisle Dispensary, founded by Dr Heysham, he has access to records of medicine as practised in Carlisle in the 18th and 19th centuries.

David Knight is Professor of History and Philosophy of Science in the University of Durham. His most recent books are *Ideas in Chemistry: a History of Science*, and *Humphrey Davy: Science and Power*. He is, this year, President of the Historical Section of the BAAS, and Vice-President of the Society for the History of Natural History. He is working on the theme of mastering nature in the early nineteenth century.

Elizabeth Lazenby BA. Department of Classics, University of Newcastle upon Tyne. Research in scientific and medical Latin.

John Le Gassicke FRCP, FRCPsych. Consultant Psychiatrist to the Northern Regional Health Authority 1964-88. Member and former member of Council of the Society of Antiquaries of Newcastle upon Tyne.

SW Stuart Menzies MB, BS, MRCGP, D Obst RCOG. For 28 years General Practitioner in North Shields. General interest in history of medicine, medical biography and medical philately. Honorary Treasurer, the Pybus Society.

F J W Miller MD, FRCP, DCH. Formerly Reader in Social Paediatrics at the University of Newcastle upon Tyne and Honorary Consultant Physician to the Children's Department, Royal Victoria Infirmary, Newcastle. Honorary Lecturer in the History of Medicine, University of Newcastle.

E A Spriggs DM, FRCP (1919-1989). Formerly Consultant Physician, Newcastle General Hospital. Joint Founder of the Pybus Club and Society. See Chapter 26.

Nicholas Wilford Medical Student, University of Newcastle upon Tyne. William Hume prizewinner 1991.

W Keith Yeates MS, FRCS. Formerly Consultant Urologist, Newcastle General Hospital and Freeman Hospital, Newcastle upon Tyne. Past President and recipient of the St Peter's medal of the British Association of Urological Surgeons. Past Editor of the British Journal of Urology. Through a long and distinguished career he made a major contribution to British and international urology. He completed work on the manuscript for this book a few days before he died on 26 July 1992.

PREFACE

The best reason for reading the history of medicine is the fun of it. But it also puts into perspective the fashions of today.

E A Spriggs

This book is the first publication of the Pybus Society for the History and Bibliography of Medicine, so both the Society and the book require some explanation.

There has been a series of clubs with an interest in the history of medicine in Newcastle at least since the early 1950s, some more ephemeral than others. The Pybus Society's origins are briefly described in the account of its principal founder, Dr E A Spriggs, in the last chapter of this book. In its present form it was revived on 26 September 1986 and since then it has met five or six times each year to discuss topics from the whole range of medical history, though often they have had a local theme. Most of the speakers have been from among our 50 or so members. In parallel, and without rivalry, our sister association, the Pybus Club, has held regular meetings since 1975, arranged by Mr James Longrigg in the Department of Classics at the University. It has no formal membership, but holds seminars three times a year, almost always with invited speakers and on medical themes from Classical or Arabian antiquity. Every year we meet jointly for the Spriggs Memorial Lecture, organised alternately by the Club and the Society.

The book was conceived as a contribution to the history of medicine in the northern counties of England (County Durham and Northumberland, with one excursion into Cumbria) to mark the 15th meeting of The British Society for the History of Medicine, to be held in Newcastle in September 1993. It is offered to those who attend the conference as a substitute for the usual volume of Proceedings in the hope that it may be of interest both to them and to a wider and less transient readership, which conference proceedings seldom seem to be.

It was plain at once that the book must be a miscellany rather than a consecutive or complete account, and we decided to try to make it of interest to local doctors and students of medicine as well as to medical historians.

The breadth of the historical interests in the Society is reflected in the fact that all but four of the contributors are members. We are particularly grateful to the four 'guests', Dr C N Armstrong and Dr Hewan Dewar whose seniority excuses them from being members of anything, and Rev John Guy and Dr Patt Honeyman who have the misfortune to live elsewhere. Dr Armstrong's contribution is mentioned below. Dr Dewar has written a personally observed account of the development of cardiology in Newcastle, one of only three such accounts of the 20th century scene in the book. His emphasis on the pioneer cardiologist Sir William Hume is particularly apposite because Hume was also one of the most notable of Newcastle's medical historians. Indeed, it was Sir William's name that the Pybus Society gave to its annual Student Essay Prize. John Guy submitted the title of a paper for the congress which was obviously right for the book and he kindly allowed us to use it without a murmur of protest. Dr Patt Honeyman presented an account of the Carlisle Dispensary at one of our meetings and kindly agreed to write a chapter about its principal founder, John Heysham.

One chapter is reprinted, with the editor's very kind permission, from *Medical History* - it seemed right to include one of Tony Spriggs' papers, although he had died before either the Congress or the book was planned. We chose his account of John Hutchinson, the inventor of the spirometer, who was a Newcastle man though his medical and scientific work was done in London. All the other chapters are new, and many of them make original contributions. Sadly, one of our contributors, Keith Yeates, died while the book was in an early stage of planning. But he had written a first draft, and we are indebted to his colleague and friend Mr Reg Hall, for completing the manuscript and indeed including information about Keith's own contributions to the development of urology in Newcastle which he himself might modestly have left out.

For some of the authors this is their first venture into print; others are experienced historians. One, Nick Wilford, is a medical student, the first winner of the Sir William Hume Prize. Another, Dr C N Armstrong, is something of a historical figure himself; he was appointed to the consultant staff of the Royal Victoria Infirmary in 1931, retired in 1962, and remains an active member of the Newcastle medical community in 1993. In July 1991 he addressed the Thyroid Club at the meeting held in Newcastle to celebrate the 100th anniversary of the first use of thyroid extract in the treatment of myxoedema, and he has kindly let us print his account of that important event in Newcastle's medical history. His chapter reproduces in full the minutes of the meetings of the Northumberland and Durham Medical Society at which Dr George Murray first presented the earliest cases in the world of effective hormone replacement therapy.

The Pybus Society exists to further not only the history, but the bibliography of medicine. To be truthful, we have never really lived up to that part of our title. But we are conscious that the Society's origin stems from a bibliophile's club of the 1950s. Joan Emmerson was later a member of that club and she has contributed a chapter on the three great collections of early medical books which we are proud and fortunate to have in the university libraries of the North East.

As editor I am grateful to many people: – To all the authors for their hard work, promptness, enthusiasm and forbearance; to my secretary Susan Robinson for her constant cheerful support, even after many long and tedious evenings of typing; to Elizabeth Lazenby for her many-talented assistance in finding missing references, designing the cover, drawing several of the illustrations, creating the index and undertaking the final stages of the production of all the 'camera-ready copy'; to Anne Hargreaves for an immense amount of help with the editing and for setting high standards which she has, and I suspect I have not, always maintained; to Peter Hughes and Terry Dobson of Alpha Word Power; and to the printers, Athenaeum Press.

DGM

Iuniperus.

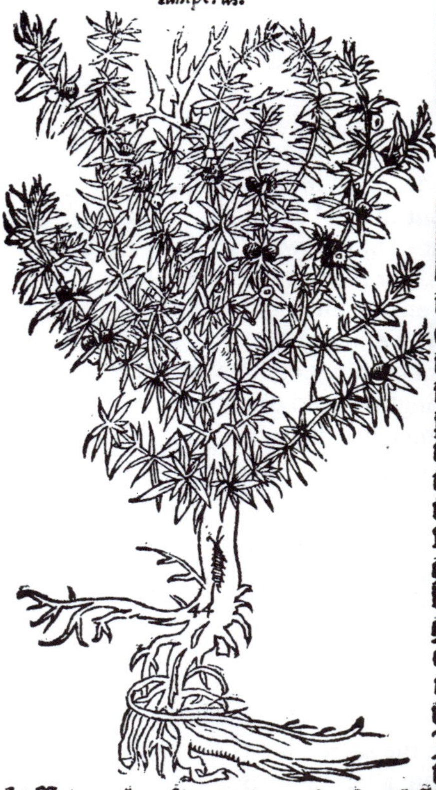

Iuniperus is called in Greke Arkēthos/in Englishe Juniper or Jeneper/in Duch wachholđ/ in Frenche du geneure.

The Description.

Dioscorides maketh ij. kindes of Juniper/the greater kinde & the lesse/ whiche only differ in bignes. Juniper both the greater & the lesse is alwayes grene & hath in the stede of leaues prickes rather thē right leaues/and euery suche leafe or pricke is very like vnto ỷ ende of the tonge/ of an hueholl or wodspike/but it is grene/the wod is redish/ whiche if it be put into the fyer/ maketh a very good smell. The berries are first grene and afterwarde black. Some holde ỷ ỷ berries are ij. yeare in ripinge vpon the tree. This tree groweth commenly in great wast & wilde mores & baron groundes/ but somtyme it groweth in metly good groundes/ In England it groweth most plentuouslye in Kent/ it groweth also in ỷ bysshopryche of Durram/ & in Northũberlande. It groweth in Germany in many places in greate plentye / but in no place in greater then a lytle from Bon/ wher as/ at the tyme of yeare the feldefares fede only of Junipers berries/the people eate the feldefares vndrawē wyth guttes and all/because they are full of the berries of Juniper.

The vertues of Iuniper.

Ther are ij. kindes of Juniper/the greater & the lesse/ they are bothe hote/ & stir men to make water/ & if ỷ they be sette a fier/ they dryue awaye serpentes. The berries do measerablely hete & binde/ & are good for the stomacke. They are good to be dronken agaynst the diseases of the brest/agaynst the cough/ agaynst winde/ gnawinges & bytinge of serpentes. They dryue fourth vrine/ they are good for places burst & shronken

The Juniper, from *The seconde parte of William Turners Herball....1568.* The leaves are likened to the tongue of the 'hueholl or wodespike' (woodpecker). There is still a juniper forest by High Force in the 'bysshopryche of Durram', but in the North East we have never shared the culinary habits of Bonn. The 44 on the stem corresponds to the page in Fuchs, possibly in his *Effigies* of 1552, on which the same figure appears in miniature and in reverse, but more probably in his *Primi de stirpium* .... of 1545, where the cuts are the same in size and orientation. The numbering differs in Fuchs' *De historia stirpium* of 1542 and *New kreuterbuch* of 1543 (cuts reversed and larger).This is a heavily disguised *corrigendum* for page 4.

For from the birth
Of mortal man, the Sovereign Maker said,
That not in humble nor in brief delight,
Not in the fading echoes of renown,
Power's purple robes, nor pleasure's flowery lap,
The soul should find enjoyment: but from these
Turning disdainful to an equal good,
Through all the ascent of things enlarge her view,
Till every bound at length should disappear,
And infinite perfection close the scene.

Book 1: 211-220

Know then, the sov'reign spirit of the world,
.... beholding in the sacred light
Of his essential reason, all the shapes
Of swift contingence, all successive ties
Of action propagated through the sum
Of possible existence, he at once
Down the long series of eventful time
So fix'd the dates of being, so dispos'd,
To every living soul of every kind
The field of motion and the hour of rest,
That all conspired to his supreme design,
To universal good: ...

Book 2: 307, 323-33

Mark Akenside, MD
The Pleasures of Imagination

Chapter 1

INTRODUCTION

'Down the Long Series of Eventful Time'

David Gardner-Medwin

'The fading echoes of renown'

Two hundred and fifty years ago, in the summer and autumn of 1743, Mark Akenside, having recently returned to Newcastle after his medical training in Edinburgh, advertised as a Surgeon and waited for work. But on his mind was his long didactic poem, *The Pleasures of Imagination*, which he completed that summer. It made his reputation and the beginning of his fortune (he sold it early in 1744, for £120). Its language and philosophy are out of tune with our own, and it never had the wisdom or the wealth of observation and experience of some other poetry of its genre, such as Erasmus Darwin's *The Temple of Nature* (1803); but it fired the public imagination of its day, and if we can not quite see why, we may still enjoy some of its more felicitous lines. With the *Pleasures* off his chest, Akenside went to Leiden to write his MD thesis. On his return he failed to establish himself in practice in Northampton before embarking on two careers in London, as a fashionable poet and as a physician, in both of which he perhaps achieved more contemporary eminence than lasting fame.[1] One notable medical contribution however was a case report presented to the College of Physicians on 6 July 1767, which is now recognised as the earliest identifiable description of neurofibromatosis.[2] It is an attractively clear account but deplorably lacking in any spirit of enquiry; von Recklinghausen's definitive clinico-pathological account in 1882 properly earned him the eponym. Mark Akenside had been born in Newcastle where his father's butcher's shop, on Butcher's Bank near All Saints Church, later became a place of pilgrimage for his admirers. The old street has gone now, but its replacement is called Akenside Hill.[3]

Akenside was one of many able doctors who were born or brought up in the North East but afterwards made their careers elsewhere, including, for example, William Turner in the 16th century, Samuel Garth (author of the poem *The Dispensary*)[4] in the 17th, Anthony Askew[5] in the 18th and Thomas Addison,[6] John Hutchinson, Samuel Fenwick,[7] John Snow and Byrom Bramwell[8] in the 19th. Turner will be mentioned shortly, and Hutchinson and Snow have chapters to themselves in this miscellany; the others must be content with footnotes. There are innumerable other interesting and indeed important people, places, events, institutions and ideas in the medical history of our area that have been passed over, by whim or circumstance, in the selection of material for this book. Some have been adequately discussed in accessible places,[9] for others we simply found no ready authors. This introduction adds a few random links to the chain.

Some medieval practitioners

After the Roman and Saxon periods, reviewed in the next three chapters, there follows a long empty quarter of our story. The names of a few medieval physicians and surgeons are known, many of them simply because their profession was stated when they signed documents or owned land. Sometimes records were kept when doctors were appointed at one of the religious houses, or attended an important patient.[10] For instance, the first known female physician in the North was Christiana, who was working at Jarrow in 1313. Nicholas Byscopton, Osbert of Laton and Thomas of Hamsterley were all physicians to the monastery of Durham in about 1321, when Geoffrey Burdon was prior. We get a hint of what was involved in such an appointment when we read that on 10 October 1348 Robertus de Ellewyke took an oath at Durham 'to serve the Prior and Convent and monks in their cells with his labour and counsel in the faculty of medicine, at their expense, for the whole term of his life.' The library available to a physician at Durham would already have been a useful one. For example, back in the 12th century Henricus had donated 26 medical books to the library at Durham, and Gervase (1165-1201), a physician and landowner at Whickham, bequeathed all his books to Durham Priory.[10]

Everyday practitioners doing the more humble work in the town would be unlikely to be recorded, unless they got into trouble. In 1375 Master Thomas de Clotton, 'a leech of Newcastle, was sued by the Earl of Chester for causing the death of Roger, son of Robert.'

Other northerners are known because of their royal connections. Patrick of Carlisle, about 1242-53, was physician and clerk to Henry III and later Peter of Newcastle was surgeon to Edward I during his infamous campaign in Scotland in 1298.[10]

Edward II was in Newcastle and Tynemouth in April 1312 where his favourite, Peter de Gaveston, Earl of Cornwall, fell ill. Master William Burntoft, physician, and Robert de Bermyngham, monk of Tynemouth, were each paid £6 13s 4d by the king's own hand for medical attendance on the earl.[11]

Yet another Northumbrian, John Chambre MD (c1470-1549), was physician to both Henry VII and VIII; in 1518 he was one of the six founding Fellows of the College of Physicians and was Censor of the College in 1523.[12]

John Malverne and St Mary's Hospital in Jesmond

One more medieval story: — Master John Malverne, who referred to himself as 'doctorem in medicina' (though from which University is unknown), was a priest whose career included appointments as Chaplain of Balliol College Oxford; Master of St Katherine's Hospital, Ledbury; Rector of St Dunstan-in-the-East; Canon of St Paul's Cathedral and Canon and Prebendary of St George's Chapel, Windsor. He was also, by 1395, physician to the Earl of Derby, who soon afterwards became King Henry IV; and he was the author of a tract on the *Spiritual and corporial remedies against the pestilence*. Six years before he died John Malverne 'exchanged his canonry of St George's for the wardenship of the free chapel of St Mary, Jesmond, Newcastle upon Tyne, which he held until his death.'[10] Why, in 1416, did this able and highly connected churchman and physician leave London for Jesmond? Did he come as a missionary? Was it a penance for some now forgotten lapse? Was he out of favour with the new King, Henry V? Was he exhausted or disabled and in need of quiet? Was he returning to his childhood home? Tantalising as our ignorance of the answers is, it is matched by the paucity of information about the Chapel of St Mary the Virgin in Jesmond itself, and its associated hospital. Another hospital of the Virgin Mary at the Westgate in Newcastle had existed at least since the reign of Henry II and survived the dissolution to continue, at least in the form of a chapel, into the early 19th century. Some of its buildings were used by the early Royal Grammar School.[13]

Dr Jonathan Miller in a radio programme early in 1992 said of Chartres Cathedral that it was 'a religious fossil from which the soft parts have long since rotted away.' How much more so at Jesmond, where the fossil itself is a mere fragment. Mackenzie informs us that the founders of the Jesmond hospital are unknown, that it existed by 1351, that after the dissolution it passed to the corporation of Newcastle by grant of Edward VI and that they immediately sold it to Sir John Brandling. Welford records that in the late 14th century the advowson of the Chapel belonged successively to Sir Alexander Hilton, to the family of Sir Bertram Monboucher and (in part) to the Middletons of Belsay Castle; by 1426 it belonged to William Harbottle; in 1483 the Chaplaincy passed from Mr Lumley to Dr Roby. Such are the known facts. But there is also a firm tradition that Pilgrim Street in Newcastle is named after the pilgrims who travelled that way to Jesmond. The street was named by 1313, so presumably the Chapel had a reputation by then.[14] No more is known. Whatever Brandling did with it, by 1769 the hospital was a dwelling house and the chapel a barn; and by 1825 only one of the little windows of the old hospital remained in the gable of a farmhouse, and the owner had tidied up the ruin of the chapel.[15] Today the chapel ruins and the reputed remains of its holy well survive in a little copse overlooking Jesmond Dene.

William Turner (c1508-1568) – scientist, rebel and physician

William Turner was the first doctor of international significance to come from Northumberland though his major importance was as a botanist, a Protestant Reformer and a pre-Shakespearian influence on the form of modern English.[16] He was born in Morpeth in about 1508, the son of a tanner; was educated there at the Chantry School; went up to Pembroke College, Cambridge in 1526 with the financial support of Thomas first Baron Wentworth; and there met Ridley (also of Pembroke, and a fellow Northumbrian), and Latimer of Clare Hall who first led Turner to become an Reformer. Religion and natural history (birds and fishes as well as plants) were the two dominant themes in his life. It is clear from his writings that they were linked in the sense that he was passionate in his efforts to rediscover the ancient truths of Christianity and to set them forth openly and in English, discarding all of what he believed to be the obscuration and distortion of the Church; and in the same spirit he sought out the original descriptions of herbs (from Dioscorides, Theophrastus and Pliny) and of birds (from Pliny and Aristotle) and used all his powers of observation to identify them in England, and later on the Continent, to describe them so that they could be recognised, or to make it clear when the herbs used by the ancients were not to be found in Western countries. His first herbal (the *Libellus*, 1538) and his book on birds (the earliest account of British birds, *Avium praecipuarum, quarum apud Plinium et Aristotelem mentio est.*.1544) were in Latin. Indeed it was his intention to publish a major herbal in Latin. In 1548 he wrote an account in English of *The names of herbes in Greke, Latin, English, Duch & Frenche wyth the commune names that Herbaries and Apotecaries use*; the preface tells how he had actually drafted the Latin herbal, but had been advised to defer setting it forth until he had explored the flora of the West Country:[16]

> that I might in my herbal declare to the greate honoure of our countre what number of sovereine & strang herbes were in Englande that were not in other nations..
>
> ....they moved me to set out an herbal in Englyshe as Fuchsius dyd in latine wyth the discriptions, figures and properties of as many herbes, as I had sene and knewe..

But he was too busy to produce the herbal at once, and so issued *The Names of Herbes* covering most of those mentioned by the ancients with their common names and the places in England where they might be found, 'that Potecaries should be excuselesse when as the ryghte herbes are required of them'.

By then Turner had already been a religious exile.[17] In June 1540 he had fled to Calais and on, probably to Cologne, then to Venice, Ferrara and Bologna where he worked for some time with Luca Ghini the 'Lecturer in Dioscorides' who, Raven suggests, influenced Turner's interest in exact identification and nomenclature. After an unknown period in Italy Turner crossed the Alps and visited Conrad Gesner in Zurich, and Leonardt Fuchs in Basel. Fuchs was in the process of publishing his great herbal *De historia stirpium* (1542) and Turner must have seen the superb wood engravings, by far the finest of their kind at that time, and he must have been thunderstruck. Somehow he managed to acquire copies within the next few years, either of the originals or of some of the many smaller scale copies that were published all over Europe in Fuchs' name in the following years. In any event Fuchs' wood engravings, exact, the same size, but reversed, are the basis of Turner's illustrations for his *A new herball* of which successive parts were published in 1551, 1562 and 1568.

From Basel he returned to Bonn and Cologne, practised there for a while and then went north to Friesland (where, for about four years, he was physician to the household of the Duke of Emden) eventually returning by way of Antwerp, Louvain and Calais to England in 1547, on the accession of young Edward VI. On his return Turner was appointed physician to the Lord Protector, Edward Seymour, Duke of Somerset, who lived at Syon House; Turner lived across the river at Kew.

It was at this stage that he wrote the first part of his English herbal, set out as the Latin draft would have been, in alphabetical order of the Latin names of the herbs. He got only as far as Faba, the bean, in this volume. Despite his deep interest in the detailed description of plants as a means of identification, he was very far from any sort of taxonomy or classification. In the preface he regrets that the 'waiting' on the Duke left him with too little time for study, and 'for these thre yeares and an halfe, I have had no more lyberty but bare .iii. wekes to bestow upon ye sekyng of herbes & markyng in what places they do grow.' So he had been unable to explore the West Country. His defence of his use of English was spirited:[18]

> Other will thinke it unwysely done, and agaynst the honor of my art that I professe, and agaynst the comon profit, to set out so muche knowledge of phisick in Englyshe. For now (say they) every man without any study of necessary artes... will become a phisician...while by occasyon of thys boke every man, nay every old wyfe will presume not without the mordre of many, to practyse phisick. To whom I make thys answer, by a questyon, how many surgianes and apothecaries are there in England, which can understande Plini in latin or Galene and Dioscorides, whereas they wryte ether in greke or translated into latin, of the names descriptions and natures of herbes. And when as they have no latin to come by the knowledge of herbes: whether all the Phisicians of England (saving very few) committ not ye knowledge of herbes unto the potecaries or no, as the potecaries do to the olde wyves, that gather herbes, & to the grossers, whylse they send all their receytes unto the potecary, not beyng present their to se, whether the potecary putteth all that shuld be in to the receyt or no. Then when as if the potecari for lack of knowledge of the latin tong, is ignorant in herbes: and putteth ether a good man by ignorance in jeopardy of his life, or marreth good medicines to the great dishonestie both of the Phisician and of Goddes worthy creatures, the herbes and the medicines: when as by havyng an herball in English all these evelles myght be avoyded.

He went on to argue that Dioscorides and Galen wrote in their native tongues without giving 'occasion for every olde wyfe to take in hand the practise of Phisick. – Dyd they give any just occasyon of murther.' ...If they gave none ..and were 'no hynderers from the study of lyberall sciences, then am I no hynderer wryting unto the English my countremen, an Englysh herball.'

It is not clear whether 'waiting on the Duke' involved a busy medical practice in the Lord Protector's household or more tediously ceremonial duties, one suspects the latter. Indeed Turner's active medical practice seems to have been confined largely to his two exiles on the continent; in England, except during this period at Syon House, his appointments were ecclesiastical, most notably, in Elizabeth's reign, as Dean of Wells. Almost all we know of Turner as a physician is indirect. There is only one actual case report, and its purpose is more defensive than educational; it appears in a letter of 21 March 1563 from Turner to the Queen's principal secretary, Sir William Cecil concerning Turner's patient, the wife of Sir Thomas Dier and 'exceedingly dear to the Queen', who fell ill after a quarrel with her husband.[19]

Our other sources of information are the prefaces of the herbals, and Turner's choice of their contents; his works on the waters at Bath, on wines and on treacles; the often very medical metaphores he uses in his religious polemics; there are scarcely more than hints (scattered through the herbal) of his actual practice on the Continent; and finally there is his hand written commonplace book in the City Library in Bath. The commonplace book is a potentially rich source, but a difficult one to harvest because of the many additions by later owners, the orthography, the often abbreviated Latin and the problems of distinguishing Turner's original statements from his unattributed quotations.[20]

Turner had a high opinion of medicine

> Phisick standeth in doyng & workinge, and is occupyed about mannys body, therefore as much better as well doyng is, then well saying, and mannys body is more precious then all other creatures: so is Phisick more noble and more worthy to be set by, then all other sciences.[21]

Whether he managed in practice to keep his well-doing up to the standards he set in his well-saying is unknown. The preface to the 1551 Herbal shows the importance he attached to what we now call pharmaceutical standards. Presumably he sometimes gathered simples to use in his practice while he botanised, or in the many gardens he mentions in his books, but there is little evidence of this, or about his personal relations with the 'potecaries' who made up his prescriptions. His principles, however, were clear:

> I went into Italy and into diverse partes of Germany, to knowe and se the herbes my self, and to knowe by practise their powers and workinge, not trustinge onlye to the olde herbe wives and apothecaryes (as manye Physiciones have done of late yeres) but in the mater of simples myne owne eyes and knowledge...[and, writing of both physicians and apothecaries and their simples,] without ye knowlege whereof they can not deuly exercise their office and vocation.[22]

There is no doubt that he relied heavily in his herbals, and presumably in his practice, on the writings of Dioscorides, Galen and Pliny. In the *Names of Herbes* virtually all of the information on the 'virtues' of the herbs is from the ancients, though rarely with a direct attribution; thus under absinthium:[16]

> Pontike wormwod, is hote in the fyrste degree and drye in the thirde. Sea wormwod is hote in the second degree and drye in the fyrste, frenche wormwod is weaker than Sea wormwod is. [He had found Sea wormwood (Artemisia maritima *L.*, [23]) 'plentuous in Northumberlande

by holy Islande,...' while the best kind of Ponticke wormwood came from Rome.][24]

Occasionally he gives an attribution; thus of Blitum [Chenopodium foliosum *Aschers*.] he says:

> ...I never saw it in England but in my lordes gardene [25], and there it was unknowen. It may be named a blete. Blete after Galen is colde & moyste in the seconde degree.

Rarely also he mentions a more recent authority as he does for capers and Nasturtium, or of the coriander:

> Coriandrum [Coriandrum sativum *L*.]
>
> ..in englishe Colander or coriander, ..It is hote in the fyrst degree after Averrhois, I thynke that he meaneth of the seede.[26]

Sometimes he seems to write of the properties of the herbs from his own experience as he does of the coriander above or of Acorus [Iris pseudacorus *L*., Yellow flag[27]]:

> Acorus groweth not in England, wherfore they are farre deceyved that use the yelowe flourdeluce, which some call gladen, for Acorus, for Acorus is hote, bytinge and opening, but gladen is colde, unsavery and astringent. I thynke that the great Galanga is the true Acorus. If they have not it they maye use Calamus aromaticus, or Asarabacca for Acorus. Acorus is hote and dry in the thirde degree.

In the *New Herball* too, the plants described in parts one and two are exclusively those known to the ancients, and only the third part (1568) 'intreats of these herbes' of which there is no mention in the old Grecian or Latin writers. Even there, however, the more trustworthy of the recent authors, Fuchs, Matthiolus, Tragus (ie Hieronymous Bock) and Dodoneus (Dodoens) are the main sources of authority, and Turner's own opinion is introduced either as an aside, or less often as a rather combative rebuttal of the opinion of others:[22]

> I taught the truthe of certeyne plantes, which these above named writers knew not at al, or ellis erred in them greatlye, as in Absintho pontico, Orobanche, Betonica Pauli, Sphondylio and divers others.

Interestingly, Turner dedicates the third part of his herbal 'To the right worshipfull Felowship and Companye of Surgeones of the citye of London chefely, and to all other that practyse Surgery within England, William Turner sendeth greting in Christ Jesu.' This presumably refers to the Barber Surgeons Company which had been founded in 1540, not a body that would have been used to cheerful greetings and praise from physicians, but Turner, despite his Royal connections, was never a member of the London establishment and, for example, was never a licentiate of the Royal College of Physicians, as his son Peter was later. Turner recommended the 'herbs found after the old writers time' to his surgical colleagues as 'very necessary for the healing of many diseases, grevous sicknesses, wounds, sores, brusinges, and breaking as well inward as outward....'.[28] On the whole the *New Herball* is disappointing in its accounts of the 'vertues' of plants, in striking contrast to the scientific approach to identification and description. Lists of uses, often seeming absurdly numerous and varied, are mere compilations from earlier works.[29] When only one use or none was recorded, Turner said so; for example, of the St Paul's betony, mentioned above, he writes: 'Paulus Egineta, who onely writeth of thys herbe, telleth no other good propertye..., but that it is good for the diseases of the kidneys'. There are rare anecdotes of personal experience, as when he warns of the dangers of the opium poppy:[30]

> For allthoughe sum be very bold in occupying of it: I taught by experience how ieperdous [jeopardous] it is, dare not w[ith]out great warnes geve it in to [the] body. For ones in East Friesland, when as I wasshed an achyng tooth w[ith] a litle opio mixed with water, and a litle of [the] same unawares went doun: w[ith] in an hour after my handes began to swell about the wrestes, and to itch, & my breath was so stopped, that if I had not taken a pece of the roote of masterwurt, called of som pilletory of Spayn with wyne, I thynck that it wold have kylled me.

It is ironic that his warning about the perils of one of the most potent and efficacious of herbs was based on a personal allergic reaction and not on the effects of overdosage or addiction.

During his second continental exile Turner practised medicine, and accompanied 'diverse seik folke in the bathes of Germanye'. Earlier, while in the Duke of Somerset's service, he had visited Bath and studied the properties of the waters there. *A Booke of the natures and properties, as well of the bathes in England as of other bathes in Germany and Italy, very necessary for all seik persones...*(1562)[31] is a vigorous promotion of the curative value of the baths and an appeal to improve the dilapidated state of the spa at Bath.

> 'I have gathered out of divers learned mennis workes, the nature and workyng of divers of the most holsom and and strong workyng bathes...in Italy or Germany, that such men as have mony to bear theyr costes, may fynd remedy for theyr diseases there.'

He lists 26 earlier authorities as his sources, and 11 baths of note (six German, one Swiss, three Italian, and Bath). Each spa's virtues are reviewed, and Bath itself is commended to those whose diseases are amenable to its waters, or who lack the means to travel further. His long list of diseases which may be healed by the baths includes some good succinct clinical descriptions:

> The castyng of children out, before the dew tyme appoynted by nature.
>
> The stoppyng of the longes & shortnes of brethe when a man can not take breth, except he sit ryght up.
>
> The hardnes and bynding of the belly, when a man can not go to the stool without Physik.

The vayn appetite of going to stoole, when a man can do nothing when he cummeth there.

The Palsey when as a man is quite num all the partes of his body & hath nether movyng nor helyng.

The trymbling of any membre, when a man can not hold it still.

The rinnyng gout which rynneth from one joynte to another.

The knobbes & hard lumpes that ar made by the french pockes.

The general dropsey throw all the body, rynnynge betwene the fell & the fleshe. [ie in the subcutaneous tissue.]

After smelling the mud from the bottom of the pools, Turner concurred with the general opinion that the main active matter in the water at Bath was brimstone, but he investigated further and walked on the surrounding hills where he found 'litle peces of marquesites and stones, menged wyth copper'. He could 'by no sense or wit perceyve' evidence of copper in the waters themselves and cautiously concluded that the baths should be tried for those diseases that were reported to respond to brimstone, making no claim for other active minerals (he was right; the water today contains 1 g/l of sulphate and less than 30 mcg/l of copper). He combined this cautious scientific approach with enthusiasm in publicising the benefits of the treatment for all who needed it, regardless of their means, likening himself to one of the flocking birds[32] which by their calls attract others to a good supply of food. He praised particularly the benefit of Bath's waters in gout and other diseases of the joints, a reputation they have enjoyed ever since. He drew up proposals for the proper restoration and development of the derelict buildings and instructions for the regimen of bathing and diet. In an interesting passage he suggests that that the beasts that serve man, particularly horses, should also benefit from the healing power of Bath's waters.

The first injunction in the regimen is that the baths should be used only when a physician has *almost* despaired of a cure (my italics), but later Turner gives advice about the use of the baths by those too poor to afford a physician. It is plain where his sympathies lie, yet he tries to maintain a kind of professional etiquette. The dilemma reflects the pattern of his life; Turner was an humane and farsighted iconoclast whose need for professional security, whether medical or ecclesiastical, confined him from time to time in a glass house of patronage. It was an uneasy life, for the patronage did not always survive his slingshots unscathed, and at times he could be querulous and even sycophantic in letters to his patrons. But when he writes for the sick and distressed, his common sense and the warmth of his personality are evident, as in the *envoi* to *The bathes*:

When as ye go homewarde, make but small iourneys, and beware of surfetinge and colde, and when ye are at home, use measurable exercise daylye, and honest myrthe and pastyme wyth honest companye. And beware of surfeting in anye wyse, and of anger, and of to muche studye or carfulnes.

The Barber-Surgeons

One omission from this miscellany is the story of the Guild of Barber Surgeons in Newcastle, which was founded on 10 Oct 1442, and survived as a remnant of two stewards and three ordinary members in 1929.[33] Two of the minute books of the Guild survive (covering only the periods 1616-86 and 1686-1778), as does a cabinet of their early 18th-century surgical instruments and a copy of the 1668 (2nd) English edition of the *Anatomy* of Thomas Bartholin (1618-1680), which was presented to the Guild by a Mr Peter Bates on 4 June 1683. There are a few brief accounts of the Guild, and extracts of the minutes were printed by Embleton (they contain little that is strictly surgical but much of interest) but the subject deserves more study.[34]

The 17th century

The activities of the Barber Surgeons, as recounted in their minute books, are a very substantial part of the fragmentary evidence about medical life in the North East during the 17th century. The dissolution of the monasteries in the previous century had removed much of the infrastructure of medical care, and the early growth of cities, particularly evident in Newcastle as the warfare with the Scots subsided, led to overcrowding and poverty. Brand records that there were 78 deaths from the pestilence in the parish of Lamesley (County Durham) in 1610; much worse was to follow in 1635-6. The plague was thought to have reached North Shields from Holland in October 1635 and spread slowly at first and then, from May, with awful ferocity so that, between 6 May and 31 Dec 1636, 5037 people died in Newcastle and, between 31 May and 17 Oct, 515 died in Gateshead. Fumigations of pitch, rosin and frankincense were tried in vain. So empty was the town of business that its streets were covered with grass.[35]

Other epidemics of 'plague' occurred in Newcastle and Gateshead in the autumn of 1642, at Tynemouth garrison (then besieged by the Scots) in October 1644, and in Darlington, Eaglescliffe, Gateshead and Newcastle in September-October 1645, though it is not always clear whether plague, typhus or some other fatal epidemic was responsible. It must have been a decade of constant anxiety. As if the visitations of the plague were not enough, a large and victorious Scots Covenanter's army occupied Newcastle in 1640-1 and the Scots appeared again in numbers during the Civil War, being turned back with difficulty from the city walls. It was at this time that the meeting place of the Barber Surgeons, the Pandon Tower on the Wall to the East of the city, was damaged so that, after a period of meeting in each others houses, they decided upon building their own hall, first used in March 1648/9. In 1675 Brand records the appearance in Newcastle and its neighbourhood of 'a dreadful pestilential disease called "the Jolly Rant" of which 924 persons died'.[35]

Two charitable hospitals were founded at the end of the century. In 1681-3 Holy Jesus Hospital was built 'at the charge of the Mayor and Burgesses' of Newcastle 'for the support of poor impotent people, being freemen and freemen's widows, or their sons and daughters that had never been married'. Then in 1700 the Keelmen's Hospital was founded, and soon after built just outside the town wall to the East, where it overlooked the busiest part of the Tyne, studded at that time with the broad stubby keels or coal barges, manhandled with a little help from a small sail, by two keelmen, a skipper and a boy.[36] Medical activity must have played a part in the life of these institutions, but principally they were to provide community care for the infirm and the destitute.

The 18th century

Few of the existing publications on the medical history of the North East have given much attention to the 18th century.[37] It is therefore particularly pleasing that several of the contributions to this book have concentrated on this interesting period, and together they give us a useful new body of information. William Hewson, Thomas Trotter and Thomas Winterbottom spent large parts of their careers away from the North East, but all had firm and lasting connections here. John Heysham in Carlisle and John Clark in Newcastle, on the other hand, were outsiders who made their careers in the North, and each made an important and lasting contribution to the health of his community by founding a Dispensary. Fred Miller has rescued Clark from undeserved oblivion by collecting information from many sources, and in particular has sifted through the minute books of the old Infirmary on the Forth to reveal a fascinating controversy between the physicians and the surgeons of the day with the not unfamiliar ingredients of jealousy over beds, cross-infection, manipulation of committees and clashes of personality. At least three 18th-century surgeons deserve more attention than they receive here – Richard Lambert (1724-81), Samuel Hallowell (1709-60) and William Ingham (1753-1817). Lambert is mentioned as the mentor of William Hewson and as the principal founder of the Infirmary, but he also deserves recognition as the first pioneer of restorative arterial surgery.[38]

Prevention of disease and the public health

Contributions to public health are, by chance, a major theme of several chapters in the book. Heysham, in addition to founding the Carlisle Dispensary, was an important pioneer in the recording of health statistics and in using them to prove the value of preventive measures such as inoculation (and later vaccination) against smallpox. Thomas Trotter's pioneering work for the health of the Navy is revealed with new clarity in Joan Carmichael's study, which includes much new material from letters in the Maritime Museum at Greenwich. John Snow, one of the very first Newcastle graduates, put to good use the experience of cholera that he gained in the North in the 1830s, when he identified the mode of spread of the epidemics in London twenty years later. Ralph Gould tells the much less well known story of a later typhoid epidemic in North Shields and the controversy that resulted. John Guy describes the prevention of sea-borne epidemics by the Port of Tyne

Authority, and its Floating Hospitals. One man, Dr Henry Armstrong, was involved both in that story and in many other pioneering aspects of public health in Newcastle,[39] but an account of him must await another occasion. Elspeth Gould shows how Newcastle made yet another pioneering contribution to preventive medicine, by the early introduction of contact tracing for venereal disease on Tyneside. But epidemics are not the only preventable causes of death and disaster; David Knight recounts the story of Davy's safety lamp, a contribution by a doctor who turned to science very early in his career, and a story not unconnected with the North East, as he makes clear. One pit disaster is mentioned in Stuart Menzies' chapter on Winterbottom; the 19th-century *Proceedings of the Northumberland and Durham Medical Society* describe the consequences of many more. It is not surprising that the earliest attempt to make lighting the mines safer was in the North East. Dr W Reid Clanny of Sunderland not only devised the first safety lamp in 1813, but also made the heroic attempt to prevent and ameliorate the 1831-2 cholera epidemic which first reached Britain from Europe at Sunderland where he was physician to the Infirmary and Dispensary and 'Chairman of the medical department of the Sunderland Board of Health'.[40] He is another figure who deserves a proper study.

Medical education in Newcastle

The story of medical teaching in Newcastle is a proud one, but also distinctly entertaining. Gordon Dale's chapter tells of the school's nine different homes and two schisms, and its many colourful characters. It is an aspect of Newcastle's medical history of which there have been several accounts (see references in the appendix) and yet deserves a deeper study. The swashbuckling, politically ambitious, larger than life figure of the surgeon, Sir John Fife, seems an improbable one to have been the seed around which the crystal of the medical school was formed. It had many ingredients. The active intellectual atmosphere of the town was one; the Literary and Philosophical Society (founded 1793) had been active for nearly 40 years, had recently moved into its fine new building (July 1825) and had gained a little space by the separation from the rapidly expanding Natural History Society of Northumberland, Durham and Newcastle upon Tyne (founded 1829). It could seek pastures new. There had been talk of founding a University in Newcastle or Durham (Durham's foundation in 1832 took the wind from Newcastle's sails, but having no medical school, Durham left the way clear for a college of medicine and science in Newcastle).[41] There was dissatisfaction with the academic standard of the old Medical Society (discussed below). Cholera had arrived from Europe in late 1831 and must have shaken everyone's confidence in the medical science of the day. And the right people were available. The result was the foundation of the new school in 1834; but by then Fife had taken the initiative and, in 1832, with a few colleagues, had started classes in his rooms in Bell's Court.

Some medical naturalists

It would have been fun to have a chapter on the medical naturalists of the North East. They have been many and, starting with William Turner, several have been distinguished. Frederick Pybus himself was a member of the Natural History Society whose lecture theatre at the Hancock Museum is named after him, and he gave that Society some notable books. Dennis Embleton, medical historian and first professor of medicine at the medical school, and his uncle Robert Embleton were both naturalists; one of the former's proudest publications was on the osteology of a fossil of a large crocodile-like amphibian found in the Northumberland coal measures (the black shale at Newsham Main colliery).[42] John Heysham of Carlisle, in addition to his medical achievements, was a competent naturalist. He was the first to publish incontrovertible evidence that the Hen Harrier and the Ringtail were male and female of the same species, and his *A catalogue of Cumberland animals* (1794)[43] (in which the description of the hen harriers appears) was the first full account of the fauna (or indeed even of the birds) of any county in Britain. The first flora of Berwick was compiled by an Army surgeon John V Thompson who later was posted to Ireland and there made far more important contributions to natural history. He showed that a small crustacean was the larval form of the Acorn Barnacle and thus that the cirripedes were not, as had been thought, molluscs but, as barnacles, a sessile adult form of crustacean. Charles Darwin (himself a medical student turned naturalist) was so excited by this discovery of Thompson's that he devoted several years to the study of cirripedes.[44] Darwin's monograph on the subject was published by the Ray Society. As Alan Binnie describes in his chapter, the Ray Society was one of the three great contributions to natural history of another Berwick doctor, George Johnston, the others being the foundation of the earliest naturalists' field club in the world, and the study and recording of a wealth of information on the inshore marine invertebrates of this country. He also wrote a second flora of Berwick. Two other naturalists who were associated with the Infirmary and the Medical School were Nathaniel Winch (1768-1838), one of the greatest botanists of his time, who was secretary to the Infirmary, and John Thornhill, co-author of Winch's earliest book, his successor as Secretary of the Natural History Society, and the Lecturer in Botany at the Neville Hall Medical School at the time of the schism.[45] One other important medical naturalist, George Stewardson Brady (1832-1921), was born in Gateshead, graduated from the Newcastle College of Medicine and practised in Sunderland from 1857-1906, including a period as physician to the Sunderland Infirmary. He was also Professor of Natural History at Armstrong College from 1875-1906. In his day he was incomparably the greatest living expert on marine plankton. His monograph on the free and semiparasitic copepods of Britain was published by the Ray Society, and he produced vast and detailed reports (1881-4) on the microscopic appearances of the ostracods and copepods collected on the *Challenger* expedition. Altogether he published 115 works in this field.[46]

Northern Medical and Surgical Societies and their publications

The North of England has a long tradition of medical and surgical societies.[47] The first to be recorded, The Philosophical and Medical Society, was founded on 1 Nov 1786 with about 39 ordinary and seven corresponding members (Secretary Mr Thomas Leighton, Jun, first President John Rotherham, MD). The members presented papers and case reports, bought and shared books, wrangled bitterly, and devised complex and restrictive rules; then renamed themselves the Medical and Philosophical Society and eventually, in 1800, dissolved themselves. The Society's property passed to The Medical Book Club, formed in 1790, and this was renamed The Medical Society. Though the rules related to its function as a small private circulating library, the Society discussed such matters as 'the Necessity and Propriety of increasing the Charges usually made in this town and neighbourhood for Medicines, Attendance, and Journeys etc.' By 1801 a long and productive tradition of presenting at each meeting 'an account of prevailing diseases' was mentioned as well as 'Medical News, Reading of Papers, Review of New Publications etc'. Mr Leighton continued as Secretary of the successive societies until 16 Dec 1846, a period of more than 60 years. Eventually his Society degenerated into a 'Supper Society' and 'died of inanition' in 1875. Meanwhile 'The Society of Physicians and Surgeons of Newcastle' had been formed in 1834 with Dr TE Headlam as President and Mr TM Greenhow as Secretary, and a medical library had been started. This new organisation first met at The Literary and Philosophical Society's rooms and it seems also to have been linked in its foundation to the School of Medicine and Surgery founded in the same year. It must have had a very different atmosphere from the old Medical Society which, from the beginning, had met in local coffee houses. Yet this Society too was short-lived; it was dissolved in 1847 and its library was transferred to the Medical School. Next was formed the 'Newcastle and Gateshead Pathological Society' in 1848, with the same President and Secretary, but this time the formula was right and the Society has survived to the present day, though with two more changes of name.[48] In 1848 too, its proceedings were published for the first time.[49] There was a break in the sequence during the first world war but otherwise the North East had its own medical journal continuously until 1971. An interesting subject for study would be an appraisal of the important contributions to medical knowledge that have first appeared in our journal. But probably none was more important than the report of the first successful treatment of myxoedema by George Redmayne Murray, reproduced in full in Chapter 22.

The 20th century

The 20th century, and indeed the earlier history of the medical specialties and of the professions allied to medicine, are only briefly represented here by accounts of the development of dental education, cardiology, pharmacy, psychiatry, urology and venereology in the North East. It need scarcely be said that equally interesting accounts could be written about every other specialty and profession, and we hope that one day they will.

Acknowledgements

I am grateful to Mr George Chapman of Morpeth for a photocopy of Turner's *Bathes*, to Dr Fred Miller for suggesting additions to the Appendix and to Susan Robinson for typing other chapters so I could concentrate on this one.

Appendix

Some sources for the History of Medicine in the North East of England (excluding individual biographies)

Bulmer W, Hodgson N. The Barber-Surgeons Company of Newcastle upon Tyne. *Archaeologia Aeliana* 1958; Ser 4, *35*:73-80.

Callcott M. The challenge of cholera: The last epidemic at Newcastle upon Tyne. *Northern Hist* 1984; *20*:167-186.

Dale G, Donald J, Wagget J. *The Fleming Memorial Hospital for Sick Children, Newcastle upon Tyne 1887-1987*. Newcastle upon Tyne: J & P Bealls, nd (1987).

Dale G, Miller FJW. *Newcastle School of Medicine 1834-1984 Sesquicentennial scrapbook*. University of Newcastle, nd (1984).

Dale G, Miller F, Bramley K. *Newcastle School of Medicine 1834-1984 Sesquicentennial celebrations: Proceedings 17-21 September 1984*. University of Newcastle, 1985.

Davison MH Armstrong. The paintings at the Royal Victoria Infirmary. *Newcastle Med J* 1965; *29*:43-7.

Embleton D. *The History of the Medical School, afterwards the Durham College of Medicine at Newcastle upon Tyne, for forty years, from 1832 to 1872*. Newcastle-upon-Tyne: Andrew Reid, 1890.

Embleton D. The Newcastle Medical Society 100 years ago. *Proc Northumb Dur Med Soc* Session 1890-91; 105-124, 155-177; *and* Biographical notices of members of the Philosophical & Medical Society of Newcastle of one hundred years ago. *Idem*; 178-210.

Embleton D. The Incorporated Company of Barber-Surgeons and Wax and Tallow Chandlers of Newcastle-upon-Tyne. *Archaeologia Aeliana* 1892; *15*:228-269.

Emmerson JS. *Catalogue of the Pybus Collection of medical books, letters and engravings, 15th-20th centuries, held in the University Library, Newcastle upon Tyne*. Manchester: Manchester University Press on behalf of the University Library, Newcastle upon Tyne, 1981.

Ferguson AJA, Prescott DT, Robertson F. *A history of medicine in South West Durham*. [Bishop Auckland]: South West Durham Health Authority, 1989. ISBN 0-9515068-0-3.

Halcrow EM. The charity for the relief of poor women lying-in at their own homes. *Archaeologia Aeliana* 1956; Ser 4, *34*:110-129.

Harley D. Pious physic for the poor: the lost Durham county medical scheme of 1655. *Med Hist* 1993; *37*:148-166.

Hibbert JC, Wells WH. A sketch of the sanitary history of Newcastle-upon-Tyne. *J Roy Sanit Instit* 1907; *28*:161-175.

Horsley PM. *Eighteenth-Century Newcastle.* Newcastle: Oriel Press, 1971. (Chapter 5 - Medical services.)

Hume GH. *The History of the Newcastle Infirmary*. Newcastle upon Tyne: Andrew Reid & Co Ltd, 1906.

Hume WE. The medical societies of Newcastle-upon-Tyne. *Newcastle Med J* 1928; *9*:1-22.

Hume WE. *The Infirmary Newcastle upon Tyne 1751-1951*. Newcastle upon Tyne: Andrew Reid & Co Ltd, [1951].

Hume WE. The origin and early history of the Infirmary of Newcastle upon Tyne. *Archeologia Aeliana* 1954, Ser 4, *32*:72-99.

Hurrell G, Harlan GP. *The History of Newcastle General Hospital*. Newcastle upon Tyne: Hindson & Reid, [1967], reprinted 1984.

Mackenzie E. *A descriptive and historical account of the Town and County of Newcastle upon Tyne, including the Borough of Gateshead*. Newcastle upon Tyne: Mackenzie and Dent, 2 vol, 1827.

McCord N. The making of modern Newcastle. *Archeologia Aeliana* 1981; Ser 5, *9*:333-346.

Miller FJW. The Infirmary on the Forth, 1753-1906. *Archaeologia Aeliana* 1986; Ser 5, *14*:143-165.

Miller FJW. The Newcastle Dispensary 1777-1976. *Archaeologia Aeliana* 1990; Ser 5, *18*:177-195.

Miller FJW, Thompson MD. The decline and fall of the Tubercle Bacillus: The Newcastle story 1882-1988. *Arch Dis Childh* 1992; *67*:251-5.

Newcastle-upon-Tyne and Northern Counties Medical Journal. Volumes *1-6*, 1920-26; and *Newcastle Medical Journal.* Volumes *7-31*, 1926-71. The journal of the Newcastle and Northern Counties Medical Society. Post-war successor to two journals closed down in 1914, the *Northumberland and Durham Medical Journal*, (no volume numbers) 1892-1914, and *The North of England Clinical Journal*, 1911-1914. These in turn were preceded by the *Proceedings of the Northumberland and Gateshead Pathological Society* 1848-60 and the *Proceedings of the Northumberland and Durham Medical Society*, 1861-92 (no volume numbers).

Pybus FC. The Company of Barber Surgeons and Tallow Chandlers of Newcastle-upon-Tyne. *Newcastle Med J* 1929; *9*:147-163.

Richardson MA. *The local historian's table book, of remarkable occurences, historical facts, traditions, legendary and descriptive ballads, etc, etc., connected with the counties of Newcastle-upon-Tyne, Northumberland and Durham. Historical Division vols.* Newcastle-upon-Tyne: MA Richardson, 4 vol, 1841-44.

Ridley U. *The Babies Hospital Newcastle upon Tyne.* Newcastle upon Tyne: Andrew Reid & Co Ltd, 1956.

Robinson W. *The story of the Royal Infirmary Sunderland: set in its social and historical background*. Sunderland: Hills and Co (Sunderland) Ltd, 1934.

Rose J Dudfield. The history of the Newcastle Medical School. *Med Illustr* 1952; *6*:187-93.

Talbot CH, Hammond EA. *The medical practitioners in medieval England: a biographical register*. London: Wellcome Historical Medical Library, 1965

Turner G Grey, Arnison WD. *The Newcastle upon Tyne School of Medicine 1834-1934.* Newcastle upon Tyne: Andrew Reid & Co Ltd, 1934.

University of Durham Medical Gazette. Volumes 1-57; 1939-1963. A source for appointments, retirements, obituaries, news and gossip, and a variety of articles on local medical history varying from flimsy to distinguished. Early issues were *Univ Durh Med School Gaz* and then *Univ Durh Med Coll Gaz.*

Wallis PJ, Wallis RV, Burnby JGL, Whittet TD. *Eighteenth century medics (subscriptions, licences, apprenticeships).* 2nd ed. Newcastle-upon Tyne: Project for historical bibliography, 1988. (1st ed 1985). ISBN 1-871768-00-4

Warrick CK. Notes on the history of the Department of Radiology of the Royal Victoria Infirmary, Newcastle upon Tyne. *Radiography* 1977; *43*:190-4.

Watts W. Progress of medicine and surgery in Newcastle upon Tyne. *Brit Med J* 1957; *3*:117-124.

Welford, R. *Men of Mark 'twixt Tyne and Tweed.* London: Walter Scott, 3 vol, 1895. Brief biographies, not always referenced, but often quite detailed and sometimes unique.

Notes and references

1. Mark Akenside (1721-1770). His curriculum vitae in London was meteoric; LRCP 1751, MD (Cantab) 1753, FRCP 1754, Censor RCP 1755 and 1760, Gulstonian lecturer 1755, Croonian lecturer 1758, Harveian orator 1759, Physician in Ordinary to Queen Charlotte 1761; all by the age of 40. *See* Charles Sir John. Mark Akenside. *Brit Med J 1957*; 2:222-3; Munk W. *The Roll of the Royal College of Physicians of London,* Vol 2. London: RCP, 1878; Welford R. *Men of mark 'twixt Tyne and Tweed.* London: Walter Scott, 1895; Akenside M. *The Pleasures of Imagination. A poem in three books.* London: 1744 and many later editions; the 1744 edition was anonymous and only in some later editions was the title 'The Pleasures of *the* Imagination'.
2. 'In the summer of the year 1761, a man of about threescore years of age came to St Thomas's hospital from a village at some distance; not with any intention of being admitted as a patient, but in order to obtain present assistance for an uncommon disorder. He was in general healthy, and apparently of a good habit of body; but he had been accustomed, during the greater part of his life, to a constant succession of wens, that shot out in several places; on his head, trunk, arms, and legs; which indisposition he inherited from his father. As often as these wens became inconvenient from their size, his method was to cut them off with a razor; at which times, he constantly found that they grew upon the part by five or six suckers, as he called them. He had not much trouble in extirpating them, except when the razor passed through those suckers; at each of which, he felt on the instant a most acute pain; but in this manner he fairly got quit of them. When I saw him , he had three such wens; one on the forehead on the edge of his hair, about the size of a horse-bean; another on the short ribs of the right side, as big as a hen's egg; and a third on the greater extremity of the os ulna of the right arm, somewhat less than a common nutmeg. This last was the occasion of his applying to me; for as it advanced in size, a numbness was produced in the fore arm and hand; so that the use of them had of late been much impaired, as with a palsy; while, from the proximity of the wen to the joint of the elbow, he was afraid of imploying his razor, as he had been used to do in other parts of his body. Upon examination, I found these wens to be hard, indolent tumours, sitting loose and moveable upon the cellular membrane. As that near the elbow differed not from the rest, and was in no degree engaged in the joint, I directed it to be cut off, and a warm saponaceous liniment to be frequently rubbed on the arm and the hand, in order more speedily to restore them to their natural feeling and activity. The man himself I never saw or heard of again.'

   Akenside M. Observations on Cancers. *Med Trans Coll Phys* 1768; *1*:64-92.

3. 'Neer the Sandhill east, is Allhallows Banck, or Butchers Banck (where most butchers dwell), the way to Allhallows church; the south side of which is many chaires or lanes that goeth down to the Key side.' Gray W. *Chorographia, or a survey of Newcastle upon Tyne.* Newcastle upon Tyne: 1649.

4. Sir Samuel Garth (c1661-1718/9). Born at Bolam, south of Bishop Auckland, Co Durham. Studied Leiden and Cambridge (MD 1691), FRCP 1693, Gulstonian and Harveian Orator. Physician to George I. See *Munk's Roll* and Garrison. *The Dispensary* (1699) deserves a revival, with minor adaptations, to show the folly that results when business interests are made to conflict with the charitable provision of health care for the disadvantaged. The 'cost-price' Dispensary set up by the College in 1687, and so strongly approved by Garth, survived till 1724.

5. Anthony Askew (1722-1774) born in Kendal, moved to Newcastle in infancy. His father Adam (1694-1773) was the first Physician to the Infirmary (1751-71). Educated Sedbergh; The Royal Free Grammar School, Newcastle; Emmanuel College, Cambridge; University of Leiden; then practised in London. Physician to St Bartholomew's Hospital 1754-74. 'As a collector of books Dr. Askew was the first who brought bibliomania into fashion' (*Munk's Roll*). Owner of The Golden-headed Cane between Mead and Pitcairn. Twice Harveian orator (1758,1762). Registrar RCP 1767-74. Died leaving 12 orphans under 20, cared for by his brother Henry to whom they later erected a fine monument in St Nicholas Church (Newcastle Cathedral). Anthony was buried at Hampstead Church.

   See Munk W. *The Roll of the Royal College of Physicians of London*. London: R Coll Phys Vol 2, 1878; McMichael W. *The Golden-headed Cane*. London: Longmans Green, 1884; Welford R. *Men of Mark 'twixt Tyne and Tweed*. London: Walter Scott, 1895. Moore N. *The history of St Bartholomew's Hospital*. London: Pearson, 1918; *II*:535-40.

6 Thomas Addison (?1795-1860). Of Guy's Hospital, pernicious anaemia and Addison's disease. Both diseases were described briefly in 1849 (*Lond Med Gaz 43*:517-8) and in his book *On the constitutional and local effects of disease of the suprarenal capsules* (London, 1855). He was born in Longbenton village, now a suburb of Newcastle, where there is a memorial window in the Parish Church which he dedicated to his parents (due to be replaced in 1993); his usually quoted birth date, 1793, conflicts with the date of his baptism (11 Oct 1795, see Pallister,1969); educated at first by the Parish Clerk, John Rutter, who later taught Robert Stephenson (son of George) the railway engineer and designer of the High Level Bridge; later at the Royal Free Grammar School. Medical training in Edinburgh. Buried at Lanercost Abbey, Cumbria near Banks House, the home of his ancestors. *See* Munk's Roll *op cit* note 1; Welford *op cit* note 1; *A collection of the published writings of the late Thomas Addison, MD, Physician to Guy's Hospital*. London: New Sydenham Society, 1868; Pallister G. Dr. Thomas Addison (1795-1860). *Archaeologia Aeliana* 1969; Ser 4 *47*:137-146.

7. Samuel Fenwick (1821-1902). Born at Earsdon; apprenticed at the Infirmary, Newcastle School of Medicine and Surgery 1839; practised at Dockwray Square, North Shields 1842-1863; Lecturer in Anatomy and Physiology at the medical school 1845 and in Pathological Anatomy 1848-63; published the outcome of almost 5000 surgical cases at the Infirmary 1848 (one in three died); moved to London 1863; Assistant Physician at the London Hospital 1868-1896; notable as an early clinical microscopist; described gastric mucosal atrophy in Addisonian (ie pernicious) anaemia 1880. *See* Gibbs DD. Samuel Fenwick MD, FRCP (1821-1902): Physician and Gastroenterologist.*Brit Med J* 1970; *3*:339-342.

8. See Chapter 23 note 2. When he left Newcastle, in April 1879, Bramwell's students presented him with a fulsome Illuminated Address, and furthermore published it in the *Brit Med J* 1879; *1*:687. Bramwell was aged 32 years!

Bramwell began the tradition of muscular dystrophy research in Newcastle; Bramwell B. *Proc Northumb Durh Med Soc* 14 Dec 1876; *Idem.* Case of pseudo-hypertrophic paralysis. *Lancet* 1879; *2*:194-5.

9. Some sources for the history of medicine in the North East are given in an appendix to this introduction.

10. Talbot CH and Hammond EA. *The medical practitioners in medieval England: A biographical register*; London: Wellcome Historical Medical Library, 1965.

11. Welford R. *History of Newcastle and Gateshead, Vol 1, Fourteenth and Fifteenth Centuries*. London: Walter Scott, 1884:22-23.

12. See *Munk's Roll* and also Clark G. *A history of the Royal College of Physicians of London*. Oxford: Clarendon, 1964; Vol 1:59, 85.

13. Mackenzie *op cit* appendix:137-145, 416.

    In this street (West-gate Street) is an hospitall, called the Spittle; in the east of that chappell is the place for electing of majors, aldermen, sheriffs, and other officers in the towne, next Munday after Michaelmas day. In which place is made of late, a famous grammer-school, writing-school, and houses within the spittle for the masters.' Gray W. (1649) *op cit* note 3.

14. Welford *op cit* note 11:29.

    In Pilgrim Street is 'an house called the Pilgrims Inn, where pilgrims lodged that came to visit the shrine in Gesmond or Jesu de Munde, which occasioned to call this street Pilgrim Street.' Gray W. *op cit* note 3:71.

15. See Wallis J. *The natural history and antiquities of Northumberland...* London: W & W Strahan, 1769; vol 2:267; Mackenzie E. *op cit* appendix:474; Welford R. *op cit* note 11; Dendy FW. Saint Mary's Chapel *in* An account of Jesmond. *Archeologia Aeliana* Ser 3 *1*:130-147.

16. For the life of Turner see Pulteney R. *Historical and Biographical Sketches of the Progress of Botany in England, from its origin to the introduction of the Linnaean system.* London: T Cadell, 1790; Vol *I*: Chapter 5;

    Raven C E. *English naturalists from Neckham to Ray*. Cambridge: C U P, 1947:48-137;

    Hodgson J. *Memoirs of the lives of Thomas Gibson MD, Jonathan Harle MD, John Horsley MA,FRS, William Turner MD.* Newcastle: CH Cook, 1831.

    Jackson B D and Stearn W T. In *William Turner: Libellus de re herbaria 1538, The names of the herbes 1548.* Facsimile edition, London: The Ray Society, 1965;

    Jones W R D. *William Turner: Tudor naturalist, physician and divine*. London: Routledge, 1988.

    For his use of English see Johnson F R. Latin versus English: the sixteenth-century debate over scientific terminology. *Studies in Philology* 1944; *41*:109-135.

    Quotations from *The names of the herbes* are from the edition above.

17. His two exiles were 1540-7 in the last part of Henry VIII's reign and 1553-8 in Mary's. During the latter he lived and practised medicine at Weissenburg, south of Nürnburg.

18. Turner W. *A new Herball, wherin are conteyned the names of Herbes in Greke, Latin, Englysh, Duch Frenche, and in the Potecaries and Herbaries Latin, with the properties degrees and naturall places of the same...* London: Steven Mierdman, 1551: preface.

    *The seconde parte...*was published in Cologne by Arnold Birckman in 1562 (not examined).

    *The first and seconde partes of the Herbal of William Turner Doctor in Physick, lately oversene, corrected and enlarged with the Thirde parte,...*Collen: Arnold Birckman, 1568.

The 1568 edition has new prefaces to parts 1 and 3 and separate title pages to all parts (see note 28).

In transcribing quotations from Turner's works I have kept the original spelling and punctuation with the exception of the following purely typographical conventions: s is used for the long s, u appears as v where appropriate, y^e and y^t as [the] and [that], w^t as w[ith], ō as on or om as appropriate, and / as , .

19. Quoted and translated in part by Chapman G T L. William Turner of Morpeth, Northumberland (1508-1568). *The Scottish Naturalist* 1986, (no vol no.):11-27. The original is British Library MS Lansdowne VII:78.

[She] complained that a tumor had arisen in the liver ...with unbearable pain in the kidneys. Jaundice set in from the abscess of the liver, which even moderately trained doctors know how difficult it is to cure. But by applying every kind of device I attacked the disease not without a happy result. But on the occasion of a fresh dispute, suddenly and contrary to all my expectations a very parching fever followed, which so prostrated the heroine that although I used all kinds of medicines I did not progress even the width of a stalk. The whole family can testify to the diligence of my efforts spent in combatting the disease. [The above translated from the Latin by Chapman]....The lorde shewed great mercy to her for her breth went out like a candle.

20. Jones *op cit* note 16 has a chapter on Turner as a physician which the present account attempts to supplement, not to precis. Neither of us has tackled the commonplace book.

Jones discusses Turner's views on the medical effects of wines, his book on treacles, and the rich medical metaphore of the religious polemics *A preservative, or triacle, agaynst the poyson of Pelagius* and *A new booke of spirituall Physik for dyverse diseases of the nobilite and gentlemen of Englande.* I have not had a chance to examine these.

21. *A new Herball* 1551, *op cit* note 18: preface.

22. Preface to the first part of *A new Herball* 1568 edition, *op cit* note 18.

23. Stearn (in Jackson *op cit* note 16) gives only two species, A.maritima would be the Northumbrian plant. The others presumably include A.pontica and A.absinthium *L.* but this leaves French wormwood unaccounted for.

24. Two other examples from *The names of Herbes. op cit* note 16:

Lepidium. [Lepidium latifolium *L.*]
Lepidium is wel knowen in Englande and is called wyth a false name Dittany,...it groweth in Morpeth in Northumberlande by a water called Wanspeke in great plentie alone without any settyng or sowyng. It is hote in the fourth degree.

Again, of Orobanche [Orobanche rapum-genistae *Thuill.*]
Orobanche is so rare an herbe in Englande, that I never sawe it in al Englande, but in Northumberlande, where as it was called newe chappel floure. It may be of his propertie called Chokeweede, because it destroyeth and choketh the herbes that it tyeth and claspeth wyth his roote. It is colde and dry in the fyrst degree.

25. The garden of the Duke of Somerset at Syon House, near Kew.

26 Not identified, but probably the Spanish Moslem physician Averroes (1126-1198), pupil of Avenzoar and Islamic interpreter of Aristotle, see Garrison FH *An introduction to the history of medicine* 4th edit; 1929. He also appears in the accounts of Capparis [Capparis spinosa *L.*] and Nasturtium [Lepidium sativum *L.*].

27. Stearn gives only I. pseudacorus here. This covers the gladen but not the great Galanga; is this the Sweet Flag, Acorus calamus *L.* introduced into Europe "by 1557" according to Clapham, Tutin and Moore?(*Flora of the British Isles* 3rd edit; Cambridge: CUP, 1987.)

28. *The thirde parte of Guilliam Turners Herball, wherein are conteined the herbes, trees, rootes and fruhtes, whereof is no mention made of Dioscorides, Galene, Plinye, and other olde authores.* Collen: Arnold Birckman, 1568.

29 An example, which gives some details of the preparations:

Cummyn as Dioscorides writeth, healeth, bindeth, & dryeth. It is good for gnawyng & for wind, both sodden & put into oyle, or laid to after the maner of an oyntment w[ith] barly mele. It is given to them that are shortwinded, in wine and water: and in wyne to them that are bitten of a serpent. Cummyn layd to with rasyns, or the floure of darnel or with litle wexe after the maner of a salve, helpeth the swellinge of ye stones. It stoppeth the overmuch abundance of weomens natural sicknes. And the same broken & laid to in vinegre, to the nosethrilles, stoppeth bloode: it maketh the coloure of them that use it muche pale. Simeon Sethy wryteth that cumyn both dryed & also springeled w[ith] vinegre, dryeth a moyst stomache, & stoppeth laxes, and [that] it is good to lay upon weomens pappes, which have clustered or clodded milke in them. Som write [that] to muche of this, ingendreth the stone, and [that] the smoke of it, driveth awaye gnattes. Pliny sayth that cumyn is good with honyed vinegre for the falling sicknes. Cumin is hote and drye in the third degree.
Herball Part I, 1568 edit: 186-7. *NB* the spelling is much changed from the 1551 edition.

30. *A new Herball* Part II, 1568 edit:78r. Masterwurt is Peucedanum ostruthium (L.) Koch, a reputed antidote to poisoning in use into the 18th Century (Grigson G. *The Englishman's flora*. London: Phoenix House, 1958.)

31. Printed at Cologne by Birckman, and usually bound with the 1562 and 1568 editions of *The new Herball.*

32. 'linnettes, goldfinches, sparrowes and twyes'

Twyes are not identified. They may be twites, or possibly twinks (chaffinches) though these names do not otherwise occur until 1681 (Grew) and 1802 (Montagu) respectively.

33. Pybus FC. *op cit* appendix:162.

34. Embleton D. (1891) *op cit* appendix; Pybus FC. *op cit* appendix; Watts W. *op cit* appendix:118; Bulmer W, Hodgson N. The Barber-Surgeons Company of Newcastle upon Tyne. *Archaeologia Aeliana* Ser 4, *35*:73-80. See also the account of the Barber Surgeons' Hall in Chapter 12 of this volume.

The few entries of surgical interest amongst Embleton's extracts are:-

> A meting houlden in sant nickholase Churche amoungs the barbares and Chiourgons Juan 22 [1637] Raph dining fiened for taking a Cuer out of Edward banbrige hend 10s a Cording to owre ornerie rec' hearof 3s 4d payd
>
> [Meeting held at Widow Archbalds 20th May 1642] Memorandu' that Robert Maultby doth acknowledge to pay unto the Company ten shillings upon the aresting of him for takeing a Cure out of Thomas Smiths hand
>
> [10 June 1642 five more cases of fines for the same offence.]
>
> [Meeting] at George Durham 4 Otober [1647] Robert Anderson is Chosen by the Company to goe to the spetell for a Elecksion. [The spetell would be St Mary's Hospital by the West Gate, then used for annual elections; *see* Bourne's *History of Newcastle* 1736 *op cit* Appendix, p 35.]
>
> [Meeting at Edward Bainebriggs 2nd Oct 1648] Thomas Smith appointed to attend the Spittell [presumably a political rather than a surgical appointment.]
>
> [9 March 1648/9 the first meeting in the newly built Barber Surgeons' Hall.]
>
> Disbursements of Edward Bainbrigg & Charles Clark [Stewards] for year ended 10 June 1650 ... Given to a poore traveller being a Chirurgion [5s]

[22 May 1676 Thomas Bierly and other members being short - that is, late - were excused] being att a patient the first dressing.

Att a meeting the 5th of January 1676[/7] Thomas Ewbanck complains of Thomas Richardson for takeing a Cure out of his hand to witt one John Waterhouse fined xxs
1 June 77 submitts

1st Janry 1676 [-7]..to three Chirurgions shipwrackt & travelrs 6s 6d

[16 June 1679] Robert Haslipp complained off by Thomas Harrison for takeing severall patients out of his hands & p'ticularly Mr William Wards child

The Accompt of Henry Shaw and Joseph Story stewards...to and with the 4th June 1683 ..pd for Carrying the Anatomy & other Charges about him 8s 6d...... Mr peter Bates have this day prsented the Company with Bartholinus his Anotamy [sic] for their use and the stewards to keep it safe & delivr it to their successors every yeare [They did, and it is now in the Tyne and Wear Archives].

[11 Oct 1683] Given Robert Ridgeway a Chirurgion that suffered shipwracke 10s in charity

January ye 16th 1683 [-4] Rob Heslope informes Against Widdow Bates for Letting of Blud. [A bit churlish if she was the same Peter Bates' widow.]

35. Brand J. *The history and antiquities of the town and county of the town of Newcastle upon Tyne.* London: B White and Son, T&I Egerton, 1789; *II*:455-6, 494 and footnote.

36. See Mackenzie *op cit* appendix:528, 550; and, for keelmen, Mitcalfe WS. The history of the keelmen and their strike in 1822. *Archaeologia Aeliana* 1937; ser 4 *14*:1-16.

37. But see Chapter 5 'Medical Services' *in* Horsley PM. *Eighteenth-Century Newcastle.* Newcastle: Oriel Press, 1971; and Hume WE (1954) *op cit* appendix.

38. Extract of a letter from Mr Lambert, Surgeon at Newcastle upon Tyne, to Dr Hunter, giving an account of a new method of treating an aneurysm. Read June 15 1761. *Med Observ Inquir* 1764; *2*:360-4. The operation, to repair a ruptured brachial aneurysm, was performed in Newcastle on 15 June 1759, with a tourniquet and ligatures above and below the lesion in place.

> ..a small steel pin, rather more than a quarter of an inch long, was passed through the two lips of the wound in the artery, and secured by twisting a thread round it, as in a hare-lip. This was found to stop the bleeding; upon which the wound was bound up, the patient put to bed and ordered to be kept quiet etc. as usual in such cases. The wound was dressed the 4th day...the pin came away in the dressings June 29th...Healed except for the two ligatures..like setons..Discharged well July 19th.

Hunter commented that, if confirmed, this would be an important discovery in surgery.

39. See Fred Miller (chapter 7) on John Clark in this book and his 'Decline and fall of the Tubercle Bacillus: the Newcastle story 1882-1988.' *Arch Dis Childh* 1992; *67*: 251-255. Also Henry E Armstrong's own account 'Sketch of the Sanitary History of Newcastle upon Tyne'. *Trans Sanitary Institute Great Brit* 1883; *4*:76-96.

40. See his booklet – Clanny WR. *Hyperanthraxis; or, the cholera of Sunderland.* London: Whittaker, Treacher, and Arnott, 1832.

Clanny was in the chair at the inaugural meeting of the Sunderland Literary and Philosophical Society on 8 Oct 1834 (Richardson MA. *Op cit* appendix, Vol 4:218).

41. Watson RS. *The history of the Literary and Philosophical Society of Newcastle-upon-Tyne (1793-1896).* London: Walter Scott, 1897: 264-7.

42. Embleton D, Atthey T. On the skull and some other bones of Loxomma allmanni. *Ann Mag Nat Hist* 1874; *14*:38-63. See also Idem. *Nat Hist Trans Northum Durh*

1873; *5*:196-226, & 1886; *8*:349- 356. He published at least 6 other notes, obituaries and articles in *Nat Hist Trans Northumb Durh* between 1873 and 1890.

43. *In* Hutchinson W. *The history and antiquities of Cumberland*. Carlisle: F Jollie, 1794.

44. Thompson JV. *A catalogue of plants growing in the vicinity of Berwick upon Tweed.* London: J White, 1807. Thompson JV. *Zoological researches and illustrations 1828-1834*. Facsimile with an introduction by A Wheeler. London: Soc Bibliogr Nat Hist, 1968.

    Darwin C. *A monograph of the sub-class Cirripedia, with figures of all the species...*2 vols. London: The Ray Society, 1851, 1854.

45. Winch was joint secretary, with William Hutton, at the foundation of the Natural History Society of Northumberland Durham and Newcastle-upon-Tyne in 1829. Thornhill was sole secretary at its rebirth as The Tyneside Naturalists' Field Club in 1846. See also Chapter 15 note 8.

    Winch NJ, Thornhill J, Waugh R. *The botanist's guide through the counties of Northumberland and Durham.* Vol 1. Newcastle: S Hodgson, 1805. Vol 2 (without Waugh) Gateshead: J Marshall, 1807.

46. Meek A. George Stewardson Brady (obituary). *Trans Nat Hist Soc Northumb Durham & Newcastle-upon-Tyne* 1923; *6*:1-14.

47. The story of the early societies was told by Professor Dennis Embleton (in *Proceedings of the Northumberland and Durham Medical Society.* Session 1890-91; 105-124 and 155-177). He had been apprenticed for five years on his sixteenth birthday, October 1st 1826, to Thomas Leighton the founding Secretary of the first Society. Leighton died aged 84 in 1848, and Embleton aged 89 in 1900. See also Hume W E (1928) *op cit* appendix.

48. 'The Northumberland and Durham Medical Society' 14 April 1859; 'The Newcastle upon Tyne and Northern Counties Medical Society' 1920 to the present.

49. For the successive local medical journals from 1848 to 1971 see under *Newcastle and Northern Counties Medical Journal* in the appendix.

Chapter 2

HEALTH CARE IN THE ROMAN NORTH

Lindsay Allason-Jones

Since 1856 when Sir James Simpson first asked the question 'was the Roman army provided with medical officers?' innumerable articles and books have been written on the subject.[1] This paper does not intend to repeat the many points already raised concerning medicine in the Roman Empire but merely to bring together the evidence for health care in the military zone of north Britain in the first four centuries of our era. Evidence from elsewhere in Britain and the Empire will be used only to clarify details, the geographical area covered being confined to north of Catterick and south of the Antonine Wall.

Personnel

The building of Hadrian's Wall by legions II Adiutrix, VI Victrix and XX Valeria Victrix, each made up of five thousand men, cannot have been completed without the need for occasional medical care. In particular, such a massive building operation will have had its fair share of industrial injuries, so it is regrettable that none of the doctors attached to the legions at that time have been recorded by name. Two doctors are known from the legionary fortress at Chester (*Deva*): Hermogenes[2] and Antiochus,[3] but it is unclear whether they were attached to the fort's garrison or were members of the legate's private entourage. It is impossible to prove on present evidence whether either ever visited the frontier.

As the legions' activities in the area diminished after the Wall was completed a discussion of their medical staff is only of passing interest in the history of the north of Britain. It is to the auxiliary units, who manned the Wall, that we must turn for the bulk of the evidence. The name of only one medical man has survived from the hundreds who must have served in the area. This is Anicius Ingenuus,[4] *medicus ordinarius* of the First Cohort of Tungrians at Housesteads. From his name, Gilson concluded that he was a freeborn son of a Greek freedman and further speculated that he may have had some connexion with Spain.[5]

There has been considerable discussion of the status of the *medicus ordinarius* in the Roman army, admirably summed up by Davies in 1969,[6] and in the absence of new evidence there is little point in rehearsing all the arguments in detail. However, a few of the comments may assist in putting Anicius Ingenuus in his context and suggest the number of medical personnel serving in the area at any one time.

The term *medicus ordinarius* has been found in legionary inscriptions throughout the Empire as well as in association with auxiliary units and one *numerus*. In each case the post-holder appears to have had Roman citizenship. Their ages range from twenty-five, in the case of Anicius Ingenuus, to

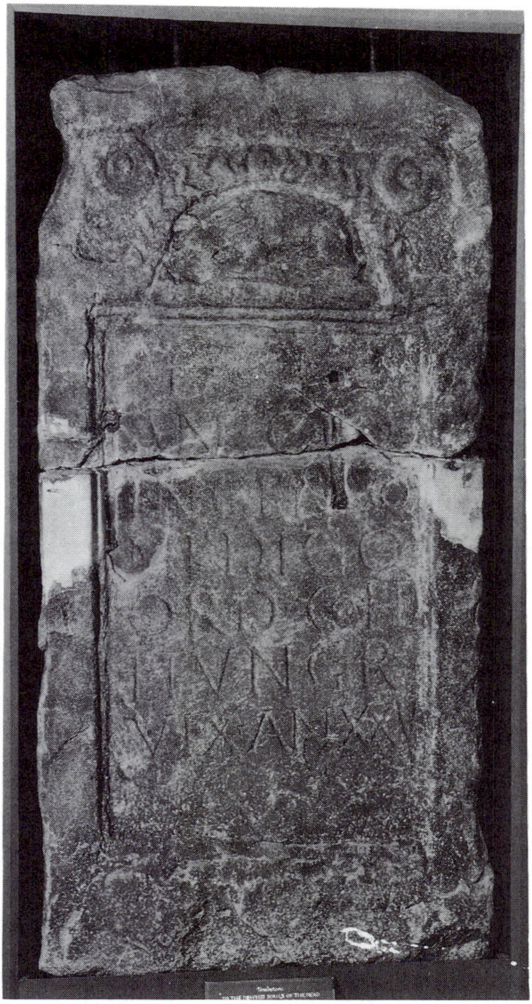

Figure 1. Tombstone of Anicius Ingenuus, *medicus ordinarius* at Houseteads.

Caius Papirius Aelianus, who died at Lambaesis in Africa at the age of eighty-five.[7] From this information we may conclude that the term did not indicate attachment to a particular sort of unit, nor a particular social status nor a stage in training. Although Anicius Ingenuus died young he was still of an age to be fully qualified according to the standards of his day. Training was often by apprenticeship, one practitioner, Thessalius, boasting that he could teach medicine in six months,[8] and anyone coming from a medical background could be considered qualified by the age of twenty.[9] C Terentius Symphorus was an acknowledged *medicus chirurgicus* (military surgeon) when he died at the age of twenty-eight,[10] while M Valerius Longinus, an

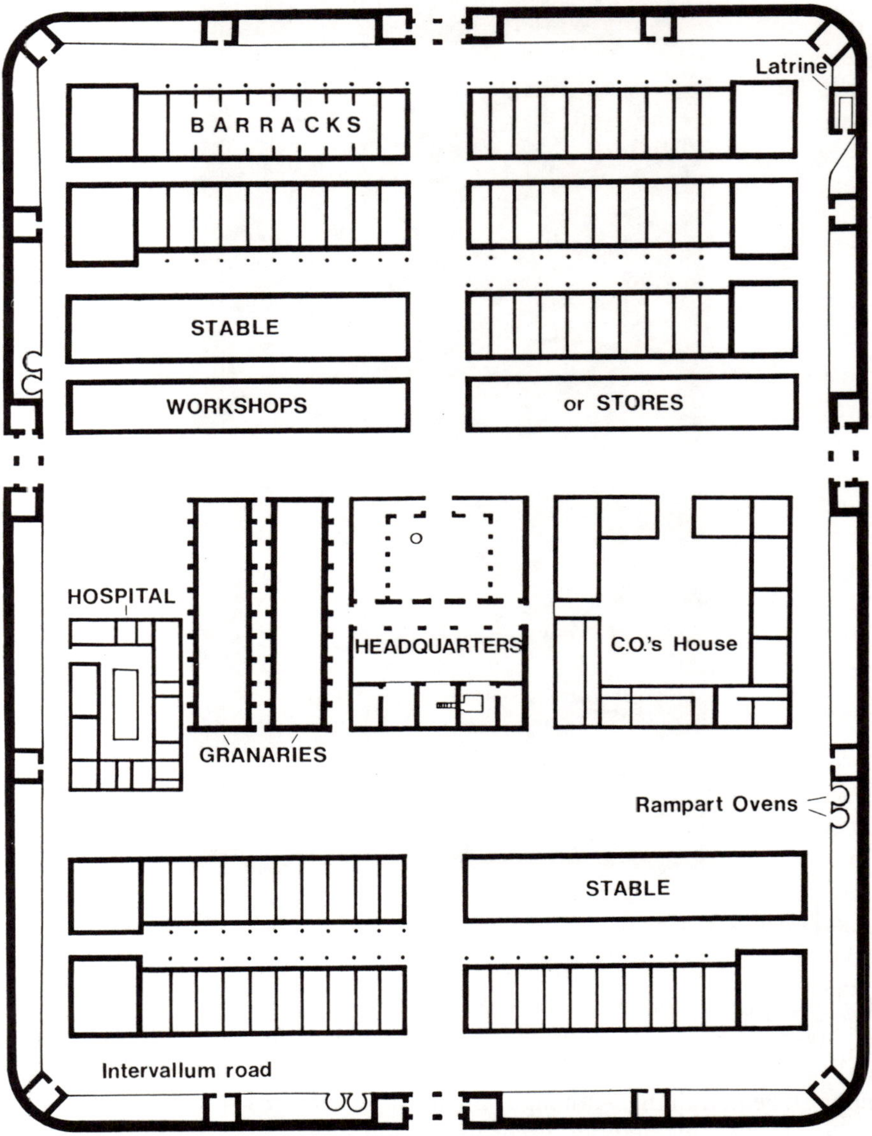

Figure 2. Plan of Houseteads Roman Fort showing the position and layout of the hospital: drawn by G. Stubbs.

established *medicus legionis*, died at the age of twenty-three at Drobeta in Dacia.[11] Anicius Ingenuus may already have been fully qualified in civilian practice before he joined the army, as were his colleagues Pedanius Dioscorides[12] or Scribonius Largus,[13] but equally he would have had plenty of time to learn the necessary skills if he joined as a recruit at the usual age of seventeen or eighteen. Davies concluded that a *medicus ordinarius* was a qualified doctor with the rank of centurion, although with purely medical responsibilities.[14] In a legion the *medicus ordinarius* would have served under the *medicus castrensis* (or *castrorum*) but in an auxiliary fort, such as Housesteads, he may have been the senior medical authority present. If each fort in the northern frontier region was provided with a *medicus ordinarius*, then at least twenty qualified doctors would have been serving at any one time, although this number will have fluctuated as forts were commissioned and decommissioned.

There is no epigraphic evidence in the area of other medical ranks, such as *miles medicus* (medical orderly)[15] or the *capsarii* whose responsibility it was to dress wounds, or any of the other medical staff who are mentioned amongst the *immunes* – those soldiers excused certain military duties and fatigues in acknowledgement of their special skills.[16] Nor are there inscriptions referring to specialists such as surgeons[17] or *medici clinici* (hospital physicians).[18] While it is possible that in the well-established frontier forts the *medicus ordinarius* was expected to act as general practitioner, hospital intern and surgeon, with little recourse to specialist advice, it is unlikely that he was without support staff to man the hospital. Each fort must have had a team of nursing staff and hospital administrators.

Hospitals

Housesteads provides the only surviving example of a hospital building (*valetudinarium*) in the region. The buildings identified as hospitals at Benwell and Wallsend are either incomplete or insufficiently excavated to offer much information,[19] while the building identified as a hospital at Corbridge is more likely to have been a storehouse or workshop.[20] The Housesteads example, excavated in 1904 and again in 1969-73,[21] is in a quiet place behind the *principia*, as recommended by Hyginus.[22] It follows the plan of the 1st and early 2nd century legionary fortress hospitals, albeit on a smaller scale, having a series of small wards arranged around a courtyard. The building underwent a series of alterations over the years; the original plan had wards opening into an adjacent room or onto a verandah overlooking the courtyard, but the verandah was later removed in order to extend the courtyard. The entrance with its well-worn threshold, was near the north end of the west wall and led into a reception room from where patients could be directed to the wards or straight into the operating theatre identified in the north range. The hospital had its own latrine in the south-west corner and possibly a plunge bath but no obvious kitchen facilities and no underfloor heating for the patients' comfort. Indeed, the building may have been damper than is consistent with good health care as there is some seepage of ground water off the whinsill in the north range, a problem solved to some extent by giving the operating theatre a raised wooden floor.

The many alterations make it difficult to judge how many rooms were used as wards at any one time but it is likely that the practice at Inchtuthil[23] and Fendoch[24] and other military *valetudinaria* was followed, whereby there was provision for one ward for each *centuria* of the cohort, which would suggest ten wards.

An accurate assessment of the number of beds available is problematic, again because of the alterations to the building. The wards appear to have been consistently smaller that the 13x14 feet available for each ward at Inchtuthil, which Pitts and St Joseph considered adequate for four beds. Figures varying from two to eight beds per ward have been proposed for other *valetudinaria* in the Empire. If one postulates ten wards with two to three beds per ward the capacity at Housesteads would be twenty or thirty beds indicating a 2-3% casualty rate, somewhat less than the 5-10% rate suggested for Inchtuthil or Fendoch.

Not all the soldiers unfit for duty on medical grounds would have been in need of hospitalization. A recently discovered writing tablet at Vindolanda, a fort on the Stanegate to the south of Hadrian's Wall, gives a military strength report.[25] Although dated to *c* AD 90, some years before the building of the Wall, it also relates to the First Cohort of Tungrians, then under the command of Iulius Verecundus. It states that, of 296 men including one centurion, 265 are fit and 31 unhealthy. On the casualty list are fifteen who are sick (*aegri*), six wounded and ten 'suffering from inflammation of the eyes' (*lippientes*). This represents approximately 10% of the available force as unfit for duty, of which half may have required hospital treatment.

As Jackson has pointed out, the military hospitals were not set up to cope with the needs of convalescents.[26] Soldiers requiring longterm care might be granted sick leave during which time they could return home, if this was feasible, or be sent somewhere suitable to recuperate, such as a coastal town or a spa. There is no written evidence as yet of the troops on Hadrian's Wall being sent away to convalesce, although the coastal forts at South Shields (*Arbeia*) and Maryport (*Alauna*) conjure up some attractive pictures to modern readers and one wonders if the curative powers of the waters at Gilsland or Haydon Spa were recognized at the time. The curse tablets found at Bath show that a third of the known visitors at the healing spring of Sulis Minerva were soldiers, including two centurions, a number of legionaries and a Spanish cavalryman.[27] During campaigns it was the practice for the Roman army to billet the sick or wounded on civilian households and it is conceivable that in more settled situations some houses in the *vici* were used as official or unofficial nursing homes.[28]

Ailments

Although imagination, backed by the medical literature of the day, can provide a list of the wounds and diseases which a frontier doctor might expect to encounter, evidence on the ground is sparse. This is largely due to the common practice of cremating the dead. The cemeteries of Petty Knowes at High Rochester[29] and Lanchester[30] can provide some information as to the sex and age of the deceased but nothing about the ailment which took him or her to the grave. The more informative tombstones are still as coy as any modern obituary when it comes to the cause of death. The few skeletons which do survive either come from late, possibly post-Roman, contexts (eg South Shields),[31] or were clearly denied medical assistance *in extremis*, such as the murdered couple buried in the floor of Building VIII in Housesteads *vicus*.[32] From other Romano-British sites we might conclude that osteoarthritis was prevalent, that broken bones were commonplace and that tuberculosis and leprosy were among the known afflictions, but the inhabitants of the military zone have only left evidence about their eyes, teeth and bowels.

The strength report from Vindolanda, already mentioned, shows that eye disorders were rife in the army. This was taken so seriously by the authorities that an eye test was included in the medical which all recruits had to pass.[33] According to Galen writing in the 2nd century AD, the *Classis Britannicus* (British Fleet), which is known to have been actively involved with building operations at Benwell, Halton Chesters and Rudchester, had its own oculist, Axius.[34] While Axius himself may have remained at the Fleet's main base at Dover, his salve, which attracted Galen's respect, will have been used widely. Its ingredients are listed as copper and zinc hydroxide, zinc carbonate, opium and mercuric sulphide, and was intended for use on 'ulcered corners of the eye, bad inflammation of the eye, intense irritation and chronic condition'.

Eye salves were made up in small solid blocks which were diluted or softened with water or egg as and when required. The blocks were identified by a text stamped on when the mixture was still malleable and a number of the stone stamps used for this purpose have been discovered. They are mostly rectangular tablets with the retrograde text cut on one or more edges. Although none have been found at a Wall fort an example is known from Watercrook in Cumbria and another from Tarent in Lothian Region, indicating that oculists were practising in the region. The stamp at Watercrook only gives a name, which may be that of the inventor of the salve or the oculist: Publius Clodius (or Clodianus),[35] but that from Tarent also gives some indication of the active ingredient and the use to which it should be put: 'Lucius Valerius Latinus's fragrant salve for scars and granulation (of the eyelids)' 'Lucius Valerius Latinus's mild saffron salve for affections (of the eye)'.[36] Saffron was also used by Quintus Iulius Martinus at Chester[37] while Iulius Alexander at York preferred 'misy', possibly identifiable as copper pyrites.[38]

Nearly 300 oculists' stamps are known in the Roman Empire[39] but Boon and Frere have both noticed that the bulk of them are to be found in the northwest provinces.[40] This is not likely to suggest that eye disease was more prevalent in this area than in the eastern or African provinces where sand provides a constant irritant, but Boon has suggested that the outlying provinces may have had to rely more heavily on prepackaged nostrums 'perhaps the stock-in-trade of itinerant general practitioners' in the absence of the well-established health provision found in the Mediterranean provinces. This does not appear to agree with the presence of a military medical service or with the fame of Axius, but it is unlikely that each frontier fort had its own oculist. It may be that doctors like Anicius Ingenuus would have ordered supplies of medications from their specialist colleagues at other forts or fortresses.

The concern of the military authorities for soldiers' eyesight does not seem to have extended to their teeth. The pre-enlistment medical was thorough but the condition of the candidate's teeth was not mentioned as one of the criteria for entry.[41] Skeletal evidence from southern cemeteries has shown that caries was less prevalent than in most modern populations, no doubt due to the lack of sugar and refined flour in the diet. The coarse stone-ground flour, however, will have worn down the biting surfaces leading to abscesses and gum infections. A few skulls have survived in the military zone which show this attrition as well as a noticeable build-up of tartar. In particular, two skeletons from late contexts at South Shields had stains of calculus on their teeth which the specialist's report has suggested 'may well have been the source of irritation and infection which has caused the reabsorption of alveolar bone which is a consequence of chronic gum disease'.[42] In the case of skeleton 49 at South Shields, an adult female, there is the possibility that 'there are two sinuses opening horizontally, which would indicate the presence of the formation of at least one abscess'. Skeleton 50 at the same site exhibited severe dental disease and had lost all the right molars *ante mortem*. The sockets had healed over but the bone was 'considerably distorted by infection'. The incisors also show evidence of disease, having lost most of their enamel with a local periodontal abscess indicated near the right front incisor.

No inscriptions survive of military dentists and it is probable that in the smaller forts the medical officer was expected to combine his role with that of dentist; military efficiency would have demanded some level of dental care even if extraction in the face of pain was the only service on offer. The civilian population may have had access to such specialists as Cascellius, who Martial described as one who 'draws or stops the decayed tooth' although it is possible that away from the big towns these specialists may have been more in the nature of the travelling tooth-drawers of medieval Britain, setting up their stalls in the markets or *vici*.[43]

In the absence of skeletons some evidence for the health of a population may be found in the analysis of cesspit material. The excavations at

Carlisle have produced the eggs of both whipworm and roundworm.[44] The whipworm has been identified as *Trichuris trichuria*, a species parasitic upon the human lower intestine and caecum, a heavy infestation of which can result in dysentery and prolapse of the rectum. The identification of the roundworm eggs is less certain but has been assumed to be from *Ascaris lumbricoides*, a slight infestation of which would lead to few, if any, symptoms but as with *Trichuris trichuria*, a heavy infestation could have led to serious complications. Excavations at York and other waterlogged sites have produced similar results, perhaps not surprising in view of the somewhat basic levels of hygiene practised at the time, particularly in regard to the storage of food stuffs. Diarrhoea and dysentery are mentioned frequently by the Roman medical writers and it is all too easy to imagine the speed at which a 'tummy bug' would travel through an army camp.

Other human parasites have been discovered at Ribchester (*Bremetenacum*), in Lancashire, where a well-preserved comb of boxwood was recovered from a waterlogged deposit. The examination of the soil residues during conservation revealed fragments of head lice (*Pediculus humanus capitis*).[45] Jackson has suggested that regular use of the bath-house as recommended by military and civic authorities alike, would have reduced the transmission of diseases carried by fleas, lice or ticks.[46] However, as most bath-houses were only cleaned out intermittently they may well have aided the transmission of bacterial or viral infections. The sharing of sponges in lavatories, such as can be seen at Housesteads, would also have played a part in the spread of disease.[47]

Medicines

The medical practitioners had a wide range of drugs available to offer their patients, many based on herbs which could be found locally. Liversidge has suggested that the courtyard of the hospital at Housesteads, later flagged, was originally used for growing medicinal herbs.[48] The analysis of deposits at Carlisle has indicated the presence of opium poppy seeds but it is unclear if these were used as a narcotic or as a culinary flavouring.[49] The opium poppy was one of the essentials of the Roman pharmacopoeia and the 1st century AD writer Celsus mentions how one opium preparation was useful for 'headache or ulceration or ophthalmia or toothache or difficulty in breathing or intestinal gripings or inflammation of the womb or pain in the hips or liver or spleen or ribs'.[50] For those patients facing a surgical procedure opium and henbane were the only available 'anaesthetics'. Henbane seeds have been found in Britain at Silchester and Carmarthen.

Carlisle apart, little evidence has emerged from seed analysis for medicinal plants in the north. There is evidence from southern sites for dock (*Rumex obtusifolius*), which Pliny recommended for the treatment of scurvy;[51] and the wild celery found in a latrine at the fort at Bearsden (Glasgow) may have been used as a diuretic.[52] Native plants such as plantains and St John's wort are commonly found in the floral remains on archaeological sites, the former beneficial in treating pulmonary tuberculosis, haemorrhage and dysentery; the latter being used to expel bladder stones.

More picturesquely, though less convincingly, Camden in 1600 was confident that the area of the Wall was ideal for the cultivation of medicinal herbs for the Roman army, in particular the wild chives (*Lilium schoenoprasum*) which still grows near Walltown Crags: 'That the Roman souldiers of the marches did plant heere every where in old time for their use, certain medicinable hearbes, for to cure wounds: whence is it that some Emperick practitioners of Chirurgery in Scotland, flock hither every yeere in the beginning of summer, to gather such simples and wound herbes; the vertue whereof they highly commend as found by long experience, and to be of singular efficacy'.[53] Although it is possible that the wild chives was introduced in the Roman period its wide distribution throughout Britain suggests that it was not confined to areas of military occupation.

Preparations of medicines are rare finds although a few inscriptions, other than collyrium stamps, survive to indicate their presence. A fort at Haltern, in East Germany, produced a lead vessel lid inscribed '*ex radice Britanica*' – 'extract of the root of Britan(n)ica'.[54] Pliny mentioned this as an anti-scorbutic but confessed himself puzzled as to why it should be named after Britain as he says 'it is certain that the plant was not named because it grew abundantly in that land'.[55] Davies, however, was of the opinion that it was the native *Rumex obtusifolius*[56] while Richmond preferred to identify it as *Rumex angustifolius*[57] although this identification is as obscure as the original inscription.

It is only recently that a possible purveyor of such preparations has been identified. A fragment of a stilus writing tablet from Carlisle refers to one '*albano seplasiario*' whom Tomlin has translated convincingly as 'Albanus the pharmacist'.[58] Whether Albanus was attached to the fort hospital or was a self-employed chemist selling his wares to the civilian population is as yet unknown.[59]

The fort at Carpow in Fife produced a fragment of an amphora with a scratched inscription indicating that it contained wine flavoured with horehound, a sovereign cure for coughs according to such authorities as Dioscorides, Celsus and Pliny.[60] The soldiers of the II Legion Augusta at Caerleon in Wales were provided with an amphora of Aminaean wine as a cure for diarrhoea and the common cold.[61] Although these are some distance from Hadrian's Wall they do indicate that some medicines were supplied in bulk to fort hospitals. Davies's suggestion that the hoard of bronze and iron objects found buried at Corbridge was for the purpose of providing the medical profession with verdigris and rust for wound salves has now been disproved.[62]

The use of the available drugs would have been widely known in the medical profession. All the doctors known by name in Britain had Greek names, as did the majority of the practitioners in the Empire, and would have been trained in the Greek tradition. A number of medical treatises were available to the profession including *Materia Medica*, compiled by the well travelled military doctor Pedanius Dioscorides. This is not the place to list the various literary texts which Anicius Ingenuus, for example, may have had to hand, but it is interesting that the cough mixture attested at Carpow, 150 miles north of the Wall and labelled in Greek, was that recommended by Dioscorides in the 1st century AD.

Instruments and equipment

Through the medical texts and from their own experience military doctors would have been aware of the latest techniques and equipment. The fort at Corbridge, on the Stanegate, has produced one of the largest collections of Roman medical and surgical instruments found in Britain,[63] although it is regrettable that the 'medical box' found there in the 1930s was lost during the Second World War.[64] Whilst not as lavishly decorated as some of the instruments found elsewhere in the Empire they indicate that the medical staff in the north had access to efficient and up-to-date tools. The scalpel handles of copper alloy, for example, had replaceable iron blades which fitted into a groove so that they did not move during use. The other ends of each handle terminated in an elliptical spatula of the type used for blunt dissection. Two tubular handles for surgical knives also survive, as well as a bone handle with a screw-thread cover which would have protected an ophthalmic needle: handled needles were used with great skill by surgeons to couch cataracts and to cauterize trichiasis.[65] One arm of a pair of epilation forceps used in this latter operation has also survived at Corbridge.

The Corbridge collection includes instruments with a specific use such as a tongue depressor for examining the throat, and a male bladder sound to deal with the common problem of bladder stones, but the majority of the instruments are probes of one sort or another. Probes were used extensively for investigating wounds but also for mixing medicines and applying them. The basic probe was the plain rod which tapered to two blunt points – the simplicity of this instrument makes it probable that many have gone unrecognized in finds and the survival of only one at Corbridge should not be taken as evidence of its rare use. Rods ending in bulbous (olivary) probes are not confined to Corbridge; examples are also known from South Shields and Carlisle, often with an elongated spoon bowl (*cyathiscomele*) at the other end.[66] Spatulate probes (*spathomele*) with a thin olivary probe at one end and a flat spatula at the other are also common.

Most of the sites in the region have produced *ligulae* with tapered circular-sectioned shanks and tiny angled flat heads.[67] These could be used for surgical purposes but were more widely used to extract ointments from bottles. *Ligulae* were also used in connexion with cosmetics and individual examples are difficult to assign to medical use with any confidence. This is also true of the long glass vessels known as *unguentaria* in which ointments and cosmetics were transported[68] and the slate palettes from South Shields and Corbridge on which they were mixed.[69] Plain tweezers, as opposed to elaborate surgical forceps, are also ambiguous despite the numbers found.

More clearly for surgical use are the two hooks found at South Shields and Housesteads.[70] The former, of bronze, is 14.8cm long with a domed head and a facetted neck while the Housesteads example is slightly shorter (13.8cm) and less elaborate, although also tapering to a hook. These can be identified as traction hooks, that from South Shields as the blunt hook (*hamus retusus*) used for dissection and raising blood vessels in the manner of the modern aneurism needle, and that from Housesteads as the sharp hook (*hamulus acutus*) which Celsus and Paulus Aegineta recommended for removing tonsils and extracting the fetus in a difficult labour.[71] The decorative facetting and moulding on these instruments, also seen on a number of the probes described above, may have been intended to prevent the hand from slipping in use.

Religion and magic in medicine

Despite the sophisticated instruments, the extensive pharmacopoeia and the extent of medical knowledge diffused through treatises, it is clear that the population had more faith in their gods than in their doctors: going to see the doctor seems to have been regarded as a last resort rather than a first call. Indeed doctors themselves did not scorn divine intervention: Abrocomas, the doctor of the Cavalry Regiment of Vettonians at Binchester (*Vinovia*) in County Durham, is known to us only because he dedicated an altar to Aesculapius and Salus.[72] Whether Titus Flavius Titianus, tribune of the First Cohort of Vardullians at Lanchester (*Longovicium*) had consulted his doctor before he dedicated an altar is unknown but his awareness of his debt to Aesculapius, god of healing, suggests that he had no doubts as to who was responsible for his cure.[73] Civilians also dedicated to healing gods, for example, the 'freedmen and slave-household of Titus Pomponius Mamilianus' at Chester.[74] There are other dedications to Aesculapius at South Shields and to Salus at Corbridge.[75]

The sick could either make offerings to a local god of healing in the hope of receiving a cure in return or could visit a shrine which combined religion with curative waters to plunge into or take internally. No major healing shrines have been identified in the north of England or Scotland – the objects found in the shrine at Coventina's Well at Carrawburgh suggest that although healing may have been one of the goddess's duties it was not her only contribution to the wellbeing of her worshippers.[76] However, the large numbers of hairpins and bracelets, traditional offerings to a deity concerned with female health, which were found in a building at Piercebridge, County Durham, may indicate that this was a shrine visited by worshippers in search of a cure for gynaecological complaints. The altars mentioned above, to Salus and Aesculapius, hint that their temples are still to be discovered at Corbridge and South Shields.

In order to ensure that illness was kept at bay amulets were worn by men and women, military and civilian, old and young. A number of bronze phalli, worn to ward off the Evil Eye have been found, although their use may have been against general bad luck rather than purely medical disasters. Two beads and an egg-shaped amulet of lithomarge found at Housesteads may have been used as pain relief aids during childbirth: the veined appearance was thought to embue the stone with apotropaic properties and holding an amulet made from the stone was thought to put the sufferer in contact with the gods.[77] Amber, 'supposed to be a prophylactic against tonsilitis and other affections of the pharynx', has been found in bead form at Housesteads and South Shields[78] but the most commonly found material with a healing connexion is jet. Pliny recommended the 'kindling of jet' for the relief of 'suffocation of the uterus'. He continued 'its fumes detect attempts to simulate a disabling illness or a state of virginity. Moreover, when thoroughly boiled with wine it cures toothache and, if combined with wax, scrofulous tumours'.[79] South Shields, in particular, has produced a wide range of objects made from jet.[80]

The patients

Academic writers are prone to compare Roman medicine with the medicine of today, pointing out where Roman practice was 'ahead of its time' and where it fell short, but it is more pertinent to consider how the contemporary population regarded the medical care on offer: the pleas for divine intervention, mentioned above, and comments in the literature of the time seem to suggest that expectations that physicians could influence the course of an illness were low. Writers, such as Martial and Juvenal, make cutting comments about the medical profession of their day, even though they had been brought up in the Graeco-Italian world and were familiar with the medical traditions of that world. It is easy to forget that the population of Britain between the first and fourth centuries AD came from a much wider geographical area: people from every province of the Empire would have been present at one time or another, people whose origins may have predisposed them to a different medical tradition. The Greek and Syrian theories and practices on which Roman medicine was based may have been viewed with some suspicion by members of, for example, the Germanic or Gallic tribes. The local British population may also have seen no reason to abandon their established methods of medical care and adopt the 'new-fangled' ideas of the Romans. Furthermore, Martial and Juvenal, living in the capital where there were many doctors, would have been in a position to judge which were the more successful practitioners and consult the physician or surgeon of their choice. Those who found themselves in a frontier zone may not only have felt uncomfortable with the medical practitioners on offer but would have had few alternatives to hand.

Much of the written evidence is limited to serving soldiers. These, however, may have been the minority in a population which would have included veterans, the families of officers, and the merchants and traders living in the *vici*. Were the skills of the *medicus ordinarius* and his staff available to the rest of the population? When the infant daughter of the commanding officer of Chesters (*Cilurnum*), Fabius Honoratus, lay fatally ill it is unlikely that he resisted the temptation to call upon the medical staff under his command for assistance.[81] If the commanding officer allowed his family this privilege, was it extended to Aelia Comindus, wife of Nobilianus, decurion at Carrawburgh (*Brocolitia*)[82] the elderly Lucius Novellius Lanuccus who died aged seventy at Great Chesters (*Aesica*)[83] or the fifteen-year-old sister of Aurelia S...illa who also died at Great Chesters?[84] The tombstones found in abundance in the area give a detailed picture of the population and their age at death as well as the names of their sorrowing relatives who would, no doubt, have sought the best medical care for them when illness struck. An inscription at Risingham suggests some degree of medical advice, although no names are given to suggest whether the family was military or civilian: it refers to a son who had been prevented by ill health from legally inheriting his parents' estate 'following the natural succession'.[85] Roman laws of inheritance were very strict and it is unlikely that the substitute heir would have had a valid claim unless an accredited doctor had declared the son unfit. The phrase 'following the natural succession' indicates that the family was following a set procedure laid down for just such a contingency. As Risingham was an outpost fort it is unlikely that any other medical authority would have been available but the fort doctor.

The excavations of the legionary fortress of Caerleon in Wales have shown that women and children were allowed to use the facilities of the bath-house.[86] An admission token found in the later levels suggests that male civilians were also admitted. There were no separate suites so any arrangements allowing women or civilians into the baths must have required an official allocation of bathing times. All the forts on Hadrian's Wall and elsewhere in the area were provided with bath-houses and on the Caerleon example it is possible to postulate that these were also open to outsiders. If this one military facility was open to the non-military then it is possible that health care facilities were also made available. The size of the hospital at Housesteads and military codes of behaviour would prohibit women and children from occupying the wards but medical advice must have been proffered. As military doctors are known to have retired into private practice it is to be presumed and hoped that their skills and experience were not confined to soldiers' ailments.[87]

From this article it is clear that the evidence for health care in the north of Britain during the Roman occupation is very uneven. The large number of basic medical instruments perhaps balances the paucity of architectural and epigraphic evidence but there are still many gaps. Some of the holes in our knowledge can be temporarily filled by comparing the evidence from other parts of the Empire and drawing upon the contemporary writers but the recent discoveries at Carlisle and South Shields indicate that much is to be hoped for from future excavation and analysis. A fuller picture of the medical services available to the military and civilian population in the 1st to 4th centuries AD is still to emerge.

Notes

1. Simpson J. *Was the Roman Army Provided with Medical Officers*? Edinburgh: privately printed, 1856.
2. Collingwood R G, Wright R P. *The Roman Inscriptions of Britain* I (*RIB*). Oxford: Clarendon Press, 1965: no 461.
3. Wright R P. Roman Britain in 1968.II.Inscriptions. *J Roman Studies* 1969; *59*:235, no 3.
4. *RIB* 1618 (*op cit* note 2). The tombstone is now on display in the Museum of Antiquities of the University and Society of Antiquaries of Newcastle upon Tyne.
5. Gilson A. A doctor at Housesteads. *Archaeol Aeliana* 1978; ser 5 *6*:162-5.
6. Davies R. The *Medici* of the Roman armed forces. *Epigraphische Studien* 1969; *8*: 83-99. See also Nutton V. Medicine and the Roman army: a further reconsideration. *Med Hist* 1969; *13*:260-70.
7. Huebner A. *Corpus Inscriptionum Latinarum* (*CIL*). Berlin: 1863-. *8* no 18314. Dessau *Inscriptiones Latinae Selectae* (*ILS*) Berlin: Weidmann, 3 vols in 5 parts, 1892-1916: no 2432.
8. Phaedrus ed Perry B E. *Fables* London: Loeb, 1965, *I*.14; Galen ed Brock A J. *On the Natural Faculties*. London: Loeb, 1916: *1*.X.804.
9. Soranus ed Temkin O. *Soranus' Gynecology*. Baltimore; 1956: 244; *CIL* no XII.533 (*op cit* note 7).
10. *Année Épigraphique* 1945:62.
11. *CIL* no III.14216.9; *ILS* no 7150a (*op cit* note 7).
12. Dioscorides ed Wellmann M. *Pedani Dioscurides anazarbein de Materia Medica*. Berlin; Weidmann, 3 vols 1906-14:*1*.4.
13. Largus ed Helmreich G *Compositiones Medicamentorum*. *Bibl. Scriptorum Graecorum et Romanorum Teubneriana*. Lipsiae: 1887:162.
14. Davies *op cit* note 6:91.
15. Cf Titus Aurelius Numerius at Aquincum: *CIL* no III.14347.5 or Marcus Sabinianius Quietus at Iversheim: *CIL* no XIII.7943 (*op cit* note 7).
16. *Digesta Justiniana* trans Mommsen T. 1866-. *L*.6.7.
17. Cf C Terentius Symphonus at Messina: *AE* 1945.62 (*op cit* note 10).
18. Cf Tiberius Claudius Iulianus: *CIL* no *VI*.2532 (*op cit* note 7).
19. Simpson F G, Richmond I A. The Roman fort on Hadrian's Wall at Benwell. *Archaeol Aeliana* 1941; ser 4 *19*:1-43.
20. Bishop M C, Dore J N. *Corbridge: Excavations of the Roman fort and town*. London: Historic Buildings and Monuments Commission Archaeological Report 8, 1988: 128.
21. Bosanquet R C. Excavations on the line of the Roman Wall in Northumberland. The Roman camp at Housesteads. *Archaeol Aeliana* 1904; ser 2 *25*:193-300; Charlesworth D. The Hospital, Housesteads. *Archaeol Aeliana* 1976; ser 5 *4*:17-30.
22. Hyginus ed von Domaszewski A. *De Munitionibus Castrorum*. 1887:4.
23. Pitts L F, St Joseph J K. *Inchtuthil. The Roman Legionary Fortress*. London: Britannia Monograph Series 6, 1985.
24. Richmond I A, McIntyre A. The Agricolan fort at Fendoch. *Proc Soc Antiq Scot* 1937-8 (1939); *73*:110-54.

25. Bowman A K, Thomas J D. A military strength report from Vindolanda. *J Roman Studies* 1991; *81*:62-73.

26. Jackson R. *Doctors and Diseases in the Roman Empire*. London: British Museum Publications, 1988:136.

27. Tomlin R S O. The curse tablets. In: Cunliffe B .*The Temple of Sulis Minerva at Bath*. II. *The finds from the sacred spring*. Oxford: Oxford University Committee for Archaeology, 1988:96.

28. Caesar ed Peskett A G. *Civil War*. London: Loeb, 1966 *III*.78.2; Caesar ed Way A G. *African War*. London: Loeb, 1964:21; ed Magie D. *Scriptores Historiae Augustae II Severus Alexander*. London: Loeb, 1967; *47*:2-3.

29. Charlton D B, Mitcheson M. The Roman cemetery at Petty Knowes, Rochester, Northumberland. *Archaeol Aeliana* 1984; ser 5 *4*:1-32.

30. Reed A, pers comm.

31. Grove R. Report on the human remains. In: Bidwell P T, Speak S C. *Excavations at the Roman fort of South Shields*. Forthcoming.

32. Birley E, Charlton J, Hedley P. Excavations at Housesteads in 1932. *Archaeol Aeliana* 1933; ser 4 *10*:82-96.

33. Davies R. Joining the Roman Army. *Bonner Jahrbucher* 1969; *169*:208-32.

34. Galen *op cit* note 8:*XII*.786K.

35. Frere S S, Tomlin R S O. *The Roman Inscriptions of* Britain *II*.4 (*RIB*) Stroud: Alan Sutton Publishing. 1992, no 2466.5.

36. *RIB* no 2466.12 (*op cit* note 35).

37. *RIB* no 2446.16 (*op cit* note 35).

38. *RIB* no 2446.1 (*op cit* note 35).

39. Voinot J.Inventaire des cachets d'oculistes gallo-Romains. *Conferences Lyonnaises d'ophthalmologie*. 1981-2 (1984); *150*:1-578.

40. Boon G C. Potters, oculists and eye-troubles. *Britannia*. 1983; *14*:1-12; *RIB* no 2446 (*op cit* note 35).

41. Vegetius trans Clark J. *The military institutions of the Romans*. Connecticut: Greenwood Press, 1985,I.

42. Grove *op cit* note 31.

43. Martial ed Ker W C A. *Epigrams*. London: Loeb, 1919; *X*:lvi.

44. Jones A K G, Hutchinson A R. Parasitological investigations. In: Caruana I. *The Roman fort at Carlisle: excavations at Annetwell Street, 1973-84*. Forthcoming.

45. Fell V, pers comm.

46. Jackson *op cit* note 26:49

47. Mann J. The Housesteads Latrine. *Archaeol Aeliana* 1989; ser 5 7:1-4.

48. Liversidge J. *Britain in the Roman Empire*. London: Routledge and Kegan Paul, 1968:329.

49. Huntley J P. Environmental synthesis. In: Caruana *op cit* note 44.

50. Celsus ed Spencer W G. *De Medicina*. London: Loeb, 1935-8; *V*:25.3.

51. Pliny trans Rackham H, Jones W H S, Eichholz D E. London: Loeb, 10 vols 1942-63; *XXV*:20.

52. Celsus *op cit* note 50; *IV*:16.3.

53. Camden W. trans. Gough R. *Britannia*. London: T Payne, 1806:470.

54. *Germania* 1928; *12*:70, fig 1.

55. Pliny *op cit* note 51; *XXV*:21.

56. Davies R. The Roman military medical service. *Saalburg Jahrbuch* 1970; *27*:84-104.

57. Richmond I A. The Roman army medical service. *Univ Durham Gaz* June 1952:2-6.

58. Tomlin R S O. Inscriptions. *Britannia* 1991; *22*:300.

59. For a military *seplasiarius* see *CIL XIII*:6778 (Mainz). For a self-employed individual see *ILS* no 7606 (Cologne) (*op cit* note 7).

60. Wright R P. Roman Britain in 1962.II. Inscriptions. *J Roman Studies*. 1963; *53*:166, no 51.

61. Celsus *op cit* note 52:*IV*.5.5; *IV*.26.3-9.

62. Davies R. A note on the hoard of Roman equipment buried at Corbridge. *Durham Univ J* 1970:177-80; Allason-Jones L, Bishop M C. *Excavations at Roman Corbridge: The Hoard*. London: Historic Buildings and Monuments Commission Archaeological Report 7, 1988.

63. Gilson A G. A group of Roman surgical and medical instruments from Corbridge. *Saalburg Jahrbuch* 1981; *37*: 5-9.

64. Prof E Birley, pers comm.

65. See Jackson *op cit* note 26:121-2 for details of the operation.

66. Allason-Jones L, Miket R F. *Catalogue of small finds from South Shields Roman fort*. Newcastle upon Tyne: Society of Antiquaries of Newcastle upon Tyne Monograph Series 2, 1984: no 3.451.

67. Eg South Shields, Chesters, Carrawburgh, Wallsend and Corbridge: Allason-Jones, Miket *op cit* note 66: no 3.458.

68. Charlesworth D. Roman glass in Northern Britain. *Archaeol Aeliana* 1959; ser 4 *37*:17-30.

69. Allason-Jones, Miket *op cit* note 67; Bishop, Dore *op cit* note 20:214, no 1.

70. Allason-Jones L. Two unrecognized Roman surgical instruments. *Archaeol Aeliana* 1979; ser 5 *7*: 239-41.

71. Celsus *op cit* note 50; *VII*:28 (tonsils); *VII*:29 (fetus).

72. *RIB* no 1028 (*op cit* note 2).

73. *RIB* no 1072 (*op cit* note 2).

74. *RIB* no 445 (*op cit* note 2).

75. *RIB* no 1052; *RIB* no 1131 (*op cit* note 2).

76. Allason-Jones L, McKay B. *Coventina's Well: A Shrine on Hadrian's Wall*. Chollerford: Trustees of the Clayton Collection, 1985.

77. Allason-Jones L. Small finds report. In: Daniels C M. Excavation report on the Roman fort at Housesteads. Forthcoming.

78. Pliny *op cit* note 51; *XXXVII*:45; Allason-Jones, Miket *op cit* note 66: Section 1; Allason-Jones L. The small finds report. In: Daniels C.M. Excavation report on the Roman fort at Wallsend. Forthcoming.

79. Pliny *op cit* note 51; *XXXVI*:141-2.

80. Allason-Jones, Miket *op cit* note 66: Section 7.

81. *RIB* no 1482 (*op cit* note 2).

82. *RIB* no 1561 (*op cit* note 2).

83. *RIB* no 1743 (*op cit* note 2).

84. *RIB* no 1745 (*op cit* note 2).

85. *RIB* no 1256 (*op cit* note 2).

86. Zienkiewicz J D. *The Legionary Fortress Baths at Caerleon*. Cardiff: National Museum of Wales, 1986.

87. *CIL* no XI.3007 (*op cit* note 7).

Chapter 3

MEDICINE IN ANGLO-SAXON NORTHUMBRIA

Rex Gardner

We have little information on the state of medical care in North East England during the six centuries between the departure of the eagles and the coming of the Normans. However, for some three or four generations after AD 634, in the blossoming of the Northumbrian springtime, we have the benefit of detailed and almost contemporary records. These, mostly written by the Venerable Bede in our Tyne/Wear heartland, are without parallel in Europe. Again, at the very close of the period in the 11th century, there is another gleam; between them, little or nothing.[1]

During this early period Northumbria was no backwater isolated from the rest of the country. Indeed, for much of the 7th century, a succession of Northumbrian kings were *Bretwalda* exercising some form of suzerainty over the other kingdoms of England; sometimes in fact over much of Britain.[2] In 9th-century Wessex, Alfred the Great was to look back to Northumbria as a centre of excellence.[3] There was inevitable diffusion of knowledge arising from a considerable amount of travel, as exemplified by the Northumbrian bishop Wilfrid. During the latter half of the 7th century, from his power-bases of Hexham and Ripon he reached out beyond his many Mercian monasteries south to Selsey in Sussex, and while commuting to Rome met up with Northumbrian missionaries in the Low Countries.[4]

Some previous medical historians have fallen into the error of imagining that our Anglo-Saxon ancestors were of limited intelligence, whose medicine was 'mere magic', and whose medical writing were 'a mass of folly and credulity'.[5] It was far otherwise.

In the 8th century the library of our joint monastery of St Peter (Wearmouth) and St Paul (Jarrow) was possibly the largest in Christendom, while Bede (672/3-735), who here spent his days worshipping, studying and writing, was recognised in his own day as the greatest contemporary European scholar. However among the volumes which Benedict Biscop in the 7th century brought by the cart-load to Sunderland from Gaul and Rome,[6] medical texts were of poor quality, for by this time the great writings of Greek physicians and surgeons had been abridged, translated into Latin, and further abridged by lesser men. Such knowledge of medicine as was contained in works such as Isodore of Seville's *Etymologies*, and in Pliny's *Natural History* was available to Bede, since they are known to have been in this library.[7] The constant alertness of his mind can be readily demonstrated. When writing his commentary on the Acts of the Apostles (at 28:8), Bede suggested that Publius had suffered from dysentery, but later, noting that Gregory of Tours in *The history of the Franks* (5:34) had given a clinical description of an outbreak of dysentery, he inserted this in his revised commentary *Retractions on Acts*.[8]

Although King Aldfrith (685-705), himself a considerable scholar, gave eight hides of land for a volume of cosmology which he coveted,[9] it is safe to assume that most books were in monastic libraries where they were copied and disseminated. In the 740s Boniface wrote from Mainz to Northumbria for copies of the writings of Bede.[10] While most of these were Biblical expositions, saints' *Lives*, or his magisterial *History of the English Church and People* (hereafter *HE*),[11] Bede also wrote scientific works of great scholarship.[12]

Although in the course of his Biblical commentaries Bede offers advice on treatment: crocus for fever and mustard for a cold in the head,[13] the only specific medical information he includes in *HE* refers to the appropriate time for that popular procedure of bleeding. He quotes an eye-witness account of Bishop John being asked to see a nun who was seriously ill:

> She had recently been bled in the arm and, while still under treatment, was seized with a sudden pain which rapidly increased. Her wounded arm grew worse and became so much swollen that it could hardly be encircled by both hands...He asked when the girl had been bled, and on hearing that it was on the fourth day of the moon, he exclaimed, "You have acted foolishly and ignorantly to bleed her on the fourth day of the moon; I remember how Archbishop Theodore of blessed memory used to say that it was very dangerous to bleed a patient when the moon is waxing and the Ocean tide flowing..." (*HE* v:3)

From that, and other sources, we learn that medicine was among the topics taught at the school started in Canterbury by Archbishop Theodore in 669 when, having walked from Rome at the age of 67, he set about his twenty-year task of firmly establishing the Church. This he did to such good effect that many of his students became as fluent in Latin and Greek as in their own tongue. The only other item of Theodore's medical teaching which can be traced is a prescription for dysentery, the gall of a hare to be mixed with pepper. Pepper was a rarity in early England. It is noteworthy that when Bede was dying he had only three possessions to give away: napkins, incense and pepper.[14] From all we know of Bede he would never have used pepper as a luxury; it was therefore presumably kept as a medicine.

There is extant a tract on the common practice of bleeding, *De minutione Sanguinis*, which has been ascribed to Bede; the ascription is probably false, although not certainly so. As no English translation appears to have been produced in modern times, one prepared for this volume by a fellow-member of the Pybus Society, is appended.[15] Bede's name is also attached to a *Penitential* in which we find confirmation that already physicians' fees could be a problem!

> He who by a wound in a quarrel renders a man weak or maimed shall pay for the physician and the fine for the scar, and make compensation for his work while he is recovering, and do penance for half a year. If indeed he does not have the means, he shall make good these things in an entire year [of penance].[16]

It is, however, from the undisputed works of Bede and his contemporaries that nuggets of information can be prised.

The Church and medical care

Medical care was largely in the hands of the church, as a work of compassion, and in obedience to its Lord's command 'Heal the sick, cleanse the lepers' (Matt.10:8). Back in the 6th century we find the sick making their way to monks, as shown by an Iona incident which Adomnan recorded to illustrate Columba's gift of prophecy.

> Also on a certain day the saint, hearing some one shouting beyond the strait, spoke in this manner: "Much to be pitied is that man who is shouting and *who has come to us to seek things suitable for physical remedies*, when today the fitter thing for him was to occupy himself with true repentance for his sins. For in the end of the this week he will die". (*AVC* I:27)[17]

When Columba's followers, led by Aidan, poured into Northumbria from 634 onwards, they must have continued such care at their Lindisfarne base. For by the end of the century at any rate, that community included physicians who co-operated with monks in treating the sick. At this time Celtic monks from Ireland were also penetrating Europe. There is extant the plan for their monastery at St Gall at Switzerland, showing a physician's house with consulting room and dispensary, two wards, an out-patient department for venesection and purging, and a garden laid out for named medicinal herbs.[18]

The men who accompanied Aidan on his missionary treks included not merely clerics but laymen (*HE* iii:5), so it is possible that there were physicians among their number. From this Northumbrian base on Holy Island almost the whole of England, from the Essex coast to the Severn, was reached by a generation of Celtic missionaries proclaiming the gospel. It may safely be assumed that they simultaneously dispensed such medical knowledge as they possessed, not merely in obedience to the Dominical command, but because the sick would certainly have looked to them for help in their sickness:

Firstly, because the best of them demonstrated a relationship with God, and therefore could be expected to intercede with heaven on behalf of the sick.[19] Secondly, because they manifested compassion. Hans Küng has noted 'The message of Jesus culminated in love of neighbour...In this light the young community of faith from the very beginning recognized active care of the suffering as a special task...'[20] Thirdly, because it would be assumed that, as these messengers had learning, they would know how to heal. These are such universal reactions that, right up to the mid-20th century, most missionaries among primitive people even if they had no medical training whatever have found it necessary to carry a stock of medicines to give to the sick who constantly thronged them.

Details of some of the medical problems faced by the monks may be gleaned from the lives of the 7th-century saints. But first we must ask whether such writings are worth looking at. How careful a writer was Bede? While Bede's claim that he wrote according to *vera lex historiae* is accepted by most historians so far as *HE* is concerned, many of them assume he adopted some quite other standard when writing his *Life of Cuthbert* (*BVC*). The evidence contradicts this, and appears unequivocal.[21]

Proof of Bede's scholarly diligence will be found in the story of a thane's servant who was healed. Cuthbert's earlier anonymous biographer had reported having been told, by an unnamed colleague still living, that the patient had been 'wretchedly afflicted with infirmity and whose life was despaired of and who was even now dying and breathing his last' (*AVC* IV:7). When, two decades later, Bede was commissioned to produce a new biography, he went to the trouble of tracking down the source of this story, 'Baldhelm, who is still alive and holding by appointment the office of priest in the church of Lindisfarne...', and obtained additional clinical details of the patient's condition: 'the extremities of his body [were] prematurely dead and he seem[ed] to draw but little breath though his mouth and nostrils' (*BVC*:25).[22]

Bede's descriptions of some diseases are so vivid that from them Weaver has distinguished between three cases of neurological disease: one as grand mal epilepsy, another as an acute febrile illness, cerebral infection, porphyria or Lesch-Nyhan syndrome, and a third as possibly the Guillain-Barré syndrome.[23] When Bede had written the *Lives of the Abbots* of his own monastery of Wearmouth/Jarrow, a few years earlier, he recorded his clinical observations of the death of Abbot Benedict Biscop: 'after three years of creeping paralysis [he] was so weakened that his lower limbs were already as good as dead and only the upper part of his body...still functioned.' (*V.Abb.*:10).

Our modern understanding of the aetiology of disease was of course as unknown to scholars of the classical era, and in the monasteries, as it was to the general populace. The latter would ascribe many cases of sudden pains or illness to the darts of malign beings: 'elf-shot'.[24] However monks, including Bede, would ascribe such cases rather to demonic attack, as so many in primitive societies do to this day. Again present evidence suggests that in occasional cases they many have been right, despite the fact that a tentative psychiatric or pathological diagnosis can usually be made in the majority of their instances.[25]

Cuthbert (c 634-687) was a monk whose training and whose heart[26] remained in the Celtic tradition, although after the changes in the Northumbrian church following the Whitby synod he went on to become Bishop of Lindisfarne in the Roman obedience. Unfortunately his biographers are not interested in the medical aspects of Cuthbert's work, but rather in the spiritual power he exhibited. However it is clear that contemporaries saw his healing ministry as an integral part of the gospel, his anonymous biographer putting it thus:

> Therefore as Saint Cuthbert excelled in virtues in his bishopric, the Lord completely and fully increased the dignity and authority of that office through him by signs and wonders; for what we read concerning the Apostles, 'Whatsoever ye shall loose on earth" etc., and "Whatsoever ye shall bind on earth", etc. was fulfilled in him with respect to men's souls *and bodies*;...' (*AVC* IV:2)

Clergy-doctor co-operation

The cases recorded in Cuthbert's Lives are of desperate cases brought to him as a last resort, and healed by God in response to his prayers: a boy *in extremis* due to plague (*AVC* IV:6), cases of madness (AVC II:8; IV:3), dysentery (AVC IV:12), a youth chronically bedridden (AVC IV:5; BVC:32). In that last case Bede specifically records, and gives credit to, the activity of medical practitioners:

> When the youth had been brought to Cuthbert and he saw his terrible affliction, he bade them all go farther off. And turning to his wonted weapon of prayer, he gave his blessing and drove away the plague *which the careful hands of the doctors could not expel with their compounds and drugs.* (*BPVC* 32)

The professional services of doctors were not despised by the monks since, as has already been noted, by the end of the 7th century at the latest, there were doctors on the staff of Lindisfarne monastery:

> a certain youth, a paralytic, who was brought in a wagon from another monastery to the skilled physicians of our monastery (*AVC* IV:17)

In that case it was only when 'after toiling long, they had no success, and gave him up altogether, despairing of curing him', that divine healing was sought and found.

Cuthbert was not unique in cooperating with doctors. There are records of John of Beverley healing a man's dumbness by prayer followed by speech-therapy, and then handing him over to the doctors for the treatment of his scabby head (*HE* v:2). Similarly Eddius Stephanus records that, after the divine resuscitation of a young man, Bothelm by name, who had fallen from a great height during the building of Hexham Abbey, St Wilfrid handed him over to the doctors for further care. Such accidents must have been an occupational hazard during the building of the monasteries, for in the Monkwearmouth excavations there is the skeleton of a man who had recovered after multiple fractures probably sustained in the same way.[27] On the other hand Bothelm may have been accident-prone, for Bede records a Hexham monk of that name fracturing his arm after slipping on the ice (*HE* iii:2).

It is worth recalling that many monasteries were among the largest communities in the country. In the earlier centuries a number, including

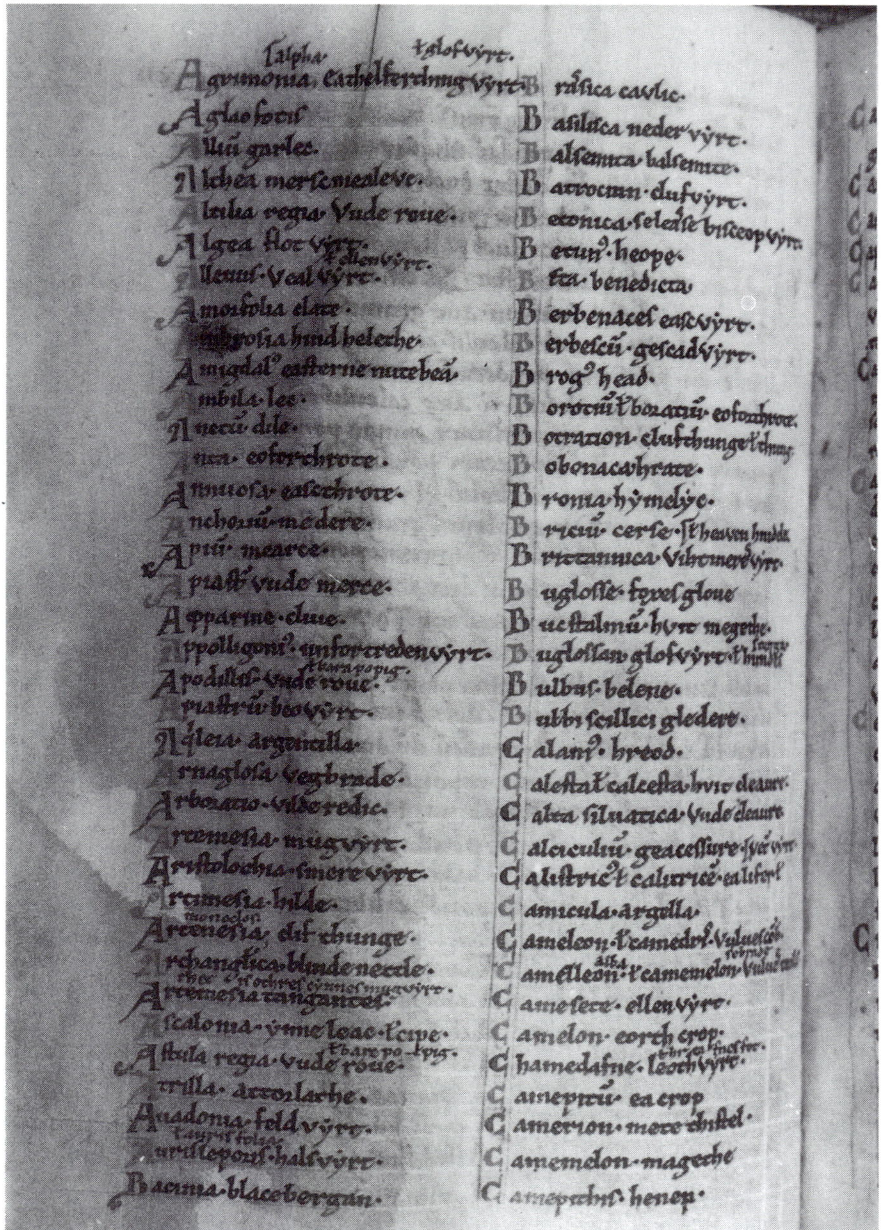

Figure 1. Latin/Anglo-Saxon glossary of plant names.
Early 12th century: *MS Durham Hunter 100.*

Coldingham and Whitby in Northumbria, were double, with houses for monks (a few of whom would be priests) and for nuns, with additionally a considerable number of laymen: tradesmen, and farm-labourers. Such double monasteries seem invariably to have been ruled by an abbess. One such, Æthelthryth, erstwhile Queen of Northumbria, died of the plague while abbess of her foundation at Ely. A few days before her death we find Cynefrith (the first doctor in our history to be named) being ordered to lance a large tumour under her jaw. He seems to have been a member of the monastic community for he was at hand when, some years later, her body was examined and found to be incorrupt.[28]

Perhaps we are guilty of an anachronism in trying to make a sharp distinction between cleric and doctor. In some, but not all, cases the causes of sickness were seen to be spiritual in origin. In these it was either self-induced by sin, or originated from outside demonic attack. The sick person required compassion and care which involved treating both body and soul. There is abundant evidence that in Anglo-Saxon England monks and priests practised as doctors, right up to the end of this period when Baldwin, Abbot of St Edmundsbury, was also personal physician to Edward the Confessor and later to William the Conqueror.[29] It was only later in the Middle Ages that ecclesiastical laws were promulgated forbidding clergy to shed blood. From then on any surgery would have to be performed by laymen, but it is unlikely that this applied in the age under discussion here.

Archaeological evidence

For the human remains found during the excavations of Monkwearmouth monastery,[30] there is fortunately a report by a medically-qualified palaeopathologist.[31] The sex and age findings suggest that the community consisted of a nucleus of monks surrounded by a population that was demographically more or less normal in structure. This view is supported by the presence of many children, for of the total skeletons 15.5% were infants, 21.4% children (1-12 yrs), and 1.4% adolescents (13-17), which is a considerably higher percentage of juvenile deaths than in most Anglo-Saxon series. Calvin Wells considered the likely causes of their deaths to have been dysentery and enteritis in the first few months of life, with bronchitis and pnuemonia as probable, and measles, diphtheria and scarlatina as possible, causes in childhood.

Interestingly, Wells found that the adults at Monkwearmouth, both men and women, lived rather longer and their mean statures were slightly taller than those in three other sites (all in East Anglia) which he had examined using the same criteria. The Monkwearmouth figures were male: mean 1725mm (range 1612-1850mm); female 1588mm (range 1539-1644mm), which are not very different from those for Northern England in the 20th century, for even with the improved nutrition of 1990 the mean figures are: males 1741mm, females 1615mm. This difference on Wearside,

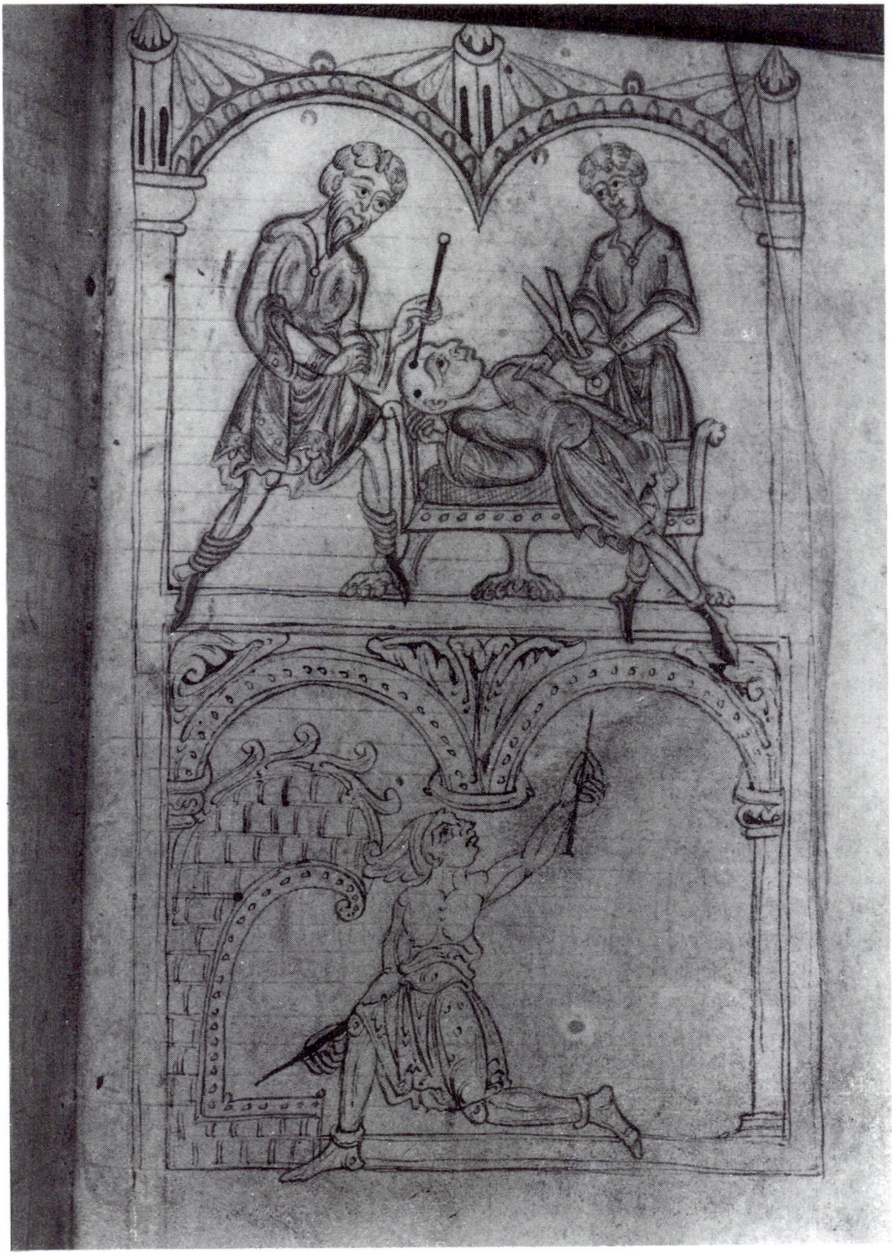

Figure 2. Cauterisation by leeches (not tonsured), and healing cauteries:
MS Durham Hunter 100.

over more than a thousand years, is no greater than that between British regions in 1990.[32]

Wells' figures for average age at death (40.8 yrs for males and 37.6 for females) must be treated with great caution. Much demographic confusion has arisen due to the estimation of the age of skeletons in this and other archaeological digs. Helen Cayton, who was involved with Calvin Wells during the excavations at the Saxon monastery of North Elmham in Norfolk, presented a dissenting report, for his figures for life expectancy there were even lower than at Monkwearmouth. She calculated from the literary record of 200 Anglo-Saxons that their overall average age at death was 57.7 years, and for ecclesiastics 64.6. These are in sharp contrast to Wells' figures based on an examination of skeletons dated by the use of the then standard palaeopathological criteria,[33] which have recently been shown to yield estimates of age which can be spuriously low.[34] It is surely a mistake to believe that life-span has altered from the 70-80 years mentioned 3000 years ago by the psalmist (Ps.90:10). To cite merely one example, it was not thought remarkable that the Mercia ruler Penda was aged 72 when killed attacking Oswy of Northumbria. It follows that the suggestion, occasionally made today, that in Saxon times folk would automatically age earlier than at present is unfounded.[35]

Nevertheless it is true that life-expectancy was much reduced, one major factor being pestilence; Bede recorded episodes of plague in 640, 661, 664, 672, 680 and 686. The nature of these outbreaks has been much debated. Despite the rarity of rat skeletons in the archaeological record it seems undeniable that some of these were bubonic plague. In the plague of 661, for instance, 'which at that time carried off very many throughout the length and breadth of England', Cuthbert was attacked but recovered, 'the swelling which appeared in his thigh gradually left the surface of his body.' (*BVC*:14). Bubonic plague appears to have occured in several waves, but the 'yellow sickness' in the previous century was almost certainly severe relapsing fever with jaundice; others may have included diphtheria and poliomyelitis, while smallpox and typhus are possibilities.[36] With bubonic plague the morbidity rate was extremely high. Coelfrith took twenty-two monks with him from Monkwearmouth to start the daughter monastery at Jarrow; after plague reached them only he and a little boy (doubtless Bede himself) were left to sing the offices.[37] Medicine had nothing to offer: when plague reached the men's part of the monastery at Barking, the Abbess gathered together the women in their part to discuss with them where they wanted be buried (*HE* iv:7).

Compared with similar skeletons examined by the same worker in Norfolk, those on Wearside (and especially the females) had much less osteoarthritis, and both men and women were slightly taller. Wells deduced, therefore, that as well as having a good food supply and farming its lands efficiently, the Wearside group in general, and their women in particular, led less physically demanding lives than the East Anglians. There were, however, a few severe arthritics with extensive eburnation of the joints, which he took to indicate that well-marked division of labour was normal here. No significant evidence of other diseases was found, and there was no malignancy.[38]

The practice of medicine

Evidence for this is found in a number of volumes, mostly Southumbrian in origin, dating from the 9th century, the best known being *The Leechbook of Bald*, and the *Lacnunga*.[39] It is the glory of Anglo-Saxon medicine that at that time these were written in the Anglo-Saxon tongue, England being the only country in Europe with a medical literature in its own language.[40] Alongside the Anglo-Saxon medical texts now treasured in the great libraries of Cambridge, Oxford and London there is one other similar document. Known as *MS Durham Hunter 100*, it is held in the north by the Dean and Chapter of Durham Cathedral.[41] Much of it is taken up with astronomy, and computational data necessary for the use of the calendar (which especially highlights, as well as Augustine, our northern St Oswald). Of medical interest are illustrations of cauterization, a lengthy glossary of plant names in Latin and Anglo-Saxon,[42] some medical material principally from Isodore and Ambrose, and some prescriptions. The relationships of the elements, seasons, humours (blood, phlegm, black bile, and yellow/red bile), and the ages of man are discussed, and illustrated in a complicated diagram of eight intersecting arcs within a circle.[43]

Underlying treatment was the theory of fours: just as there were four seasons of the year (spring, summer, autumn, winter), four elements (earth, air, fire, water), and four ages of man (childhood, youth, maturity, old age), so there are four humours of the body. As Bede explained:[44]

> Man himself, who is called by wisemen a microcosm, this is a little world, has all these qualities in the temperament of his body, and each individual humour dominates the body at different time. Blood, which governs the spring, is wet and warm; red choler which rules the summer, is hot and dry; black bile which rules the autumn, is dry and cold; and phlegm, which governs winter, is cold and wet. Also blood is strongest in infancy, red choler in youth, melancholia in maturity, that is bile mixed with black blood, and phlegm in old men.

The basic concept behind the doctrine of the four humours is one of a balance of forces within the body. When the four humours are in harmony the body is healthy, but disruption of the balance results in disease which can be cured only when the natural order is restored. It was thus possible to work out the correct means of treating an illness by considering the date of birth and the innate temperament of the patient, together with the time of the year at which the illness occured. Once the particular humour causing the disease had been identified, the treatment was perfectly straightforward, and consisted of means to reduce the dominance of that humour. If, for instance, blood was in excess then bloodletting was required.[45]

The literature does, nevertheless, give a description of various presenting symptoms and their management: 'half-dead disease' is a good description of hemiplegia. Talbot has challenged 'the accepted view among all medical historians that the emergence of Salerno and Salernitan medicine brought a new and rational element into the hitherto debased practice of the West' He shows that the texts used and published by the earliest Salernitan writers of the 11th century were known and read in Anglo-Saxon England almost two centuries before.[46]

The major part of Anglo-Saxon medical literature, however, is taken up with a description of herbs ('worts'), the herbals containing many illustrations by which the herbs could be recognised. One of King Alfred's proverbs says that there is no herb which grows in the woods or the fields which does not promote health.[47] Some knowledge of them must have been handed down from the dim past. We await the result of current genetic research, but blood-group studies on the present population of north Northumberland suggests that the great majority of the population remained of British (Celtic, originally 'Welsh'-speaking) stock, despite the assumption of power by Anglian rulers from the mid-6th century.[48] It may be assumed that both in-coming Angle and native Briton (a distinction largely lost during the course of the 7th century) would have a wide-spread knowledge of herbal medicine from their Celtic or Teutonic forbears. It is an error to assume that such 'native remedies' are all ineffectual as was demonstrated to the present writer in Eastern Uganda by the dire results of the hyper-efficient oxytocic brews employed by traditional birth attendants, two cases of ruptured uterus being admitted to his unit in a single evening.

A discussion of the Anglo-Saxon pharmacopoeia occupies a major part of Helen Cayton's thesis, one of the problems being the identification of each herb from its Anglo-Saxon name.[49] The major Saxon medical texts include a total of 327 herbs and spices, of which 62 herbs were regarded as positively identified, and 59 were probably reliably identified. In regular use were 191 herbs, but 25 of them made up a nucleus of half of the usage, presumably being of proven effectiveness. The most popular herb was betony (*Betonica officinalis*) being first choice for 'sore of the side' (?pleurisy) and lung diseases. It was also employed for fever and for nausea as well as for 'devilsickness' and other mental disorders and ailments of the head: 'For broken head, take betony, bruise it and lay it on the head above, then it unites the wound and healeth it'.[50] Second in popularity was rue (*Ruta graveolens*), probably introduced to Britain by the Romans from Southern Europe. Its active principles have been identified and it still appears in modern herbals.[51] In Anglo-Saxon times it was used for abdominal conditions: of the wamb and the maw (parts of the stomach) and the milt (spleen), for the eyes, and for the head: 'For head wark, take rue and wormwood, pound them and mingle with vinegar and oil, strain through a cloth, smear the head with it; or work a paste of the same, lay it on the head and swathe it up well, then thou will to bed.'[52]

Many of the prescriptions in the Leechbooks were, however, translated from textbooks of Mediterranean origin.[53] Their origin is sometimes displayed by their demand for exotic substances which could have been obtained in England only with considerable difficulty, if at all. For instance the Anglo-Saxon Leechbook describes the use of *petraoleum* (petroleum), a word not recorded in Latin or Greek. It, like balsam in the same recipe, came from the Near East. However there is record of the Patriarch of Jerusalem sending a present of these, together with a white stone, to King Alfred the Great, of whose ill-health he probably heard from Anglo- Saxon pilgrims to the Holy Land.[54]

Frequently these volumes direct that the worts are to be gathered, or the mixture compounded, to the saying of charms or the performance of ritual.[55] This applies to some of those copied from classical sources, as well as to others invoking Teutonic or Celtic deities. There is also occasional mumbo-jumbo containing Irish words, a reminder that the Irish Sea was not so much a barrier as a Celtic Mediterranean bustling with traffic. In many cases we find Christian prayers or rituals associated with the gathering, compounding, or administration of medicines. Karen Jolly has made a valuable contribution to understanding them:[56]

> Late 19th and early 20th century scholars interpreted charms as a clear statement of pagan sentiments, and their Christian elements have been suppressed. Yet in the form in which they appear in late-Saxon medical manuscripts the charms constitute an inseparable blend of Christian and pre-Christian ideas. They have been assimilated into a Christian framework much as Pope Gregory the First advised Archbishop Mellitus and Augustine of Canterbury to adapt pagan temples and practices to Christian uses...Thus we get a spectrum: Magic (bad) → charms → other medical remedies → Christian ritual → miracle (good).... By separating the charm remedies from 'non-magical' remedies the editors of charm books are creating a false distinction which leads to a distortion of the medical text's unity and a misunderstanding of the charm's function in the Christian society of Anglo-Saxon England.

They can be seen as seeking God's blessing on the treatment. In Cayton's view:[57]

> An ecclesiastic giving a blessing to a sick man, or pronouncing an exorcism, was performing a ritual of healing as well as a normal clerical function. A doctor who recited a charm over a sick man or who added the names of the Evangelists or a few Pater Nosters to increase the efficacy of a remedy seemed to be acting in much the same way.

In addition to herbs, substances of animal origin were also sometimes prescribed: *eg* bull's gall and honey instilled into the ears was recommended for earache, and new goat's cheese bound to the head was employed for headache. The principal descriptions of these are in the *Medicina de Quadrupedibus* of Sextus Placitus.[58]

Surgery was by no means unknown. As Bonser pointed out, the number of men with such epithets as 'wooden-leg' indicated a certain skill in amputation and the substitution of wooden legs.[59] These often followed battle wounds, but the Leechbooks give the very sound advice that when amputation is performed for gangrene, the incision is not to be at the junction of dead and living tissue, but through healthy and quick tissue. Wisely, but surprisingly in view of its expense and rarity, silk is recommended as suture material, eg for hair-lip (Lkbk xiii). Cauterization was widely employed. Its use has been considered by some historians as being largely a superstition 'as evident from the fact that one part of the body was often cauterized for a complaint in another or opposite portion or member'.[60] In these days of acupuncture few would wish to make so scathing a judgment. Of great interest in the Durham manuscript is an illustration of cauterization points.[61]

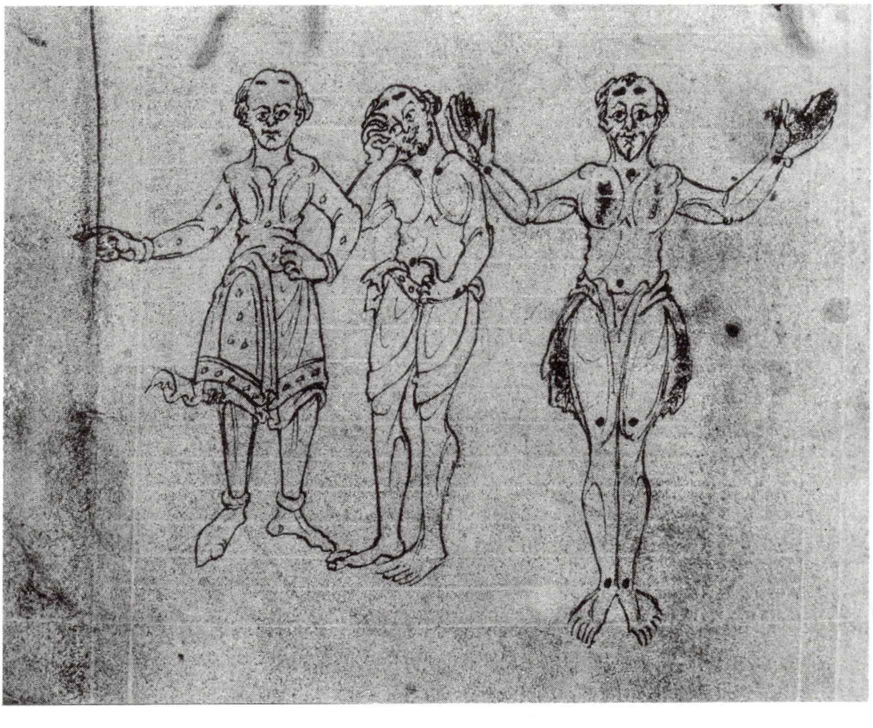

Figure 3. Cauterisation points. *MS Durham Hunter 100.*

Descriptions of this *MS Durham Hunter 100* may give the wrong impression, for unlike the large, splendidly illuminated Bible manuscripts which are the glory of our Northumbrian renaissance, this is a handy manual (even in its modern handsome binding it could be squeezed into a coat pocket), obviously meant to be carried round. The tiny writing is beautifully legible, but the pages rather grubby from much use. As one handles it with consummate awe and respect, it is not difficult to picture some colleague, now dead these eight hundred years, anxiously poring over it when faced with a difficult clinical problem, nor — aware as we are of all the ancillary aids he lacked — to sympathise with him.

Acknowledgments

I am grateful to Mrs Jill Ivy, Dean and Chapter Library, for making available illustrations from MS Durham Hunter 100.

References

1. No attempt can be made here to discuss Anglo-Saxon medicine in general. For this consult Bonser W. *The medical background of Anglo-Saxon England*. London: Wellcome Historical Medical Library, 1963; Rubin S. *Medieval English Medicine* Newton Abbott: David & Charles, 1974; or Helen Cayton's PhD thesis *Anglo-Saxon medicine in its social context*, 1978, Durham. Regrettably this valuable work has not been published.
2. *HE* (see note 11) ii:9; iii:6; iii:24.
3. King Alfred's Preface to his Anglo-Saxon translation of Gregory's Pastoral Care. Keynes S, Lapidge M. *Alfred the Great*. Harmondsworth: Penguin, 1983:125.
4. Colgrave B. *The Life of Bishop Wilfrid by Eddius Stephanus*. Cambridge: Univ Press, 1927:85.
5. Such quotations from Singer's writings (Grattan JHG, Singer C. *Anglo-Saxon Magic and Medicine*. Oxford: Wellcome Historical Medical Museum, 1952: 38,92) are discussed by Denton P, Beyond the book: Charles Singer and Anglo-Saxon medicine revisited. *Canadian bull med hist* 1986; *3*:263-70.
6. Bede. *Lives of the Abbots of Wearmouth and Jarrow* (V.Abb.: 4,6). This is conveniently found in Farmer DH. *The Age of Bede*. Harmondsworth: Penguin, 1983:185-210. Bishop Stubbs wrote: 'The debt which England owes to Benedict Biscop is a very great one, and has scarcely ever been fully recognised....the civilization and learning of the 8th century rested on the monastery [at Wearmouth, modern Sunderland] which he founded, which produced Bede and through him the school of York, Alcuin and the Carolingian school, on which the culture of the Middle Ages was based.' (Quoted by Fletcher E. *Benedict Biscop*, Jarrow Lecture, 1981).
7. The medical literature available in this period is listed by Bonser *op cit* note 1:24-27. For discussion see Cayton *op cit* note 1:31-49.
8. Laistner MLW. The library of the Venerable Bede. In Thompson AH, ed. *Bede: his life, times, and writings*. Oxford: Clarendon, 1935:237-66. Bede's original *Commentary of the Acts* (but unfortunately not his *Retractions*) has been translated into English by Martin L, 1989, Kalamazoo: Cistercian Studies. The description of dysentery is in Gregory of Tours' *History of the Franks* (in the Penguin Classics edition. Harmondsworth 1974:96); however Helen Cayton cites this as coming from an unsourced writing of Cassius Felix (*op cit* note 1:36).
9. Bede *V. Abb.*:15.
10. Levison W. *England and the Continent in the eighth century.* Oxford: Clarendon, 1946:140.
11. *Historia ecclesiastica gentis Anglorum*. The standard edition (Latin and English) is that of Colgrave B and Mynors RAB, Oxford: Univ Press, 1969. There is also an English translation by Sherley- Price L. in a Penguin Classics edition, recently re-edited by Farmer DH.

12. Stevens WM. *Bede's scientific achievement*. Jarrow Lecture, 1985. Jones CW. *Bedae opera de temporibus*. Cambridge, Mass: Mediaeval Academy of America:1943.

13. Cayton *op cit* note 1:37, quoting Bede's *Cantica Canticorum Allegorica Exposito* iv:14, and his *In Lucae Evangelium Exposito* v:17.

14. Lapidge M. The school of Theodore and Hadrian. *Anglo-Saxon England* 1986; *15*:45-71. Lapidge here quotes Theodore as giving, in his *Laws*, the prescription for dysentery. For Bede's pepper see the account of his death written by a fellow monk (confusingly named Cuthbert) in Colgrave and Mynors: 580-87 (see note 11).

15. I am most grateful to Elizabeth Lazenby, Dept. of Classics, University of Newcastle on Tyne, for preparing this. Payne (see note 40):19-20 mentions that there is in the British Museum an English ms translation, which he supposes to be 14th century, entitled 'Medesyns approbate for mortal Sekenesses by Saynte Bede'. My endeavours to obtain a copy of this have been unrewarded.

16. McNeill JT, Gamer HM. *Medieval handbooks of Penance*. New York: Columbia Univ Press, 1938,1990:225. A much later law no longer fixes the amount of the fine arbitrarily. The wounder must first pay the victim the cost of his leech, as much as is required for the curing of the wound, but must swear on relics that he could not be cured for less, and that he has not increased the amount due (quoted by Bonser *op cit* note 1:107). Fraudulent claims were obviously a problem even then; human nature has not changed!

17. *Adomnan's Life of Columba (AVC)*. Critical ed. Anderson AO,Anderson MO. Edinburgh: Nelson, 1961. English translation only, Lampeter: Llanerch, 1989. Although not written until about a century after Columba's time, Adomnan (who was one of his successors as Abbot of Iona), repeatedly refers to named eyewitness as the source of his statements.

18. The plan of the monastery at St Gall in Switzerland will be found conveniently described by Rubin (*op cit* note 1:175-76).

19. We can glimpse these 7th-century missionaries in an 1918 eye-witness account of Christian Sadhu in India: 'whenever he appeared in public wondering crowds followed him. Even the children gathered behind him that they might touch his yellow robe, and the sick were brought that he might pray with them. It is almost impossible to convince the people that he does not heal the sick, even when the assurance comes from his own lips' (Parker A. *Sadhu Sundar Singh*. London: Christian literature society for India, 1918: xiv).

20. Quoted by Davey in Introduction. In Browne SG, Davey F, Thomson WAR. *Heralds of Health: the saga of Christian medical initiatives*. London: Christian Medical Fellowship, 1985:8. That volume, and *The Church and Healing* vol 19 of *Studies in Church History* (1982), will introduce a vast literature.

21. An English translation by Webb JF will be found in Farmer DH. ed. *The age of Bede*:41-104 (see note 6). Bede also wrote a metrical version of the *Life of Cuthbert* which adds nothing new; it has not been translated into English. The original *Life of Cuthbert (AVC)* had been written 20 years earlier by an anonymous monk of Cuthbert's own monastery of Lindisfarne. In 721 Bede uses this as a foundation for his own work, written at the request of Lindisfarne. He takes great care to assure his reader that 'I have not presumed to write down anything concerning so great a man without the most rigorous investigation of the facts nor, at the end, to hand on what I had written to be copied for general use, without the scrupulous examination of credible witnesses.' He goes on at length to spell out the steps he took: obtaining accounts, making notes, having the notes checked by eye-witnesses, re-writing, and then the reading of the whole before the leaders at Lindisfarne for final confirmation (*BVCP* prologue). For a critical edition of both the anonymous and Bede's prose *Life* see Colgrave B. *Two lives of Saint Cuthbert*. Cambridge: Univ Press, 1940, 1985.

22. Despite Bede's care, many workers write off these records as worthless, as mere hagiography – in effect puffs for the reputation of some 'saint', written to draw pilgrims and therefore revenues to a shrine. While that criticism is often valid for writings in the later Middle Ages, at this time there were no cults, no financial ulterior motive, and the pilgrimage industry had not been founded. Moreover there is not the slightest evidence that Bede would have accepted that his historical writings could be divided into different genre. In any case current evidence is that accounts of 'miracles' cannot be discarded as readily as as hitherto been the case. It is noteworthy that the scholars who reject the veracity of Bede's *Life of Cuthbert* happily believe his *Lives of the Abbots of Wearmouth and Jarrow*, thus demonstrating that in fact their criterion is not 'hagiography' but the presence (*BVC*) or absence (*V.Abb.*) of 'miracles' in his account. In later centuries manufactured 'relics', faked healings, and charlatans will abound, but not yet. Despite gross exaggeration in some present day reports, also modern fraudulent healings and financial rogues on the American TV scene (Randi J. *The Faith Healers*. New York: Prometheus Press, 1987), there is enough current evidence of genuine healings, in reponse to prayer, to entitle us to treat these 8th-century records with a certain amount of respect (Gardner RFR. Miracles of healing in Anglo-Celtic Northumbria as recorded by the Venerable Bede and his contemporaries. A reappraisal in the light of twentieth century experience. *Brit med J* 1983; *287*:927-33; *idem, Healing miracles: a doctor investigates*. London: Darton, Longman and Todd, 1986). Bede names his sources, which is a dangerous thing to do if the story is untrue or exaggerated. The present writer has likewise named sources and had a TV crew come from Australia to interview them for confirmation.

23. Weaver LT. Medicine in the time of Saint Cuthbert. *Perspectives in biology and medicine* (Chicago) 1989; *32*:387-97.

24. The evidence for Anglo-Saxon beliefs was collected by Oswald Cockayne in three large volumes for the Rolls Series, *Leechdoms, wortcunning, and starcraft of Early England* London: Longman Green, 1866. For an anthropological study see Barley N. Anglo-Saxon Magico-medicine. *J Anthrop soc Oxf* 1972; *3*:67-76.

25. See Nevius JL. *Demon possession*. Grand Rapids: Kregel, 8th ed, 1968 (1st pub 1894). That Bede's diagnosis should not be automatically rejected out of hand is further suggested by the work of the modern American psychiatrist M Scott Peck (*People of the lie*. London: Rider, 1986:182-211), and by the report of the Bishop of Exeter's Commission, *Exorcism*. London: SPCK, 1972. Following this each Church of England Diocese has appointed an exorcist. Bede would have been interested to know that it was the Rural Dean of *Wearmouth* (Canon Granville Gibson), being one of these, who re-enacted an exorcism for the serious, low-key, TV programme *Deliverance* (Network ITV August 26 1992).

26. Colgrave *Two lives* (see note 21):5.

27. *The life of Bishop Wilfrid by Eddius Stephanus* c.23. Critical edition: Colgrave B. Cambridge: Univ Press, 1927,1985:47. There is another English translation by Webb JF in *The age of Bede* (see note 6):105-84. The case of survival after multiple fracture sustained probably by falling from a building, found in the Monkwearmouth excavations, was reported by Calvin Wells. Une fracture rare chez un ancient Anglo-Saxon. *Helium* 1975; *15*:237-43.

28. Cuthbert's body was found to be incorrupt, and to have remained such at least until the time of the dissolution of the monasteries in the 16th century. (*Rites of Durham* (Surtees Soc. 107:102-03)). For a discussion of this phenomenon see Colgrave's *Two Lives*...:338-39. The suggestions that incorruption, which was taken as an evidence of sanctity, was either due to an air-tight tomb, or was fraudulently pre-arranged by embalming techniques (Rollason D. *Saints and relics in Anglo-Saxon England*. Oxford: Blackwell 1989:39-41), may not be acceptable as an adequate explanation in every case. This is shown by a passing reference (where the writer obviously has no idea of historical implications, and a time when medieval ideas of 'saints' were

abhorrent) to the body of one of the early Scottish reformers being found incorrupt, eighty years after his burial (Wodrow J. Collections for the Life of the Rev Robert Bruce. In Cunningham W. *The sermons of the Rev Robert Bruce*. Edinburgh: Wodrow Society, 1842:150).

29. Bonser *op cit* note 1:6. In the 10th century Aelfric, in one of his Anglo-Saxon sermons, wrote: 'Medicine is granted for bodily infirmity, and holy prayers, with God's blessing', adding the warning 'all other aids are hateful to God'. Skeat WW. *Aelfric's Lives of Saints*. London: Early Eng Text Soc, 1881; I:379.

30. The full report of this, by Professor Rosemary Cramp, is in the press

31. Wells C. *Report on human remains from Monkwearmouth, Durham County*. nd. I am grateful to Dr Cayton for making a copy of this typescript available to me.

32. I am grateful to Dr Albert Martin, Director of Public Health for Sunderland, for making these statistics available to me.

33. For instance, whereas Calvin Wells judged the life-expectancy of Anglo-Saxon adults to be 37, Cayton suggested a truer figure would be 49. Wells C, and Cayton H. The human bones. In Wade-Martin P, ed. *Excavations in North Elmham Park 1967-72*. Norwich: East Anglian Archaeological Report *9* 1980; 2:247-314.

34. Acsádi G, Nemeskéri J. *History of human life-span and mortality* Budapest: Académiai Kiadó, 1970. Kunitz S. Making a long story short: a note on men's height and mortality in England from the first through the nineteenth centuries. *Med Hist* 1987; *31*:269-80.

35. Even Stanley Rubin (*op cit* note 1) fell into the trap. Discussing arthritis he wrote 'While it is now generally regarded as a disease of 'aging', *and as the Anglo-Saxon average age at death was low, it follows that* osteoarthritis became active at a much earlier age than is now the case' (italics added).

36. McArthur W. The identification of some pestilences recorded in the Irish annals. *Irish historical studies* 1949; *6*:169-88.

37. Anonymous. *Life of Coelfrith*. In Whitelock D, ed. *English Historical Documents: I c.500-1042* London: Eyre and Spottiswoode, 1955: 695-708; there is an earlier translation by Boutflower DS, Sunderland: Hills, 1912, reprinted Lampeter: Llanerch 1990.

38. Wells C. *Report on human remains from Monkwearmouth, Durham County. Op cit* note 31.

39. These documents are among those reprinted by Cockayne (*op cit* note 24); an edition of the *Lacnunga* makes up the second part of Grattan and Singer (*op cit* note 5:95-227). Bald's *Leechbook* has been reconsidered in two papers by Cameron ML. Bald's *Leechbook*: its sources and their use in its compilation. *Anglo Saxon England* 1983; *12*:153-82; Bald's *Leechbook* and cultural interaction in Anglo-Saxon England, *ibid* 1990; *19*:5-12.

40. Payne JF. *English medicine in the Anglo-Saxon times* (The Fitzpatrick lectures for 1903). Oxford: Clarendon, 1904:30.

41. I am greatly indebted to Mr Ralph Norris, Deputy Librarian of the Dean and Chapter Library, for allowing me to examine this volume. It is described in Mynors RAB. *Durham Cathedral Manuscripts*. Durham: Dean and Chapter, 1939, item 57. A detailed manuscript summary of its contents was prepared earlier in this century and is filed as MS Durham Hunter 100A.

42. Now folios 85-101 (originally at the beginning of the volume before it was wrongly rebound). This list is to be found in Cockayne (*op cit* note 24 *iii*: 299-305).

43. The section of MS Durham Hunter 100 which deals with this is discussed by Bonser *op cit* note 1:35-37.

44. Cayton *op cit* note 1:52. The passage from Bede is her translation of a passage which will be found in Jones CW. *Bedæ: Opera de Temporibus* Cambridge Mass,: Mediaeval Academy of America, 1943: 247.

45. Cayton *op cit* note 1.

46. Talbot CH. Some notes on Anglo-Saxon medicine. *Med hist* 1965; *9*:156-69.

47. Bonser *op cit* note 1:306.

48. Potts WTW. History and blood-groups in the British Isles. In Sawyer PH, ed. *Medieval settlements*. London: Arnold, 1976: 236-53; but note criticism of this paper by Sunderland E. Comment on W.T.W. Pott's paper, *ibid*: 254-61.

49. Cayton H *op cit* note 1:76-116. Less valuable and briefer but more accessible accounts are in Singer C. Early English Magic and Medicine. *Proc Brit Acad* 1919-20; *9*:341-76 at 365 fol; and Payne JF. *English medicine in the Anglo Saxon Times*; 39-82, plus 22 figures at the end of the volume.

50. *Leechbook of Bald* (see notes 24,39) I,i,14.

51. 'Among the medically active constituents are a volatile oil, a little tannin, alkaloids, derivatives of coumarin, and the flavonoid glycoside rutoside.' Cayton H *op cit* note 1:83.

52. *Leechbook of Bald* (see notes 24,39) I,i,2.

53. Principally the 5th-century North African *Herbarium* of Pseudo-Apuleius, and the Latin version of the *Herbarium Dioscorides*, the chief Greek work on pharmacology.

54. Meaney AL. Alfred, the Patriarch and the white stone. *J Australasian Univ Language and Literature* 1978; *49*:65-79 (I am grateful to Dr Iain Gardner of Perth, for obtaining this for me). This stone was sent by the patriarch both as a source of medicinal scrapings, and obviously as a charm. For the significance of white stones see Lebour N. White quartz pebbles and their archaeological significance. *Trans Dumfriesshire & Galloway Antiquarian & Nat Hist Soc* 1914; *2*:121-34. Also the present writer's *The Church of Christ in Early Bernicia: forerunners and foundation*. Durham Univ MA thesis 1992 (excursus on white stones pp 79-80).

55. Saints' relics were frequently turned to as a place of contact with heaven, the earthly end of a divine power-arc. It is not a concept that appeals to us today, but an attempt at understanding was made in the present writer's *Healing miracles...* (see note 22):78-80.

56. Jolly KL. Anglo-Saxon charms in the context of a Christian world view. *J med hist* 1985; *11*:279-93.

57. Cayton *op cit* note 1:44.

58. In English manuscripts this is found in association with the *Herbal* of pseudo-Apuleius.

59. Bonser *op cit* note 1:101-03.

60. Quoted by Bonser (*op cit* note 1:303) from Thorndike L. *History of magic and experimental science* 1923; *1*:723.

61. One of these is reproduced in Singer C, Early English Magic and Medicine. *Proc Brit Acad*. 1919-20; *9*:344.

Chapter 4

DE MINUTIONE SANGUINIS, SIVE DE PHLEBOTOMIA: ON BLOOD-LETTING OR PHLEBOTOMY, BY THE VENERABLE BEDE:

A translation and commentary

Elizabeth Lazenby

Translation:

At any time, day and night, if necessity compels it, when sufferings are severe, one ought to use phlebotomy; especially in the period from 25th March[a] to 26th May[b] it is useful to draw off blood because then the blood increases in quantity. But later the conditions of the times and the phases of the moon are to be observed, that is, the fifth, tenth, fifteenth, twentieth, twenty-fifth and thirtieth phases of the moon.[1] On these days one ought not to practise phlebotomy, because on these days many doctors declare that untold numbers of men have died through this sort of negligence, that is by not observing the conditions of the times and the phases of the moon. For in every respect care must be taken when practising phlebotomy from 18th July[c] to 5th September,[d] which are called the Dog Days.[2] At that time one should not take a purge, because all the humours are then mixed, except when (as we have said already)[3] a blow has led to severe sufferings, which could not otherwise happen unless the patient is beaten, and the copiousness or badness of the blood must then be dispersed.

But a purge is useful at one particular time, say from 24th September[e] to 24th November,[f] because, since the body has accumulated choler and phlegm during the winter and summer, it befits it to be purged at the time already mentioned. For if the purge is carefully done the patient can be freed from choler. He must only watch carefully his intake of food and drink, take what is beneficial, and abstain from those things by which he could be hurt.

What is a phlebotomy except the correct cutting of a vein? In which places or because of which sufferings do we perform a phlebotomy, or what vein must we cut? In the case of a complaint of the head and attack of

NB. All notes, apart from Roman dates, relevant to this translation may be found with the notes at the end of the chapter.

a *ab octavo Kal. April.*: eight days before the Kalends of April = 25th March.
b *in septimum Kal. Junii*: seven days before the Kalends of June = 26th May.
c *a quindecimo Kal. August*: the fifteenth day before the Kalends of August = 18th July.
d *in Nonas Septemb.*: the Nones of September = 5th September.
e *ab octavo Kal. Octobr.*: eight days before the Kalends of October = 24th September.
f *in octavum Kal. Decembris*: eight days before the Kalends of December = 24th November.

madness the arterial veins at the back of the head [are to be cut] on a line towards the mouth in a measure of four fingers from the ear. We cut both temples in the case of an effusion of the eyes; two veins below the tongue in the case of flux of the gums, or ailments of the mouth and tooth-ache; three veins in the forehead in the case of headache and retreat into complete delirium; from the nostrils two veins in the case of heaviness of the head and eyes; from the neck two veins in the case of water on the brain. From the arm three veins are cut, because they carry the blood through the whole body, the three being the vein to the head, the maternal vein and the box vein.[4] From the hand two veins are cut, one above the thumb for a swelling of the lung, and another from the little finger for a swelling of the spleen. From underneath the ankle veins are cut for gout in the foot, delirium, and sciatica for example of the loins, and in the case of women whose periods do not come and who do not conceive. From the region of the orifices two veins are cut for pain in the kidneys, and from above the big toe two are cut for sores of the testicles.

There are many Egyptian days[5] on which by no means nor for any reason is it allowed to draw blood from man or beast, nor to give a draught, *// but of these, three are especially to be observed: 6th April,*[a] *the first Monday in August, and the last Monday in December; on that particular Monday much diligence is to be observed because all the veins are then full.*

Whoever cuts a man or beast on those days //[6] [the patient] will die either immediately or on that very day or on the third day, or he will not last until the seventh day. And if anyone has taken a draught he will die on the fifteenth day following; and if either a male or a female child is born on one of those days, he or she will die a bad death; and if anyone eats goose on those days he will die after fifteen days.[7]

In the month of January, beginning with the first day and ending with the seventh, and on the first, fourth, fifth, eighth and fifteenth day after the new moon of this same month, one must abstain from phlebotomy and purging, indeed from any sort of incision.

In the month of February also, beginning with the eighth day and ending with the seventh,[8] and on the seventeenth, nineteenth and twenty-fifth day after the new moon of this same month.

In the month of March also, beginning with the third day and ending with the seventh, and on the fifteenth, sixteenth, seventeenth and eighteenth day after the new moon of this same month.

In April also, beginning with the tenth day and ending with the eleventh, and on the ninth, seventh and twentieth day after the new moon of this same month.

a *octavo Idus April*: eight days before the Ides of April = 6th April.

In May also, beginning with the fourth day and ending with the seventh, and on the fifth, twelfth and sixteenth day after the new moon of this same month.

In June also, beginning with the eighth day and ending with the fifth,[9] and on the fifth, sixth and seventh day after the new moon of this same month.

In July also, beginning with the seventeenth day and ending with the tenth,[10] and on the sixteenth, seventeenth, eighteenth and twenty-seventh day after the new moon of this same month.

In August also, beginning with the fifth day and ending with the fifteenth, and on the nineteenth, twentieth and twenty-first day after the new moon of this same month.

In September also, beginning with the ninth day and ending with the ninth, and on the fifth, fifteenth and twenty-fifth day after the new moon of this same month.

In October also, beginning with the ninth day and ending with the tenth, and on the sixth and seventh day after the new moon of this same month.

In November also, beginning with the fifth day and ending with the sixth, and on the fourteenth and twenty-fifth day after the new moon of this same month.

In December also, beginning with the fifteenth day and ending with the eighth,[11] and on the first, fifteenth and seventeenth day after the new moon of this same month.

Besides the days to be carefully observed are in each month the first, fifth, ninth and fifteenth day after the new moon and the three days at the beginning and the three before the aforesaid abstinence ends.

The first day of the lunar month is good all day.

The second day of the lunar month is not good.

The third day of the lunar month is good.

The fourth day of the lunar month is good in the morning.

The fifth day of the lunar month is not good.

The sixth day of the lunar month is not good.

The seventh day of the lunar month is good all day.

The eighth day of the lunar month is good from the ninth hour until late.

The ninth day of the lunar month is not good.

The tenth day of the lunar month is good.

The eleventh day of the lunar month is not good.

The twelfth day of the lunar month is good.

The thirteenth day of the lunar month is good to the ninth hour.

The fourteenth day of the lunar month is good.

The fifteenth day of the lunar month is not good.

The sixteenth day of the lunar month is useless.

The seventeenth day of the lunar month is good all day.

The eighteenth day of the lunar month is not good.

The nineteenth day of the lunar month is better.

The twentieth day of the lunar month is good all day.
The twenty-first day of the lunar month is good in the morning.
The twenty-second day of the lunar month is good from the sixth hour.
The twenty-third day of the lunar month is good from the eighth hour.
The twenty-fourth day of the lunar month is good.
The twenty-fifth day of the lunar month is not good.
The twenty-sixth day of the lunar month is not good.
The twenty-seventh day of the lunar month is good all day.
The twenty-eighth day of the lunar month is not good.
The twenty-ninth day of the lunar month is not good.
The thirtieth day of the lunar month is not good.

On the fifth, fifteenth, twentieth,[12] twenty-fifth and thirtieth days of the lunar month phlebotomy is forbidden. The days from 18th July[a] to 5th September[b] are called the Dog Days, on which phlebotomy must not be practised or a draught given. However, a draught is useful from 24th September[c] to 24th November[d].

At all times, if it is absolutely necessary, phlebotomy can be performed. However the most useful time for drawing off blood is from 25th March[e] to 25th May[f] because then the blood in man increases in quantity. Later on careful observation must be made of the times and course of the moon.

The Latin text, from which this translation was made, is given in full in J P Migne, *Patrologiae cursus completus*.[13]

a *a decimo quinto Kalen. Augusti*: fifteen days before the Kalends of August = 18th July.
b *in Nonas Septemb.*: the Nones of September = 5th September.
c *ab octavo Kal. Octob.*: eight days before the Kalends of October = 24th September.
d *ad octavum Kal. Decembr.*: eight days before the Kalends of December = 24th November.
e *ab octavo Kal. April.*: eight days before the Kalends of April = 25th March.
f *ad octavum Kal. Jun.*: eight days before the Kalends of June = 25th May.

Commentary

As the eastern Roman empire was overrun by Moslem invaders in the seventh century, the western empire lost its main reservoir of Greek learning. Much Greek scholarship was preserved, however, in the monasteries of the west, including that of Bede (673-735 AD) at Monkwearmouth and Jarrow, although few original contributions to knowledge were made in this period.

Before the 13th century scholars seem mainly to have been preoccupied with the magical and astrological properties of natural objects and phenomena. Bede's writings are representative of the state of Latin scientific knowledge before translations of Greek and Arabic works became available in the west. Bede based his work mainly on Latin sources, the works of Pliny the Elder, Isidore of Seville, St Ambrose, St Augustine, St Basil the Great and St Gregory the Great, and on Latin writings on the calendar. He wrote two scientific books: a general cosmology, the *De rerum natura*, written about the year 700 and based largely on the works of Isidore and Pliny, and a more original work on specific problems connected with the calendar, the *De temporibus* of 703, which he later rewrote in 725 in an enlarged form as the *De temporum ratione*.

The only medical work attributed to Bede is the *De Minutione Sanguinis sive de Phlebotomia*, On Blood-letting or Phlebotomy. There has been considerable discussion about the authorship of this work, the consensus of opinion being in favour of attributing it to Bede. The text itself was printed by J P Migne in 1862.[13] Giles, the editor of Bede's works, thought it genuine and included it in his standard edition.[14] C W Jones was scathing in his denunciation of the attribution,[15] but Charles Plummer considered it 'less obviously spurious, might possibly be by Bede'.[16] Wilfrid Bonser settles for 'attributed to Bede'.[17]

That medical writings were available in England in the 8th century is shown in a letter written by Cyneheard, Bishop of Winchester, to Lull, Bishop of Mainz, about 754; he asks Lull to let him know if he acquires any new medical books because 'we have some medical books, but the foreign ingredients we find prescribed in them are unknown to us and difficult to obtain'.[18] English libraries obviously had medical books, although many may have been in an epitomised form, and would have included Latin and Greek works such as those by Dioscorides, Pliny, Philumenus, Oribasius, Vindicianus, Pseudo-Apuleius and Isidore. There is also a large quantity of mostly unedited and unpublished work of the type edited by Sigerist, including tracts on the four humours and blood-letting.[19] A manuscript of late eleventh century date[20] but almost certainly a copy of an earlier Anglo-Saxon work, contains amongst other things part of book IV of the *Etymologiae* of Isidore of Seville,[21] and also works known as *Lunary* and *The Egyptian Days*. This manuscript is, like the work attributed to Bede, a mixture of medical treatise and calendar *cum* astrological writings. There is also another work of this kind surviving from the ninth century,[22] which lists among its contents: *Lunaria cursus: Epistula de fleotomia Gallieni: Egyptian Days: Lunary* and two works entitled *Epistula de phlebotomia.* A mediæval practitioner, especially in a monastery, would have had such works in his library.

The subject of this paper, the *De minutione sanguinis*, is a Latin text of 929 words, concerned mainly with giving suitable, and unsuitable, times for the practice of blood-letting or phlebotomy. The tract, however, both begins and ends with the injunction that phlebotomy is permissible at all times, 'si necessitas urget'. There is also a short section which lists the veins to be opened for specific ailments. Before the discovery of its circulation, the blood was thought to be either static or just to ebb and flow. Thus it was thought that particular veins related to particular diseases and so should be opened for their cure. In early mediæval times much emphasis was placed on the calendar and on astrological signs related to the calendar for the performance of most functions in life, celestial forces both causing and curing illness. Many problems arose in trying to work out various dates at this time, as the calendar then in use was a combination of the Roman Julian calendar, based on the annual movement of the earth relative to the sun, and the Hebrew calendar, based on the monthly phases of the moon. Bede attempted to reduce this to some sort of order for his pupils at Jarrow in his *De temporibus* of 703; his treatises on the calendar remained standard textbooks for five centuries, and were used even after the Gregorian reform of 1582. The *De temporum ratione* is still one of the clearest expositions of the principles of the Christian calendar.

De minutione sanguinis emphasises in great detail not only the days of each month on which phlebotomy can be practised but also the precise time of day; that this was a usual preoccupation of the era can be seen from the place blood-letting played in the calendars, which took the place of almanacs in the seventh and eighth centuries. We must suppose that Bede based his lunar month on a synodic month (of 29.53 days), rather than a sidereal month (of 27.32 days), as he lists the times for and against blood-letting for *thirty days* in a month (called also '*phases of the moon*' in this text). He makes particular mention of the Dog Days and the Egyptian days, on which under no circumstances should there be any blood- letting.

There were various early superstitions that there were certain days, including the Egyptian days, which were not only unlucky generally, but on which it was especially dangerous to let blood or undergo any medical treatment. They were presumably called 'Egyptian' because the Egyptians to date were the most accurate calculators of astronomical computations necessary for drawing up the calendar. The Egyptians also had a list of lucky and unlucky days, which are specified in the *Papyrus Sallier iv*, which dates from the time of Rameses II (*circa* 1279-1212 BC).[23] The name '*Ægyptiaci dies*' dates from the first half of the fourth century, when twenty-five such days were marked as Egyptian; Grattan and Singer[24] believe that 'these unlucky days originally corresponded to the days succeeding the days for senatorial meetings'. The earliest extant mention is by Saint Augustine of Hippo (354-430 AD) who says that such days should not be observed, 'Non observetis dies qui dicuntur *Ægyptiaci*'. Bede may have derived the term 'Egyptian days' from Augustine, but he could also have derived it from the *Herbarium* of Pseudo-Apuleius, which probably dates to the late fourth century and was well known throughout the mediæval period;[25] there are some twenty Latin texts and three Old English texts of Pseudo-Apuleius still extant.[26] Bede, himself, in *De temporum ratione* of 725, gives directions as to the proper days of the moon for various actions.

In the passage of the *De minutione sanguinis* under discussion, Bede mentions three formidable Egyptian days to be avoided at all costs; this passage is almost exactly reproduced in one of the 'Anglo-Saxon Leechdoms', which can probably be dated to about the year 1000:[27]

> Þry da3as syndon on 3eare Þe we e3iptiaci hatað, þæt is on ure 3eþeode plihtlice da3as, on Þam natoþæshwon for nanre ne mannes ne neates blod sy to wanienne; þæt is þon*ne* ut3an[3]end*um* þam monþe þe we aprelis hatað se nhysta monan dæ3 an; þon*ne* is oþer in3an3endum þam monþe þe we a3ustus hatað se æresta monan dæ3; þon*ne* is se þridda se æresta monan dæ3 æfter ut3an3e þæs / monþes decembris. Se þe on þysum þrim da3um his blod 3ewani3e, sy hit man. sy hit nyten, þæs þe we sec3an 3ehyrdan þæt sona on þam forman dæ3e oþþe þam feorþam dæ3e his lif 3eændað; oþþe 3if his lif læn3re bið, þæt to þam seofoþan dæ3e ne becymð; oððe 3if he hwilcne drænc drincð þ*am* þr*im* da3um his lif he 3eændað binnan XV da3um; 3ifhwa on þis[um] da3um acænned bið, yfelum deaðe he his lif 3eændað; *7* se þe on þys[um] ylcum þrim da3u*m* 3ose flæsces onbyri3eð, binnan feowerti3es da3a fyrste he his lif 3eændað.

> There are three days in the year which we call Ægyptiaci, that is, in our tongue, dangerous days; in which by no means, for no occasion, neither man's nor beast's blood must be diminished; that is, the last Monday in April, the first Monday in August, and the first Monday in January. Whosoever on these three days diminish his blood, be it man, be it beast, shall, as we have heard said, soon on the first day or the fourth day end his life; or if his life is longer he shall not reach the seventh day; or if he taketh any draught on those three days he shall end his life within fifteen days. If anyone is born on these days he shall end his life by an evil death. And he that on these days tasteth flesh of goose, within a space of forty days he shall end his life.

Here the days are different but the principle is the same; the text of the *De minutione sanguinis* may indeed have been almost identical originally, as the Latin in Bede's text does not construe (marked in the translation //------// and in *italics*): I quote here the text as we now have it with, in parenthesis, the correct grammatical form of the dubious words: '*sed ex his tribus* (the scribe has copied incorrectly, giving an ablative plural to agree with *his*; it should read *tres* in the nominative case) *maxime observandi, octavo Idus April, illo die lunis* (dative or ablative plural given here, but it should be *lunae* in the genitive singular case), *intrante Augusto: illo die lunis* (*lunae* as above) *exeunte Decembri; illo die lunis* (*lunae* as above), *cum multa diligentia observandum est, quia omnes venae tunc plenae sunt.*'

The text of the Bede tract, '*Qui in istis diebus hominem aut pecus inciderit*', continues to be corrupt here, as it seems to imply that the person performing the phlebotomy will die, when surely it is intended to mean that the patient will die.

In another 'Leechdom' there is a more detailed account which, although it does not mention Egyptian days by name, is another parallel for the Bede, indicating that there was at this period almost a formula for medical doctrine of this type. I quote the translation given by Cockayne in full:[28]

> The old leeches laid it down in Latin books that in every month there are ever two days which are very dangerous for drinking any medical potion, or for blood-letting; because there is one hour on each of those days, in which if any vein is opened, it is loss of life, or long disease. A leech tested this doctrine, and let his horse blood on that hour, and it soon lay dead.
>
> Now here are the days as is said here.
>
> The first day in March, that is, in the month of Hlyda, and the fourth day before the end of it.
>
> In the next month, which we call April, the tenth day is mischievous, and the eleventh before its end.
>
> In the month of May, the third day is mischievous, and the seventh before the end of it.
>
> In the month of June, the tenth day, and the fifteenth before the end of it.
>
> In July, the twelfth, and the tenth before the end.
>
> In August, the first day, and the second before the end.
>
> In September, the third day, and the tenth before the end.
>
> In October, the third, and the tenth from the end.
>
> In November, the fifth, and the third from the end.
>
> In December, the seventh, and the tenth from the end.
>
> In January, the first, and the seventh from the end.
>
> In February, the fourth, and the third from the end.
>
> In the commencement of this series we have put the month of March, which men call Hlyda, since it is the beginning, after right reckoning, of all the year, and the Almighty God on that month created all creation.
>
> Now again of the moon: it is much to be observed that none let blood on the fourth night of the moon's age, or on the fifth, as books tell us, before the moon and the sea be in harmony. We have further heard a man say, that no man should live, who had blood let from him on All Hallows day; nor if he were then wounded. This is no sorcery, but wise

men have made experiment of it, through the holy wisdom, as God Almighty dictated to them.

There are three days in the twelvemonth, with three nights, on which no woman is born; and whatever man is born on those days never putrefies in body in the earth, nor turns foul till doom's day. Now one of those days is in the latter part of December, and the remaining two are in the early part of January, and few there are who know or understand these mysteries.

Another such list, which exactly parallels the first paragraph of *De minutione sanguinis*, is, 'A man shall forego blood-letting on each of the six fives of the month' (that is, on the 5th, 10th, 15th, 20th, 25th and 30th). 'Leeches teach that no man on the five nights old moon, and again on the ten nights [old], and fifteen, and twenty and twenty-five and thirty nights old moon should let blood, but between each of the six fives'.[29]

There is a good example of the link between Egyptian days, venesection and the relationship of days of illness to the prospect of recovery in a small Anglo-Saxon manuscript by Ælfwine, Abbot of New Minster, Winchester, from 1035 to 1052.[30] There is similar material in another manuscript from the same collection[31] and also other material of this type published by R T Hampson in *Medii aevi Kalendarium* (London 1841).

The Welsh documents of the Anglo-Saxon period also list dangerous days:[32]

The third Monday in January, the first Monday in February, and the second Monday in October: whoever is bled on these days will be in danger of death. There are three days in the year on which no-one should be bled, or take any medicinal potion [the Egyptian days?]. These are the last day of April, the first Monday of August, and the last Monday in the month of September. Whosoever is bled on one of those days will die by the fifteenth or seventh day.... And he who shall eat of the flesh of a goose, will die in three days time.

Although the actual dates differ we have here yet another parallel for *De minutione sanguinis*, which also gives warnings against bleeding on certain days and the length of life left to those who are bled on these days: like the Bede passage, this one too warns against the taking of medicines and the eating of goose flesh on the three dangerous days. The eating of goose flesh was a Celtic taboo perhaps brought to England by Irish missionaries.[33] Another interesting coincidence is that in both documents some of the dates appear to be going backwards in time: the Welsh document states that 'whosoever is bled on one of those days will die by the fifteenth or seventh day': the section of *De minutione sanguinis* listing the days of each month which are harmful includes reversed dates in February, June, July and December. Egyptian Days were held to be generally unlucky: for example, it was unlucky to hold a feast, go on a journey, get married or even to plant a vineyard on such days. In the *Lacnunga* the three days listed above were also considered to be unlucky, 'he that on these days tasteth flesh of goose, within a space of forty days he shall end his life'.[34] The *Lacnunga, Meddygon Myddfai* and the *De minutione sanguinis* all give the same warning against eating goose flesh although predicting death after a different number of days.

In the British Museum there is what purports to be a translation made in the fourteenth century of *De minutione sanguinis*.[35] Although it, like the passages given above from the *Lacnunga* and *Meddygon Myddfai*, corresponds in part with the text given by Migne,[36] it is not an exact translation, as can be seen here: its title is *Medesyns approbate for mortal Sekenesses by Saynte Bede* and a selection from the translation is as follows, '(Whoever) of mankynde letteth hyme blode upon any of these iii dayes he shall be dede withynne five dayes nexte that followyn. These be iii forbode dayes; the firste is the last daye of Averil, the secunde is the firste daye of Auguste, the thirde is the firste daye of September.'

In Arabic literature, Wednesdays in which a number four occurs will be unlucky (that is, 4th, 14th, 24th of the month).[37] Phlebotomy was also often banned on holy days such as All Saints' Day (1st November) as is seen here, 'no man should live who had blood let from him on All-Hallows Mass-Day, or if he were then wounded'.[38]

However, the Anglo-Saxons believed some days were especially suitable for blood-letting as in the *Leechbook*,[39] where we find the following: 'the Kalends of April best of all, when trees and herbs first up-sprout and when the evil phlegm increases, and the evil blood in the hollow parts of the body'. There were also 'lucky' days for bleeding in Wales: 'whosoever is bled in the right arm on the eighteenth day of March, and the twentieth day of the month of April in the left arm will never be blind, for it has been often proved'.[40] Like the Bede which gives as a suitable time for phlebotomy 'the period from 25th March to 26th May', both documents recommend spring time for blood-letting.[41]

Bede mentions blood-letting in *Historia Ecclesiastica* V. 3 in conjunction with the report of a miracle:[42]

> She [the abbess] told us that the nun had recently been bled in the arm....and that the wounded arm grew worse and became so swollen that it could hardly be encircled with two hands. [A case of surgical sepsis?] The abbess therefore begged the bishop [John of Hexham] to visit the nun and give her his blessing, being sure that she would improve if the bishop blessed or touched her. He enquired when the girl had been bled, and when he learned that it had been on the fourth day of the moon, he said: 'You have acted most foolishly and unwisely to carry out blood-letting on the fourth day of the moon. I remember that Archbishop Theodore, of blessed memory, said that it was very dangerous to bleed at a time when the light of the moon and the pull of the tide is increasing'.

The nuns may have used a bleeding chart similar to one found in a psalter of the Old English period, which says for the fourth day, 'in matutina bona est'.[43] Despite a grammatical error in the Latin in the quotation from the psalter, this is an exact parallel with the Bede, which says, 'Luna quarta, in matutino bona est'. (The scribe has written *matutina* to agree with bona following, but it should read *matutino* [that is, *in* plus the ablative of *matutinum* – the morning].) Apart from the necessity for paying attention to the phases of the moon, there is a marked similarity with *De minutione sanguinis* in the instruction to bleed from the arm.

Bede, although he is scarcely known as a medical writer, mentions many items of medical interest in his works, mainly miracles, such as that mentioned above, when Bishop John restored a nun to health; the stories he gives in his *Ecclesiastical History* of individual cures by saints in person or by means of their relics tells us much about 'general practice' in his day, which was by and large in the hands of the church. In his *The Lives of the Holy Abbots of Wearmouth and Jarrow* and *The Life and Miracles of Saint Cuthbert, Bishop of Lindisfarne*, he also gives many examples of saintly cures. Cameron points out that Bede does however deal with medical matters directly on several occasions.[44] Part of chapter 30, *De Aequinoctiis et Solstitiis*, of his *De temporum ratione* deals with the physical and physiological fours, the relationship between the four winds, seasons and elements of the physical world and the four ages and humours of man. Bede names as his source here the *Epistula Hippocratis ad Antiochum Regem*;[45] [note that, although there were many rulers called Antiochus, the first ruled Syria from 280-261 BC, so Hippocrates living in the fifth century BC could hardly have written to any of them!] In his commentary on the Acts of the Apostles [Acts XXVIII 8], the *Retractatio in Actus Apostolorum*,[46] when he discusses the fever and dysentery suffered by Publius' father, Bede explains the symptoms of dysentery by quoting lines from Cassius Felix *De Medicina* ch.48 (*Ad dysenteriam*),[47] which in turn were quoted from Hippocrates.

Bede's concern with medicine can also be deduced from a letter sent by his pupil, Cuthbert, to a fellow pupil concerning the last hours of Bede's life; Bede, shortly before his death in 735 shared out his possessions among his companions in the monastery; these included linen (used for bandages), and pepper and incense (both used in mediæval medicines).

Dating back to at least the beginning of the ninth century is the *Epistula de phlebotomia* or *Phlebotomia Hippocratis* mentioned earlier,[48] which was perhaps the closest to a systematic medical phlebotomy available in mediæval times. It lists the veins from which a patient can be bled, especially the three great veins in the arm. It was widely distributed in monastic libraries, such as that of St Gallen mentioned above, and would have served as a guide to the prophylactic blood-letting, which was an annual monastic event. From this period there is also a parallel document, the *Epistula de sanguine cognoscendo*,[49] which presumed a knowledge of, or availability of, a more practical document such as the *De minutione sanguinis* or the *Epistula de phlebotomia*; this treatise explains how an examination of the consistency and colour of the blood could help in the patient's prognosis. Interestingly there is a somewhat later work[50] dated by Singer[51] to about 1110, which seems to consist of Bede's *De minutione sanguinis* with, inserted into it, extracts from the *Epistula de phlebotomia*.

Bede's medical knowledge was also passed on directly in the 11th century in the *Enchiridion* of Byrhtferth of Ramsey; in this work everything of medical interest seems to have been taken from Bede's *De Temporum Ratione*.[52]

Blood-letting [in Anglo-Saxon *blód-læswu: blód- lætan*, to bleed] was an established and very frequently used medical practice for the reduction or correction of excessive or corrupt humours from ancient times until the 19th century. Each of the four humours, all concentrated in the blood, was capable of being transformed into a harmful secondary humour, which had to be removed for the maintenance of good health. Phlebotomy was used by the Greeks as a cure for wounds: it is mentioned in the Hippocratic corpus in connection with a description of a tourniquet.[53] The Chinese did not practise phlebotomy, although acupuncture may originally have been a form of surgical drainage to remove blood or pus; whereas the Greeks believed that the humours causing infection were in the blood, the Chinese believed in a set of imaginary or spiritual vessels or 'meridians' containing not blood but *ch'i*.[54] Venesection was also regularly practised in India, where it was said that 'Venesection properly performed is half the treatment in surgery'.[55] There is also a possible reference to blood-letting in the Ebers Papyrus (c 1555 BC): 'a remedy for curing the *irft* disease — let him be given the knife treatment on the lower thigh'.[56] Galen (129 — c 199 AD) believed in bleeding for almost every disease, even to cure hæmorrhage; he wrote a book *On Venesection against Erisistratos*, because Erisistratos and his followers did not believe in practising venesection.[57]

The ideas for the treatment of wounds remained static for almost a thousand years after Galen, who endorsed and elaborated the Hippocratic concept of the four humours. This theory in the Middle Ages became an attempt to fit man into the universe by a scheme of fours, in the same way as the Chinese were trying to do by a scheme of fives. The astrological and chronological basis for the treatment of illness, which was followed at the time of Bede, can be seen emerging here as Majno argues.[58]

There are many parallels to the *De minutione sanguinis* of Bede in the *Leech Book of Bald*, which although it contains allusions to King Alfred (10th century), seems to be a copy of an earlier work already existing in Anglo-Saxon and is probably 9th century in date. In it are the following references to venesection:

Leech Book II, iii, 181-183:

> of swelling and sore of the maw: if the man have the strength to bear it, let him blood....

Leech Book II, vii, 187:

> and when one lets him blood on a vein, on those days let none other leechdom be done to him, except about five days later or more....

Leech Book II, xviii, 201:

> For swelling or puffing up of the liver: if the outgoing lodge, the man must first be let blood on a vein, on the left side.....[59]

Leech Book I, xlvii.1, gives another parallel for *De minutione sanguinis*, where it recommends that blood-letting for *peór-ádl* (a 'dry disease' or swelling of the chest) should be performed below the ankle.

Leech Book 63, *περι διδαξεων* gives as a remedy for vomiting:

> Let him blood from both feet below the ankle; let the blood be so let that the sick man faint not....and the second blood-letting, by which thou shalt cure the sick, is that thou shalt let him blood under the tongue....and after the blood-letting has been performed, thou shalt scarify him; then take salt and rub the wounds with it.

Leech Book II, xliii also shows the importance of the correct time for blood-letting:

> It is good to let blood in early Lent from the left arm.

The *Leech Book*, although it seems to be just a list of remedies, was intended as a practical manual and not a complete medical textbook of anatomy and physiology; it would assume its reader could gain this knowledge elsewhere.[60]

Between the 12th and 15th centuries many tracts on blood-letting were circulating in Europe.[61] One such is the 13th century eleven page treatise *Of Phlebotomie*,[62] which although it could be Salernitan in origin, is usually attributed to Henry of Winchester, who was a master at the medical school of Montpellier. It is a vernacular English translation of an earlier Latin phlebotomy, which in turn was probably written by an academic physician in the late 12th century.[63] This treatise lists diseases and the veins to be opened for their cure, but, like the earlier Bede passage, only if all other conditions are suitable. *Of Phlebotomie* shows something of the difficulties of an English translator of the period in trying to turn technical medical/scientific Latin into English prose, as the following parallels with the *De minutione sanguinis* show:

1. In tempore enim calidissimo non debet fieri flebotomia nec frigidissimo nec luna recenti, et est ratio in estate et maxime circa dies caniculares ultra modum dissolvitur corpus humanum et per dissolutionem multum inanitur. [lines 60-64]

   In moste hoote tyme forsoþ it owiþ not to be donne ne ful cold tyme ne in recent or newe mone. Þe reson or skelis is redi spede: in somere & moste aboute þe caniculere dayes mannys bodi ouer mersure is disoluyd; by dissoluyng it is moche inaynte or anantisiþ.

   [Phlebotomy ought not to be practised at the hottest or coldest times nor at the time of the new moon; for in summer and especially around the time of the Dog Days the body is weakened and emptied by too much blood-letting.]

2. posteriora capitis dolentia, recta vena incisa in fronte. [lines 256-257]

> Þe hyndere partie of þe heed akynge, þe ry3t strey3te veyne þat is in þe myddis of þe fronte ikutt.

[If the back part of the head aches, cut the right vein in the front of the head.]

3. Laborans podagra, minuat prius de basilica, postmodum de sophena. Laborans sciatica, et maxime de calida causa, minuat sibi de sophena exteriori. [lines 270-272]

> Laborynge of þe potagre, mynusch firste of basilica, after of sophena. Laboryng of sciati[c]a & moost of hoot cause, mynusche hym of sophena wiþout forþ.

[For gout, blood should first be let from the basilica, then from the saphenous vein. For sciatica, particularly that of hot origin, bleeding should be done from the exterior saphena.]

By the 14th century a change in the format of phlebotomy tracts circulating in western Europe perhaps indicates their use by a wider readership than the earlier monastic one; such manuscripts began to include illustrations and charts to show exactly where to bleed for each ailment, and at what time such treatment could be given. Sudhoff[64] gives a chart from a fourteenth century manuscript,[65] which despite its later date, is probably a good indicator of Anglo-Saxon practice in blood-letting; it shows the patient being bled from the right arm, with his right foot in a blood-letting basin. His right hand holds a stick, presumably as a support and to prevent contractions of the arm muscles; there is a bandage round the arm to control the flow of blood. Thorwald gives a phlebotomy table of AD 1480, based on the Babylonian doctrine of the relationship of every part of the human body to the signs of the zodiac, showing that blood-letting was allowed only at specific times for specific parts of the body.[66]

The places for blood-letting were outlined in calendars, charts and illustrations; often there were notations of lucky and unlucky days, seasons and even hours given. There were also many illustrations of a 'bleeding man' showing the veins and arteries to be opened for specific ailments; the actual position for drawing blood was important as the blood system was believed to be static or to ebb and flow rather than to circulate. It is noteworthy that there were many bleeding points near the elbow, presumably because of the numerous blood vessels easily accessible there. Most of the actual blood-letting illustrations show a surgeon or his assistant making an incision near the elbow, in the ante-cubital flexure. The *De minutione sanguinis* mentions three veins to be cut in the arm, the capitanea linea, the matricaria and the capsale, but does not specify which ailment cutting them could cure: is this because they were the veins chosen for curing many different ailments rather than a specific one? The most commonly opened veins in all the tracts and diagrams seem to have been the cephalic, median basilic and basilic veins in the arm. The futility of trying to specify where to open a vein is seen in the following fourteenth century saying:[67]

> Pro lapide....lete hym bloud in the grete to, ȝif þou myȝt vynde any veyne þer-Inne; and ȝif þou myȝt fynde non, lete hym bloud in þe arme.

Here we see that if a specific vein in the big toe cannot be found then the arm should be bled.

As can be seen from the extant literature and from illustrations, the most favoured place for blood-letting was at the bend of the elbow, and as a matter of practice the largest vein here was usually chosen. This is generally the median basilic, although there are both advantages and disadvantages in choosing this vein. It is often chosen because, in addition to being the largest vein and thus providing the greatest amount of blood, it is the least movable and can be steadied on the bicipital fascia on which it rests. However as it is separated from the brachial artery only by the bicipital fascia, one of the early disadvantages of phlebotomy would have been the risk of an arterio-venous aneurism. Also the median basilic is crossed by some of the branches of the internal cutaneous nerve, which could be divided in the process of phlebotomy, leading to what, according to Henry Gray,[68] Tillaux calls 'traumatic neuralgia of extreme intensity'.

The study of the Bible also played a part in mediæval medicine as no doubt it had in Bede's time; the therapeutic treatment of disease involved an interest in astrology, a magical interest in incantation, and a linguistic and metaphysical interest in the Hebrew language. Jews had arrived in England shortly after William the Conqueror, and although they remain largely anonymous, they had a considerable influence on Christian scholars, who began to learn Hebrew. As with incantations from the *Lacnunga*, recitation of psalms and prayers would have accompanied Mediæval medical treatment. A Hebrew Codex of psalms from the thirteenth century gives instructions for the chanting of Hebrew psalms as an aid to medical healing;[69] for example Psalm 79 is cited as an accompaniment to blood-letting: '......Before our eyes let it be known among the nations that You avenge the spilled blood of Your servants....'

By the 14th century medical education was becoming more formalised with rules and licensing in some countries, which led to standardization of practices. For example, a decree issued in 1332 by King Alfonso of Aragon followed the advice of technical manuals on phlebotomy in forbidding barber-surgeons in Valencia to practice blood-letting in the heat of summer (the Dog Days) except 'when evidently necessary or by advice of the medici'.[70] This again parallels the *De minutione sanguinis* in stating that blood-letting should not be practised during the Dog Days except when absolutely necessary, 'si necessitas urget'.

Caniculares dies or Dog Days are the days about the time of the heliacal rising of the Dog-star, and are some of the hottest and most unpleasant days of the year. Bede gives the dates for the Dog Days as from 18th July to 5th September. These dates for avoiding blood- letting at the time of the Dog Days are almost exactly paralleled in *Leechbook I*, lxxii:

> Blodlæs is to forganne fiftyne nihtum ær Hlafmæsse ⁊ æfter fif ⁊ þritig nihtum forþon þonne ealle æterno þing fleogaþ ⁊ mannum swiþe deriað.

> Blood-letting is to be foregone fifteen nights before Lammas, and after it for five and thirty nights, since then all poisonous things fly and injure men.

Cockayne,[71] although he lived before the days of modern viral theory,[72] seems to believe these 'flyers' to be epidemic viruses, which passing from one person to another could be assumed to blow about in the air. Payne, writing in 1904, says that 'the word translated "flying venom" or in modern language "air-borne contagion", seems to refer to epidemic diseases generally.'[73] Perhaps the linking of 'flying' poison with swelling, discoloration, and sores in these texts would point rather to bacterial infection, which is air-borne in dirt and dust, and affects some wounds but not others. The date of Lammas is the 1st August, in the heat of summer, at the time of the Dog Days as given by Bede. At the present time the Dog Days are calculated on the rising of either the greater dog-star (*Sirius*) or the lesser dog-star (*Procyon*), and on the heliacal or cosmical rising of either of these; their duration varies from 30 to 54 days. At Greenwich the cosmical rising of Sirius takes place around August 11th and that of Procyon around July 27th; the heliacal rising is several days later. In current almanacs the Dog Days begin on July 3rd and end on August 11th.

From the time of Galen until the Renaissance, physicians, although willing to criticise their predecessors, did not advance medical knowledge. They regarded their main task as being one of interpreting and understanding earlier concepts and therapeutic methods, especially the theory of humours and the practice of blood-letting to rid the body of bad humours. Phlebotomy continued to be used regularly in the same way as in Bede's time for many centuries. In the 14th century one of the treatments for the plague was to bleed the patient. In the 16th century Andreas Vesalius supported the classical procedure of blood-letting in his *Epistola docens venam axillarem dextri cubiti in dolore laterali secundam*. Specifically he rejected the then more commonly used Muslim method of taking blood from a location distant from the injured part, encouraging the classical procedure of taking it from near the lesion; furthermore he introduced a new, more scientific method of determining the precise location for blood-letting. In the *De minutione sanguinis* Bede recommends that for problems concerning the head, veins in the head are to be opened, but otherwise the veins should be generally far from the source of the complaint.

Although 17th-century England saw many developments in medical knowledge, the traditional humoral theories and practice of venesection continued. Even William Harvey (1578-1657), after his discovery of the circulation of the blood in 1628, still believed in venesection; he prescribed it as a treatment in 1653 for John Aubrey: 'Postera die emittatur sanguis ex vena hepatica dextri brachii ad 3ij'.[74] Again a parallel for Bede in recommending venesection from a vein in the arm.

The casebooks of Joseph Binns (surgeon at St Bartholomew's Hospital from 1647-1664) show the continued use of blood-letting, although he only advocated it for certain cases: for example, in two direct parallels with the *De Minutione Sanguinis*, he recommended it for headaches[75] and also for amenorrhoea, where he drew blood from the saphenous vein in the foot to draw the menses down.[76]

Also in the 17th century John Symcotts, a rural physician and contemporary of Binns, believed in the body's humoral balance, and as part of his treatments he ordered bleeding.[77] Phlebotomy was a fashionable treatment for all manner of ailments at this time, being often requested by the patients themselves. Two direct parallels with the *De Minutione Sanguinis* are the bleeding of John Evelyn on four occasions in May 1640 for sore eyes[78], and that of Samuel Pepys in July 1668, who was bled fourteen ounces of blood 'towards curing my eyes'.[79]

In the 18th century, apart from the ailment itself, the position of the vein to be opened, the position of the planets and the time of day were all still considered before phlebotomy could be practised, as can be seen in the work of Thomas Palmer (c 1666-1743). His work, *The Admirable Secrets of Physick and Chyrurgery*,[80] is a notebook of current medical theory and practice written when he was a young Massachusetts practitioner, giving the information most important in his daily rounds. Illness was still regarded as an imbalance of humours, which could be corrected by bleeding; Palmer says that he would have considered the patient's age, the location of the ailment and thus the appropriate vein to be opened. He recommends that the site for blood-letting be far from the affected part, presumably for complaints other than those of the head, since, like Bede, he advises that migraine could be eased by 'opening of a vein in the forehead or nostrils'.[81] Palmer also says that he would have considered the planet which controlled the particular part of the body and the planets then in ascendance. He repeats, albeit in a slightly different form, Bede's advice as to the time of year when phlebotomy may be used; Bede uses months and days, whereas Palmer gives zodiacal signs, but both place great emphasis on the importance of timing, such as Bede's warning against using phlebotomy on Egyptian days. He gives his rules for *Phlebotomy and Admin[istering] Physick* in similar terms to those of the *De minutione sanguinis*,[82] mentioning specifically:

> Again in Dog-dayes it is very hurtfull to take Physick at all unless there be great need. In such a case the Disease being desperate, the cure must be adventured.

Palmer is here re-iterating what Bede says in the first paragraph and the last two of the *De minutione sanguinis*.

Palmer again closely parallels Bede when he talks of the veins to be opened in the arm:

> The veins in the arm opened are Cephalica or head vein: Basilica or lower vein: Mediana or the vein between the two former.
>
> The Mediana is formed of the branches of Cephalica & Basilica, running both in one. Note: that vein that narrows most is to be bound. Cephalica hath neither Artery nor Sinew near it. The Mediana hath a Sinew just under it. Note that Cephalica sometimes doth not appear, & so sometimes some of the other Veins and sometimes neither of them. In some cases blood-letting saves life, and in some cases destroys it. In abundance of blood and in inflammation of blood, open a vein.

Phlebotomy has continued into the modern era; for instance, it is believed that excessive blood-letting rather than his actual ailment killed George Washington! Venesection is still used on occasion today, for example in cases of polycythæmia rubra vera, where there is an increase in all the cellular elements of the bone marrow – red cells, granulocytes and blood platelets. Treatment, which can alleviate but not completely cure the condition, is either by repeated venesection or by radioactive phosphorus.

For thousands of years phlebotomy was used curatively or prophylactically as a specifically surgical method of freeing the body of disease or evil humours. Before 1200 blood-letting was relied upon in an almost irrational way, not just for specific ailments, but as a 'cure-all' as the *De minutione sanguinis* shows. It was prescribed almost to a set formula in technical phlebotomies, as I have tried to show in this paper by referring to various documents similar to the *De minutione sanguinis sive de Phlebotomia* of Bede. Not only the documents of the Anglo-Saxon period but also those of much later, such as the Commonplace book of Thomas Palmer written in the early 18th century, one thousand years after Bede, emphasize particularly both that the time of year must be taken into account before phlebotomy is practised and that the site for phlebotomy be carefully chosen. The following passage from the 12th century shows what were believed to be the all-embracing powers of phlebotomy:[83]

> It contains the beginning of health, it makes the mind sincere, it aids the memory, it purges the brain, it reforms the bladder, it warms the marrow, it opens the hearing, it checks tears, it removes nausea, it benefits the stomach, it invites digestion, it evokes the voice, it builds up the sense, it moves the bowels, it enriches sleep, it removes anxiety, it nourishes good health.

William Harvey, in his *De generatione animalium* of 1651, perhaps best sums up the mystical and divine attitude to the powers of the blood and to phlebotomy, which had continued to be held from ancient times, through the Anglo-Saxon period of Bede, up to his own century:[84]

> But when I assert that the soul resides first and principally in the blood, I would not have any man hastily conclude from this that all phlebotomy is dangerous or injurious, or believe with the common herd that for so

much blood taken off, the same amount of life is taken away with it, because the Scriptures locate life in the blood. For it is well known from daily experience that blood-letting is a safe relief in many diseases and the chief among universal remedies, in that the vitiation or superabundance of the blood constitutes the greatest breeding-ground of diseases, and a timely letting of blood often rescues men from desperate diseases and even death itself. For so much blood that is taken off according to the art, the same amount is added to life and health.

Further reading for the Anglo-Saxon and Mediæval periods.

Bonser W. *The Medical Background of Anglo-Saxon England*. London: The Wellcome Historical Medical Library, 1963.

Campbell S, Hall B, Klausner D (Eds.). *Health, Disease and Healing in Medieval Culture*. London: (Centre for Medieval Studies, University of Toronto), MacMillan Academic and Professional Ltd, 1992.

Cockayne T O. *Leechdoms, Wortcunning and Starcraft of Early England:* 3 volumes. London: Longman Green, 1866.

Colgrave B. *Two lives of St. Cuthbert: a life by an anonymous monk of Lindisfarne and Bede's prose life.* Cambridge: University Press, 1940.

Crombie A C. *Mediæval and Early Modern Science, Volume I: Science in the Middle Ages: V-XIII Centuries.* New York: Doubleday/Anchor, 1959 (2nd edition).

Giles A (Ed.). *Complete Works of the Venerable Bede*. London: 1843.

Grattan J H G and Singer C. *Anglo-Saxon Magic and Medicine*. London: Wellcome Historical Medical Museum: Geoffrey Cumberledge, Oxford University Press, 1952.

Grattan J H G and Singer C. *"Lacnunga" A Magico-Medical Commonplace Book*. London: Oxford University Press, 1952.

Jones C W. *Bedae Pseudoepigrapha: Scientific Writings Falsely Attributed to Bede*. Ithaca, New York: Cornell University Press, 1939.

Jones C W. *Bedae Opera de Temporibus.* Cambridge, Mass.: The Mediæval Academy of America, 1943.

Laistner M L W (Ed.). *Bedae Venerabilis Expositio Actuum Apostolorum et Retractatio*. Cambridge, Mass: Harvard University Press, 1939.

Migne J P. *Patrologiae cursus completus: Latin Series Volume 90.* Paris: Turnholt, 1862.

Payne J F. *The Fitz-Patrick Lectures for 1903: English Medicine in the Anglo-Saxon Times*. Oxford: Clarendon Press, 1904.

Plummer C. *Venerabilis Bædae: Historia ecclesiastica gentis Anglorum*. Oxford: Clarendon Press, 1896: Volume I: clviii.

Plummer C. *Bædae opera historica*. Oxford: Clarendon Press, 1896.

Sherley-Price L (Trans). *Bede: A History of the English Church and People*. London: Penguin Books, 1955.

Singer C. A Review of the Medical Literature of the Dark Ages, with a New Text of about 1110. *Proc Roy Soc Med* (Section on the History of Medicine) 1917; *10*:107-60.

Singer C and Underwood E A. *A Short History of Medicine*. Oxford: Clarendon Press, 1962.

Siraisi N G. *Medieval and Early Renaissance Medicine*. Chicago: The University of Chicago Press, 1990.

Stenton F. *Anglo-Saxon England c550-1087*, [The Oxford History of England, Volume 2]. Oxford: Clarendon Press, 1985 [Third edition].

Talbot C H. Some Notes of Anglo-Saxon Medicine. *Med Hist* 1965; *9*:156-169.

Notes and references.

1. Bede uses the term 'phases of the moon' for the days of the month: see commentary, pages 63-67.
2. For Dog Days see commentary, pages 72-73 *et passim*.
3. Presumably this is referring back to line 1 of this text, or possibly to an earlier reference, no longer extant.
4. *capitanea linea, matricaria* and *capsale* or box vein: see commentary, pages 71-72.
5. For Egyptian Days see commentary, page 63 *et passim*. Further information on the Egyptian Days can be found in: Steele R. Dies Aegyptiaci; *Proc Roy Soc Med* London: 1919; *13* Suppl:108-121. Also in Du Cange C de F. *Glossarium*. Paris: c.1660.
6. //-----// indicates that the text is corrupt at this point: see commentary, pages 64-65.
7. For the prohibition of the consumption of goose flesh on Egyptian Days see commentary, pages 64 and 66-67.
8. For a discussion on the list of days given by Bede, which are forbidden for phlebotomy, and which seem to go backwards in time, see commentary, page 66.
9. *ibid.*
10. *ibid.*
11. *ibid.*
12. Although this conflicts with the earlier list, the Latin text is quite clear in both instances. Unless the scribe has omitted a word following *vigesima*, we must accept the text and contradiction as it stands. If there is an omission, then, according to the earlier list, Bede could have been prohibiting phlebotomy on the twenty-sixth, twenty-eighth or twenty-ninth days of the month.
13. Migne J P. *Patrologiae cursus completus: Latin series Volume 90.* Paris: Turnholt, 1862:959-962.
14. Giles A (Ed). *Complete works of the Venerable Bede*. London: 1843; *4*:349.
15. Jones C W. *Bedae Pseudoepigrapha: Scientific Writings Falsely Attributed to Bede*. Ithaca, New York: Cornell University Press, 1939:88-89.
16. Plummer C. *Baedae opera historica*. Oxford: Clarendon Press, 1896.
17. Bonser W. *The Medical Background of Anglo-Saxon England*. London: The Wellcome Historical Medical Library, 1963.
18. Tangi M. *S. Bonifati et Lullii Epistolae*. Berlin: 1955; MGH, Epistolae Selectae *I*:247.
19. Sigerist H E. *Studien und Texte zur Frühmittelalterlichen Rezeptliteratur*. Leipzig: Studien zur Geschichte der Medizin, 1923.
20. British Library Manuscript: *Sloane* 475: folios 125-231.
21. Sharpe W D. Isidore of Seville: The Medical Writings. Philadelphia: *Trans Amer Philosoph Soc* 1964; *New Series 54*: Part 2.
22. S. Gallen Manuscript: *Stiftsbibliothek* 751.
23. Chabas F. *Le Calendrier des jours fastes et néfastes de l'année Égyptienne*. Paris: 1891.
24. Grattan J H G and Singer C. *Anglo-Saxon Magic and Medicine*. London: Wellcome Historical Medical Museum: Geoffrey Cumberledge, Oxford University Press, 1952:43.

25. The standard edition is Howald F and Sigerist H E (Eds). *Antonii Musae de Herba Vettonica Liber, Pseudo-Apulei Herbarius, Anonymi de Taxone Liber, Sexti Placiti Liber Medicinae ex Animalibus etc*. Leipzig: Corpus Medicorum Latinorum, 1927.
26. Beccaria Manuscript. *Codici*: 441-485.
27. British Museum Manuscript: *Harley 585* includes *The Lacnunga*. This passage comes from folios 190a and 190b.
28. British Museum Manuscript: *Cotton Caligula A XV*: folio 126b. quoted also in Cockayne T O. *Leechdoms, Wortcunning and Starcraft of Early England*. London: Longman Green, 1866; the three volumes of this work include both text and translation of the three *Leechbooks*.
29. Cockayne op cit note 28; 1:72.
30. British Museum Manuscript: *Cotton Titus DXXVI*.
31. British Museum Manuscript: *Cotton Titus DXXVII*.
32. Pughe J (Tr.). *The Physicians of Myddfai (Meddygon Myddfai)*. Llandovery: Welsh MSS Society, 1861: I:91-92. See also: Diverres, P. *Le plus ancien texte des Meddygon Myddveu*. Paris: 1913; this contains only Part 1 of the *Meddygon Myddfai*.
33. Halm F. *Gans* in Hoop's *Reallexikon der germanischen Altertumskunde*.
34. *Harley 585 op cit* note 27; folio 118: CLXXXIX.
35. British Museum Manuscript: *Additional 5467*: folio 71, 72.
36. Migne *op cit* note 13:959-962.
37. de Meynard and de Couteille (Eds). *Maçoudi [Ali Ibn Husain, al-Mas'udi] Les Prairies d'or*. Paris: 1864: *3*: cap.lviii:416.
38. *Cotton Caligula op cit* note 28; folio 127a.
39. Cockayne: *op cit* note 28; *1*:72.
40. Pughe *op cit* note 32; *I*:91-92.
41. See note 4: Steele *op cit* note 5 and Du Cange *op cit* note 5.
42. Taken from the translation by Sherley-Price L. *Bede: A History of the English Church and People*. London: Penguin Books, 1955:268- 269.
43. British Museum Manuscript: *Arundel 60*: 1r.
44. Cameron M L. The Sources of Medical Knowledge in Anglo- Saxon England. In: *Anglo-Saxon England*. Cambridge: 1983; *11*:146.
45. Jones C W. *Bedae Opera de Temporibus*. Cambridge, Mass.: The Mediæval Academy of America, 1943:235-237.
46. Laistner M L W (Ed). *Bedae Venerabilis Expositio Actuum Apostolorum et Retractatio*. Cambridge, Mass.: Harvard University Press, 1939:145.
47. Rose (Ed). *Casii Felicis de Medicina*: 122.
48. *Stiftsbibliothek* 751 *op cit* note 22.
49. Brussels Manuscript *3701-15 (3702):* folios 13r-14v.
50. Oxford: *St. John's College Manuscript 17.*
51. Singer C. A Review of the Medical Literature of the Dark Ages, with a New Text of about 1110. *Proc Roy Soc Med* (Section on the History of Medicine) 1917; *10*:107-60.
52. Crawford S J. *Byrhtferth's Manual*. London: EETS, 1929.
53. Littré edition of *Hippocrates V:* 117; *Epidemics II*, #14. Also: Jones W H S and Withington E T (Trans.). *Hippocrates*. Cambridge, Mass.: Loeb Classical Library, Harvard University Press, 1923.
54. Chamfrault and Ung Kang Sam (Tr.): *Les Livres sacrés de médicin chinoise: a translation of Huang Ti Nei Ching.* Veith: 1966.
55. Bhishagratna K L. *Sushruta Samhita*. Chowkamba Sanskrit Series Ofice, Varanasi, India: 1907-1911 (re-printed 1963): *II*:207.

56. Ebell B. *The Papyrus Ebers: The Greatest Egyptian Medical Document*. Copenhagen: 1937.

57. Kühn C G. *Claudii Galeni Opera Omnia*. Ed. Lipsiae: 1821-1833. Off. Libr. C.Cnoblochii: Greek text with Latin translation [22 volumes].

58. Majno G. *The Healing Hand: Man and Wound in the Ancient World*. Cambridge, Mass.: Harvard University Press, 1975:418.

59. British Library Manuscript *Royal 12:* D.xvii.

60. Wright C E. *Bald's Leechbook: British Museum Royal Manuscript 2.D. XVII*. Copenhagen: 1955.

61. Kibre P. *Hippocrates Latinus: Repertorium of Hippocratic Writings in the Latin Middle Ages*. 1979: *V Traditio* 35.

62. Cambridge: *Gonville and Caius College Manuscript 176/97.*

63. The Latin text from which 'Henry of Winchester' worked has not been positively identified, but, according to Voights and McVaugh, the closest found so far seems to be Madrid, *Bibliotheca Nacional Manuscript 3066*: folios 5v-7v. Voights L and McVaugh M R. A Latin Technical Phlebotomy and Its Middle English Translation. *Trans Amer Philosoph Soc.* 1984; *New Series 74*:9.

64. Sudhoff K. *Beitrage zur Geschichte der Chirurgie im Mittelalter*. Leipzig: 1914; *1*: plate 54 (4).

65. British Museum Manuscript *Harley 3719.*

66. Thorwald J. *Science and Secrets of Early Medicine*. London: Thames and Hudson, 1962:152.

67. Henslow: *Medical Works of the Fourteenth Century*. London: 1899:42.

68. Gray H. *Anatomy, Descriptive and Surgical*. New York: Crown Publishers, 1977:608.

69. Bodleian Library, Oxford Manuscript *Laud Or. 174.*

70. Ballester L G and McVaugh M R. *Nota sobre el control de la actividad medica y quirurgica de los barberos en los Furs de Valencia de 1329*. Valencia: 1988.

71. Cockayne *op cit* note 28: *I*:38.

72. The term '*virus*' was used as early as 1728 for 'a morbid principle.... capable of being introduced into other persons or animals by inoculation or otherwise and of developing the same disease in them' (OED).

73. Payne J F. *The Fitzpatrick Lectures for 1903: English Medicine in the Anglo-Saxon Times*. Oxford: Clarendon Press, 1904:43.

74. Cule J. *A Doctor for the People*. London: Update Books, 1980:55. Cule states, without giving the actual reference, that this prescription of Harvey's is from a transcription and annotation by Gweneth Whitteridge.

75. British Library Manuscript *Sloane 153:* 6 (case number 17) and 10 (case number 25); this manuscript comprises Joseph Binns' surgical casebook.

76. *ibid*, 192 (case number 379).

77. Beier L McC. *Sufferers and Healers*. London: Routledge and Kegan Paul, 1987:104.

78. De Beer E S. *The Diaries of John Evelyn* (six volumes). Oxford: Clarendon Press, 1959; *2*:271. See also: Bowle, John: *John Evelyn and his World: A Biography*. London: Routledge and Kegan Paul, 1981.

79. Latham R and Matthews W (Eds) *The Diary of Samuel Pepys*. Cambridge: Bell and Hyman, 1978; *9*:261. See also: Bryant A. *Samuel Pepys*. Glasgow: Collins, 1949.

80. Palmer T (Ed. Forbes T R) *The Admirable Secrets of Physick and Chyrurgery*. New Haven: Yale University Press, 1984 [originally begun about 1696].

81. *ibid*, 126.

82. *ibid*, 176 for Palmer's rules for phlebotomy.

83. Bibliotheque Nationale Manuscript *Nouv. acq.229:* folios 1a-10a. Also Thorndike L. *A History of Magic and Experimental Science During the First Thirteen Centuries of Our Era.* New York: 1923; *I*:728.

84. Whitteridge G (Trans). *William Harvey: Disputations Touching The Generation of Animals*. Oxford: Blackwell Scientific Publications, 1981:257.

Chapter 5

LOCAL SOURCES FOR THE STUDY OF MEDICAL HISTORY

Joan S Emmerson

Students of medical history in the North East have available to them source material of some importance. While not as extensive as the Wellcome Library or other large metropolitan libraries, the Robinson Library in the University of Newcastle and the Library of the University of Durham nevertheless together contain several valuable collections of early medical books. The chief of these in each of the libraries have been presented or bequeathed by local medical men.

Newcastle has been fortunate to receive two particularly notable acquisitions. The first, a major bequest, was made in the nineteenth century, originally to the old Infirmary; the other, a donation made in its owner's lifetime, came to the University Library in 1965. The donors both lived to a great age, the one, Thomas Masterman Winterbottom died in 1859 at 93 years old (see also Chapter 11); the other, Frederick Charles Pybus in 1975 at 92. Each in his own time contributed much to his chosen profession and left a valuable literary legacy for succeeding generations.

Dr Thomas Winterbottom and his collection

Dr T M Winterbottom of South Shields bequeathed 'all my books, in every language on medical and surgical subjects to ..the Library of the General Infirmary of Newcastle upon Tyne....'. A substantial number of non-medical works was bequeathed to the University of Durham.

When in 1906 the Royal Victoria Infirmary came to its present building from the old Forth Banks, its library, a valuable collection of old books, was also brought and housed in the basement. Among these was Dr Winterbottom's legacy. Nothing more was heard of these books until 1921 when a fire occurred. Firemen, breaking open what they thought to be a wooden partition, discovered that it was composed of the backs of several bookcases, many of the contents having been already damaged or destroyed. The remainder (about 340 volumes) were subsequently (1926) transferred to the University Library where, together with the more valuable books from the old College of Medicine, they became our first historical Medical Collection. Some of them show the marks of fire and water and undoubtedly many of the original 3000 medical volumes must have perished altogether.

Winterbottom presented his MD thesis *De morbo puerperali* in Glasgow in 1792. From August of that year until April 1796 he served as physician to the Sierra Leone Colony. There he wrote his first book, published in 1798, *Medical directions for the use of navigators and settlers in hot climates*. It was written at the request of the Chairman and directors of the Sierra Leone Company to whom it is dedicated, and was first described as 'Medical directions for the use of the vessels of the Sierra Leone Company'. In the early years of the colony a large proportion of the Europeans who went out died from fevers within a few months of their arrival and the company was obliged to take steps to ensure the well-being of its officials.

The book is an expansion of certain medical directions originally written for the guidance of trading vessels which carried no medical officer. To these original instructions has been added an account of various diseases, and their treatment, to which Europeans in hot countries are particularly prone. The book is written throughout in the clearest terms, understandable to the layman, and technical expressions have been entirely avoided. It is addressed primarily to the captains of trading vessels advising in the first instance how diseases and undue discomfort in tropical conditions may be avoided by the proper regulation of diet, clothing and exercise, and giving the precautions to be taken when it is impossible to avoid anchoring the ship off a marshy shore where disease is likely to be contracted. As always, Winterbottom is concerned for sailors and their welfare, and exhorts captains to observe their men closely and if they show signs of fatigue and weakness to allow them to rest and be cared for; and later, when speaking of vaccination 'the author earnestly recommends the practice to the serious consideration of every benevolent commander of a vessel....'. Treatment for seasickness and scurvy is next described, advice given to intending passengers on the kind of food and drink to take with them, and on methods of preserving food and water. There is even advice for the shipwrecked on how to quench thirst by dipping clothes twice a day in the sea and putting them on wet, when the skin will absorb the needed moisture; and on how to still the pangs of hunger by imitating the American Indians who, when likely to be without food for some time, 'compress the stomach by means of flat-boards laced round them, which they draw tighter every day'. After this there are directions on how to care for men rescued at sea.

The second part of the book describes not only the diseases which most frequently occurred in Sierra Leone and to which Europeans were most liable – fevers, remitting and intermittent, yellow fever, dysentery, etc, – but almost every mishap which might befall, from wounds and fractures to the effects of poisons and insect bites, and their remedies.

Dr Winterbottom concludes his book with a list of the weights used in medicine and a list of suitable medicines with the quantity sufficient for twenty men for one year, directions as to their use and for keeping in well-labelled containers in a locked medicine chest. It was a book intended for practical every day use and admirably fulfils its purpose; many of its recommendations, in fact, would be equally valid in similar conditions today.

Despite his very full life in the colony – in addition to his medical duties, which largely involved him in treating the fevers of both settlers, colleagues and natives, he assisted the Governor, Zachary Macaulay, by acting as a magistrate – he embarked in 1794 on his major work *An account of the native Africans in the neighbourhood of Sierra Leone to which is added an account of the present state of medicine among them*. 'It was resorted to,' he says, 'with the view of restoring some degree of activity to a mind broken down by sickness and afflicted by the scenes of distress which daily presented themselves'. Two events particularly, added to his unceasing efforts to look after his patients, had contributed to Dr Winterbottom's depression at this time. In 1794 one of his brothers, also employed by the Sierra Leone Company, was accidentally drowned; and at much the same time considerable hardship and suffering was inflicted on the inhabitants of the colony by a French invasion.

Macaulay therefore, in order to cheer him and to distract his mind from these misfortunes, encouraged him to record his investigations into the life and the diseases of the native Africans. The book was published in 1803 by Mr Hatchard, who first published the *Christian Observer* with which Macaulay was closely connected. The work was published in two volumes, the first of which, reviewed by Sidney Smith in the *Edinburgh Review*, gives a general account of the country, its inhabitants and their language, with details of customs, climate, agriculture and trade. It bears evidence throughout of Winterbottom's wide reading and he quotes profusely from a great variety of authors, so much in fact, that Sidney Smith was constrained to remark that 'upon the whole, it must be rather considered as a compilation from previous writers than as the result of the author's experience'. He does, however, acknowledge that '[the author] is extensively acquainted with the subjects on which he writes, and has a talent of selecting important matter and adorning it', and ends a long and favourable review by saying that 'this.... volume may be safely purchased'. The second volume of the work is devoted to 'the present state of medicine' among the Africans and again shows Winterbottom's extensive reading. Following an introduction which is a brief survey of the origins of medicine in primitive races, the work is divided into three sections:

1. General diseases
2. Diseases of women
3. Diseases of children

Detailed descriptions are given of diseases observed and treated by Winterbottom with descriptions and comparisons as given by other medical writers, and it is in the first section of this volume that occurs his classic description of sleeping sickness:

> The Africans are very subject to a species of lethargy, which they are much afraid of, as it proves fatal in every instance. (Here he gives native names for the disease from various tribes)..... it is called by the Soosoos, Kee Killee Kindee, or sleepy sickness..... It is said to be much more common in the interior parts of the country than upon the sea coast. Children are very rarely, or never, affected with this complaint, nor is it more common among slaves than among free people..... At the commencement of the disease the patient has commonly a ravenous appetite, eating twice the quantity of food he was accustomed to take when in health and becoming very fat. When the disease has continued

some time the appetite declines and the patient gradually wastes away. Squinting occurs sometimes, though very seldom in this disease and in some rare instances the patient is carried off in convulsions. Small glandular tumors are sometimes observed in the neck a little before the commencement of this complaint, though probably depending rather upon accidental circumstances than upon the disease itself. Slave traders, however, appear to consider these tumors as a symptom indicating a disposition to lethargy, and they either never buy such slaves or get quit of them as soon as they observe any such appearances. The disposition to sleep is so strong as scarcely to leave a sufficient respite for the taking of food, even the repeated application of a whip, a remedy which has been frequently used, is hardly sufficient to keep the poor wretch awake. The repeated application of blisters and setons has been employed by European surgeons without avail, as the disease under every mode of treatment usually proves fatal within three or four months. The natives are totally at a loss to what cause this complaint ought to be attributed....'

In trypanosomiasis today, enlargement of the cervical lymph glands is known as Winterbottom's sign.

Throughout his time in Sierra Leone Winterbottom, despite his very full medical duties, found time to carry out research on various subjects and to communicate numerous papers, notably to *Medical Facts and Observations* from 1792 onwards.

Dr Winterbottom left Sierra Leone in 1796 to take over his father's practice in South Shields. From that time until he retired in 1822 he 'was only absent from Shields one day, and then because he had a subpoena for a trial at Durham'. However after his retirement, until his sight began to fail in 1855, he made an annual journey to the continent and it was during these journeys that he acquired much of his considerable library. In speaking of a voyage from Italy in 1822 during which the ship was held up for some time in quarantine he says 'Having laid in a good store of books at Leghorn I was independent of time'.

His interest in books was wide and varied and he was an accomplished linguist; the non-medical portion of his library, consisting of some two thousand volumes, all that remain of a much larger collection, is in the University Library at Durham. They cover almost every subject on which books have been written from the earliest classics to contemporary books of travel, particularly in West Africa and other tropical countries. He had gathered together also a number of works of considerable philological interest, especially in the German language, as well as novels, books on chess and on 'equestrian education'.

The medical portion of the library is equally extensive and varied, both in date and subject matter. The earliest work is the *Opus de Peste* of Jacobus Soldus, published in 1478, which bears on the flyleaf the words 'libro rarissimo' – possibly a 'find' by Dr Winterbottom while browsing in some continental bookshop. There are early editions of Hippocrates, Galen, Celsus and other classical writers.

Sixteenth and seventeenth medicine is represented by, among others, Ingrassia, G F – *Informatione del pestifero*, Palermo, 1576; Susio, G B – *La pestilenza*, Mantova, 1576; Gerarde, J – *Herball*, London 1633; and William Harvey – *De generatione animalium*, Amsterdam, 1651. Joseph Fox's *Diseases of the teeth*, published in 1806, indicates that Dr Winterbottom kept well up to date with current literature. Indeed he was very much concerned with the medical discoveries and developments of his own day, not less than with the history of his subject. As might be expected, there are a number of books on diseases in hot climates, on fevers of all kinds and on quarantine and contagion, and many volumes of contemporary medical periodicals. He was a staunch supporter of vaccination for smallpox. In his *Medical Directions for the use of navigators.... in hot climates*, he writes 'Those who wish to confer a benefit upon mankind, and to make some reparation to those unhappy nations who have derived only misery from their acquaintance with Europeans, and who have suffered so dreadfully from the Small-Pox, will endeavour to convey to them the blessing of the Cow-Pox Inoculation', and goes on to give the address of the Vaccine Institute in Golden Square from which cow-pox matter could be obtained. Nor did he neglect subjects ancillary to medicine and his library contained many works on chemistry (Black, Fourcroy, Neumann), on botany and all the natural sciences.

Several of Dr Winterbottom's books contain the signature of his father James and these are often pharmacopoeias or dispensatories which it may be supposed were in almost daily use. Others were given to him by their authors, notably some from Robert Willan. Apart from the two books already described, Dr Winterbottom's own writings were limited to a number of letters written to Willan from Sierra Leone and later published in *Medical Facts and Observations*, and to several papers on quarantine and contagion in the *Edinburgh Medical and Surgical Journal* during the years 1828-29.

The Winterbottom books are now incorporated in the Medical Collection of the Robinson Library, which includes also other books and periodicals from the library of the Infirmary (together with its original MS catalogue) and from the old College of Medicine. These libraries themselves held numerous important volumes. A first edition (1798) of Jenner's treatise on vaccination, early editions of Laennec on auscultation (1821), John Hunter on inflammation and gun-shot wounds (1794), on venereal disease (1786) and on the natural history of teeth (1771), Heberden's commentaries (1802) containing his original description of angina pectoris and Morgagni's great work *The seats and causes of diseases* (1761) which has been called the 'high-water mark of clinico-pathological description' are chosen at random to illustrate the extent of the Collection. Representative American works are Benjamin Rush's classic account of yellow fever (1794) and William Beaumont on the physiology of digestion (1838).

Frederick Pybus and his collection

The Medical Collection supplements and complements the Pybus Collection and together they provide a valuable source of historical importance. Professor F C Pybus was born in Stockton on Tees in November 1883. He entered the Newcastle Medical School in October 1900 to embark on the five-year degree course. In his third student year his first clinical attachment was as a dresser in Professor Rutherford Morison's surgical ward and in 1907 he became House Surgeon to Morison. While still a House Surgeon his interest in medical history was aroused, primarily by discussions with George Grey Turner (then a Registrar) on anatomy and physiology and of historical figures in medicine and surgery.

Professor Pybus had a long association with the RVI. Following his original appointment as House Surgeon to Rutherford Morison he studied in London at Barts (for a special Final Fellowship Course), at the Gordon Hospital and the Cancer Hospital (Royal Marsden), returning to Newcastle as Registrar in various departments of the hospital. He became a private assistant to the Senior Surgeon (Mr Martin) and made drawings for Rutherford Morison's book, *An introduction to Surgery* (1910). During the early days of the First World War Pybus organised the 1st Northern General Hospital, located in Armstrong College (now the Armstrong Building of the University). In 1915 he was in Egypt in charge of the surgical division of the 17th General Hospital from where he was invalided home. Appointed Assistant Surgeon to the RVI in 1920, he was Senior Surgeon in 1938 and became Professor of Surgery in the University in 1941.

Professor Pybus published one book, *The surgical diseases of children*, a handbook for students and practitioners which appeared in 1932. Throughout his life, however, for fifty years or more he was greatly concerned about the causes of cancer, particularly of the lung. For many years he conducted research on mice; he bred strains which produced spontaneous cancer, induced it in others and studied the effects of different treatments. He wrote many articles on the subject and conducted a voluminous correspondence, waging almost a one-man campaign against air pollution from the gases produced by the burning of coal, from diesel and from bonfires and maintained the most important cause of lung cancer to be soot containing benzpyrene and sulphur. He was particularly proud of his copy of the first edition of John Evelyn's *Fumifugium: or the inconvenience of the aer and smoak of London dissipated ....* (1661), and of the various reprints from 1772 to that of 1933 published for the National Smoke Abatement Society with an introduction by Rose Macaulay. One copy of this is bound in a volume containing the report of the Committee on Air Pollution 1953 and Parliamentary proceedings leading to the Clean Air Act of 1956. Like Dr Winterbottom, Professor Pybus cared for his patients and was frequently impatient of conditions and administrations which seemed to him unnecessary or ill-suited to the needs of the sick.

About 1913-14 in Edinburgh, Pybus met Douglas Guthrie, founder of the Scottish Society of the History of Medicine, through whom his interest in medical history was re-awakened. In subsequent years he began to collect portraits of the eponymous characters of medicine and medical science who had interested him in his early days at the RVI. This eventually led to the acquisition of the books and MS letters which with some 2000 portraits make up the Pybus Collection. In his early days of collecting, about 1920-21, Professor Pybus being, as he says, 'hard-up' decided to limit his collection to the 'few English Masters – Harvey, Hunter, Jenner and Sydenham'. However, while in Edinburgh for the second meeting of the Association of Surgeons he first saw a copy of Vesalius' *De humani corporis fabrica* which so inspired him that he began to extend his collecting interest, first to anatomical and surgical texts and eventually to books on all the medical specialties and, like Dr Winterbottom before him, including important works in related sciences. The Collection contains many editions of the classical Greek and Roman authors with examples of seminal works in all branches of medicine up to and including the 19th century.

There is much to interest students of printing and illustrative techniques; there are many fine examples of early printing, including several incunabula and the methods of illustration used range from the early woodcuts as seen in Mundinus and Vesalius, through copper and brass engravings to the lithographic techniques of the 19th century.

The earliest published work in the Collection is the 14th-century manuscript of the works of John of Arderne (1307-1390). He was an English military surgeon during the Hundred Years War, who subsequently practised in Newark and his writings on various surgical subjects were widely read and copied over many years. The Pybus copy is about 1380. The instruments used and his method of treatment for *fistula in ano*, an operation for which he was justly famed, are well illustrated.

Of the early printed works in the Collection one of the most attractive is *De medicina* of Celsus, printed in Florence in 1478. This is a particularly interesting copy of one of the first medical books to be printed. Apart from the interest of its subject matter – the first use of the term 'insanity' (*insania*) occurs in the third book – this work is a rich compendium of the medical knowledge of his time (about 30 AD). It is a specially fine example of early printing, with hand-coloured initial letters, and contains a section in manuscript apparently in a contemporary hand. As in Winterbottom's collection, the early classical writers are well represented. There are excellent copies of the collected works of Hippocrates and Galen, each published in Basle in 1538, as well as later editions both in Greek and Latin and also a small volume of Hippocrates edited by Rabelais, printed in Leiden in 1532. The great tradition of Arabian medicine is represented by editions of Rhazes, Avicenna, Haly ben Abbas and of Albucasis.

Of the many anatomical and surgical works to be expected in the library of a surgeon some of the more important may be mentioned. The work of

Mundinus who flourished towards the end of the 13th century and the early part of the 14th is perhaps of most interest. It is a remarkable forerunner to the work of Vesalius some 200 years later and though the dissection may be crude and the illustrations simplistic, Mundinus begins to lay the foundations of modern anatomy. The work was originally published in 1316 as a guide for students; the Pybus copy is dated 1541 – an indication of the long popularity of the work. Vesalius follows in direct line from Mundinus; Pybus has a fine copy of the second edition (1555) of the *De humani corporis fabrica.* Fabricius ab Aquapendente (1533-1619) who taught William Harvey in Padua and built the famous anatomy theatre there is represented by many of his writings on anatomy and embryology, notably *De formato foetu* (1600) and *De venarum ostiolis* (1603) and other works all illustrated with fine copper-plate engravings. There are several editions of Harvey's *De motu cordis* and a specially interesting association copy of his *De generatione animalium* (1651) containing the signature of Elias Harvey, William's brother, and notes in William's own hand marked with his distinctive delta sign and the initials WH.

Surgical works to be noted are those of Ambroise Paré (1510-1590), Gasparo Tagliacozzi (1545-1599) and, in more modern times, of course John Hunter. In addition to copies of Hunter's numerous works there are several volumes of students' manuscript copies of his lectures.

Some interesting provenances

Many of the books in these special collections have inscriptions, signatures and bookplates indicating their often distinguished provenance. Some of them, particularly those from the RVI and the College of Medicine have come from founders of the RVI and early members of hospital and College staff. The Winterbottom pharmacopoeias and dispensatories mostly belonged to Winterbottom *père* but one other notable signature may be mentioned, that of Robert Willan. Following his graduation Dr Winterbottom went to London as assistant to Willan with whom he formed a close and long-lasting friendship based not only on shared professional interests but on the charitable instincts they had in common. Willan was a member of the Society of Friends and became physician to the Public Dispensary in London. Dr Winterbottom's copy of Willan's book *On vaccine inoculation* (1806) bears the inscription 'In amicitio atq. observantio testimonium R.W.'.

Of the many Pybus books indicating provenance one of the most interesting, in addition to the Harvey already noted, is a copy of François Mauriceau *Des maladies des femmes grosses et accouchées*, 1668. The inscription, so far as it can be deciphered, reads, 'J'apartenes sidevant a Marie Forbec et après son desès a Marie Gillain d.l.v. sa fille faut (?) L'esperence de le pouvoir posesder'. Marie Gillain, to whom the book passed after the death of Marie Forbec was probably Marie Anne Victoire Boivin née Gillain, one of the most famous Paris midwives of the 19th century. A copy of her important work *Mémorial de l'art des accouchements* (1812) is also in the Pybus Collection.

Very recently, to augment these two major collections, the Robinson Library has received from Dr Edwin Clarke a generous donation of books from his own library of important medical works. These have yet to be catalogued and incorporated into the Library's stock. Dr Clarke, lately Director of the Wellcome Institute of the History of Medicine, graduated MBBS 1945 and MD 1954 at the University of Durham, of which the Medical School and King's College in Newcastle were then constituent parts; together in 1963 they became the University of Newcastle. This valuable addition to the Library will undoubtedly prove to be a major contribution to the considerable collection already available.

Durham – the Kellett Collection

Shortly before his death in 1978 Dr C E Kellett of Shotley Bridge in County Durham began to hand over to the University Library in Durham his library of medical works. Unlike the Pybus Collection which, though weighted towards anatomy and surgery, includes all branches of medicine over many centuries, the theme of the Kellett Collection is essentially the development of European medicine in the 16th and early 17th centuries.

Dr Kellett was born at St Helen Auckland in 1903. His early education was at Bow School in Durham and at Rossall, followed by medical education at Cambridge and at University College Hospital in London. He gained his MRCP in 1928 and was elected FRCP in 1949. His early medical practice was in paediatrics, at the Hospital for Sick Children, Great Ormond Street, at Johns Hopkins University, Baltimore and, on his return to the North East, he worked with Sir James Spence at the Fleming Hospital for Sick Children in Newcastle. He turned to general medicine and eventually became Senior Physician at Newcastle General Hospital from where he retired in 1967. In addition to holding consultant posts at other hospitals in the Region he lectured in clinical medicine and on the history of medicine to dental students at the University.

Dr Kellett was an excellent linguist, fluent in French and Latin, and his published writings on the history of medicine illustrate his love and special knowledge of 16th and 17th-century European culture. In particular his writings *Medical illustration and the school of Fontainebleau* (1957) and *Mannerism and medical illustration. Lectures on the iconography of the Chirurgia of Vidus Vidius and the De dissectione of Charles Estienne and Riviere given at the University of California, Los Angeles, October 1961* illustrate the cultivated background which he brought to his Collection and the use to which he put his books.

The Collection consists of about 200 pre-1801 books, with modern facsimiles of some others and several hundred 19th and 20th century books and offprints – secondary literature on medical history or modern editions of early texts.

In addition other more general collections within the University Library contain may pre-1850 books of medical and related interest. A typed list, an 'exploratory survey of holdings of medical interest' produced in 1978 contains items from the 16th to the 19th century arranged in alphabetical order of author, together with a subject list and a list of the particular Collections in which the books are held. Of particular specialised interest may be a number of medieval manuscripts in Bishop Cosin's Library, some of which relate in some way to medicine.

Each of the three major Collections described has its own characteristics. Winterbottom is largely composed of more or less contemporary medical publications, illustrating its original owner's preoccupations with the practical welfare of his patients and current developments of value in his clinical practice.

The Pybus Collection, that of a general surgeon, is particularly strong in anatomical and surgical works of historic interest with important works in all branches of medicine and related sciences; added interest is provided by the numerous portraits of scientists and medical men and a collection of MS letters.

The Kellett Collection, built around the writings of the 16th-century French physician, Jean Fernel, provides a source of primary texts for the study of 16th and 17th-century medicine, texts in which Dr Kellett found expressed the principles of good medical practice to which he was devoted and regarded as universally applicable.

All three men exemplified in their lives these sound principles, regarding their patients as individuals with special needs, not as examples of particular disorders. In Dr Kellett's view the study of the history of medicine should be concerned with the interpretation of medical knowledge for the benefit of the patient and not simply as a narration for the development of theories and systems. Professor Pybus envisaged medical history as part of a cultural whole. On the occasion of the official handing over of his Library to the University he said ..... 'I hope it will be a stimulus to the study of medical history, which I think is becoming more and more realised as an important part of both national and social history'.

Acknowledgements

I am indebted to Miss Beth Rainey, Keeper of Rare Books in the University Library, Durham, for permission to use material from her catalogue *The practical art of Medicine: Early books from the Kellett Collection: an exhibition*, 1989 Durham University Library.

Further reading

Emmerson JS. Thomas Winterbottom MD, 1766-1859. *Univ Durh Coll Med Gaz* 1955; *49*: 23-27.

Emmerson JS. *Catalogue of the Pybus Collection of Medical books, letters and engravings, 15th to 20th centuries, held in the University Library, Newcastle upon Tyne*. Manchester: Manchester University Press, on behalf of the University Library, Newcastle upon Tyne, 1981.

Emmerson JS. FC Pybus: the man and his books. In: Dale G, Miller F, Bramley K, eds. *Newcastle School of Medicine 1834-1984: Sesquicentennial Proceedings.* Newcastle: University of Newcastle, 1985.

Chapter 6

DENTAL SERVICES IN NEWCASTLE FROM 1790 TO 1799

A S Hargreaves

Poised between the old town and the new, and chafing to expand beyond the perimeter of its mediaeval walls, Newcastle, in the closing decade of the 18th century, was slowly awakening to the new tempo of the Industrial Revolution, and growing economically and commercially. Clearance of the old walls and gates and other old property had already begun, since deliberate town planning had commenced in the mid-eighties, with the construction of new streets, widening of the old ones, and the building of the new Theatre Royal. Improvements in transport meant that regular mail coach services had begun to run both north and south from the town in 1786 – the London coach went via Leeds and took 45 hours, for a fare of 4gns. There were three regular weekly newspapers (the *Newcastle Advertiser*, *Chronicle* and *Courant*), and the Literary and Philosophical Society was founded in 1793 to promote interest in literary and scientific subjects. Yet the population of approximately 24 000 in 1770 had risen only to 28 294 by the time of the 1801 census, with a further 8 597 inhabitants in Gateshead and 12 412 in Sunderland. The explosions in population and building were yet to come.

The health care of the inhabitants came mainly from those eight physicians and twenty or so surgeons, resident and practising in the town.[1] The Infirmary had been established in 1751, to be followed in 1777 by the Dispensary, which dealt with a mass of disease that was undoubtedly due to infection, whether respiratory or intestinal.[2] Dentistry in mid-century was generally of low priority and confined mainly to relief from pain, but this did not necessarily mean that treatment was limited solely to crude extractions by the pelican or the key. As early as 1724, the mathematical and musical instrument-maker in the Side, William Prior (also Assay Master to the goldsmiths), was utilising his manual dexterity and aesthetic skills in the construction and fitting of artificial teeth, 'so neatly as not to be discernable from natural ones'. This must have proved a lucrative side to his business, since by 1739, when he had moved to the foot of Westgate, his advertisement was dominated by the teeth and the instruments relegated almost to a footnote.[3]

As provincial dentistry expanded, improvements in road transport enabled the London dentists, both indigenous and from overseas, to make more extensive forays outside the capital, to practise and to promote their own proprietary tinctures, dentifrices and tooth-brushes. Spas such as Bath and the Hot Wells at Bristol, where could be found the fashionable and the wealthy, the nobility and the gentry, had been the earliest venues for these excursions, before the itineraries extended to include the Midlands and then slowly the rest of the country as urban development proceeded apace. Dentistry, and particularly restorative dentistry (artificial teeth and, later on, fillings) was not cheap, but such were the demands of vanity in some sections of the public that the charges rarely proved a major deterrent.

Visiting dentists had appeared in Newcastle from about 1760, ranging from Michael Whitlock and Nathaniel Lee (who claimed to be present 'by the King's authority') to Mrs Bernard from Berlin and Brandenberg in 1773, the Huguenot descendent Jacob Hemet in 1776, Hemet Hart from Mannheim in 1778, Mr Marks, dentist and operator for the teeth, in 1780 and Mr Crawcour in 1783.[4] These were all short-stay callers, who seem to have confined themselves to a single visit, but from 1790 there were to be further developments in the pattern of treatment provision.

These providers were to number no more than nine men, but they nonetheless covered the gamut of the differing skills and services that were available in England at that period. Thus they included both resident and visiting practitioners, some of whom combined dentistry with another trade or activity, with the visitors in attendance on either a regular basis or on a single flying visit that comprised part of a northern tour or a sales-drive for a particular proprietary preparation.

The only man to be resident over the whole period was the surgeon Frederick Horn, who had been naval surgeon successively on the *Lynx*, *Medway*, *Grafton* and *Crown* from May 1777 until December 1782. His earlier attendance upon 'the most eminent professors in London in the surgical and medical line' had then been augmented in 1786 with instruction by an eminent (but unnamed) practitioner 'in the business of a DENTIST' in London, before his return to Newcastle.[5] This was to support his claim that

> He scales and cleans and performs all the operations on the teeth, makes and fixes artificial and removes or prevents the irregularities which take place in the teeth of young people at the time of getting their second set.

Despite offering virtually all the clinical techniques then available (although there is no direct mention of extractions or transplantation), general surgery remained his main area of concentration. He was listed simply as 'surgeon' in the local directories for 1787-9, 1790 and 1795, and was appointed surgeon to the Infirmary in 1800, but his entry in Mitchell's directory for 1801 describes him firmly as 'surgeon and dentist', so his interest in the mouth and dental ills had been maintained.

In his advertisement of 1786, Horn had stated an intention of attending Durham, Sunderland, North and South Shields in addition to his dental practice in Newcastle, but the frequency of these visits would have been regulated by the number of those requiring his assistance. Being resident in Newcastle and well-known — he was president of the local Medical Society in 1796, and was also surgeon to the Dispensary — he had scant need to advertise his presence or services in the local press, so there is little indication now of whether his enthusiasm for matters dental was sufficient for him to offer the lately-developed all-porcelain dentures or other advancing restorative techniques.

The other resident dentist in Newcastle, Mr Lesec, is a more interesting individual by virtue of his obviously single-minded determination to pursue dentistry on its own as a profitable career, by combining good training with an alertness to advances in clinical practice and the development of good business skills.

M Lesec (subsequently listed in the London trade directories as John Lesec) announced his intention of residing for some time in Newcastle and its vicinity in mid-July 1790, when he could be applied to at Mr Powell's, the Close.[6] Claims about having been trained by a royal operator or of attendance upon royalty were a not uncommon advertising ploy in the 18th century, but Lesec's claim that he had been a pupil of 'M.Burdet, Dentist to the Queen of France' cannot be as easily dismissed as those of some other men, since Étienne Bourdet (1722-1789) had certainly been appointed as *Dentiste du Roi* in 1760. Paris was generally regarded as a centre of excellence for dentistry at this period, so although Bourdet's 2-volume *Recherches et Observations sur toutes les Parties de l'Art du Dentiste*, published in 1757, may have been strongly influenced by Pierre Fauchard's pioneering *Le Chirurgien Dentiste* of 1728 and its expanded second edition of 1746, he had pushed the technical and clinical boundaries of operative dentistry yet further, showing particular concern for the design of palatal obturators.

With the assumption that his training had genuinely been under Bourdet, and therefore to a reasonable level of competence, Lesec's early advertisements (which follow the standard pattern of offering to clean and whiten teeth, reset natural teeth or replace with artificial ones when they are decayed, and undertake some very simple re-alignment at the transition from the deciduous to the permanent dentition) show an initial modesty while he assessed the potential scope of practice in this new neighbourhood. The public's response must have been favourable, however, since he had moved into his own lodgings in Newgate-street, near the White-cross, with his name over the door, only one month later. As his confidence grew, he sought to widen his practice still further:[7]

> **MR LESEC,**
>
> **DENTIST**
>
> (Removed to the Bigg-Market, near the High-Bridge)
>
> RETURNS his most sincere Thanks to the Nobility, Gentry, and the Public in general, for the many Favours already conferred upon him. Being now a Resident in Newcastle, he will undertake to attend Families and Boarding-Schools, both in Town and Country; and flatters himself the Benefit arising from his Attention and Care, will fully answer the Confidence of those who may honour him with their Favours.
>
> Mr LESEC, having studied Surgery when with Mons. BURDET, Surgeon-Dentist to the Queen of France, at Paris, does not confine himself to the Operations of the Teeth, but relieves and cures all

Diseases incident to the Mouth and Gums, as those confess who have done him the Honor to consult him upon such Occasions.

Mr LESEC places artificial Teeth, which look quite natural, and without any Pain whatever. Begs leave to recommend his DENTIFRICE for the Teeth, and his TINCTURE for the Scurvy.

Yet Newcastle on its own does not seem to have provided Lesec with sufficient custom to satisfy his drive. There had been a professional visit to Durham in December 1790, but it was not until January 1792 that he announced his intention of being in that city the first Monday in every month, although this had to be changed to Wednesday 1 August on account of the Assizes, before reverting again to Mondays, and the November visit was postponed from the 5th to the 12th of that month. This expansion was then extended to cover Sunderland, at Mr Jowsey's, High-street, where after an initial reconnoitre for a few days from Wed 6 Feb 1793, he would attend the first Wednesday of every month thereafter. By May that year, he had decided to assess Stockton as a further venue on his regular itinerary, but his growing links with the more southern county of Yorkshire began to become more apparent. Not only had he commenced visiting York regularly but the footnotes to his advertisements which listed the retail suppliers for his tooth-powder and improved tooth-brushes also included a Mr Craggs at Richmond.

In November 1794 he had come to a decision. Newcastle was no longer to be his professional base but York,[8]

> the centrical Situation of that Place affording him an Opportunity of observing more punctually, the Orders of his numerous Friends and Patrons THERE, in NEWCASTLE, and the various intermediate and adjacent TOWNS.

Nevertheless, he deemed it also particularly necessary to inform the

> LADIES of NEWCASTLE, that he still purposes visiting this TOWN occasionally; and will at all Times be happy in attending to their Commands, as usual; that he will ever, with heartfelt Gratitude, remember their past kind Patronage and Favour, and feel himself peculiarly honoured in the Continuance thereof.

He kept his word. Twice a year thereafter he returned north, usually in May or June and again in October or November, carefully and politely giving advance notice in all three weekly newspapers of the proposed date of arrival and particular lodgings, and usually followed by confirmation of his arrival, with an indication of his planned length of stay.

Although the York newspapers have not been presently studied for more details of his activities there in the latter half of the decade, yet there are signs that this city was still not sufficiently fulfilling. Even though he did not move to London until 1801, an advertisement in the Newcastle press for 29 June 1799 reveals that he had been keeping up to date and refining his techniques in the provision of artificial teeth. Not only did he supply the usual ivory-based appliances, but he was now prepared to offer all-porcelain dentures. These had initially been developed some ten years earlier by Nicholas Dubois de Chemant in Paris and patented there, but they were also patented in England once de Chemant had moved to London, away from the uncomfortable atmosphere generated by the other Parisian dentists who resented his virtual theft of the original idea from the apothecary Duchâteau. In this country, the porcelain paste was provided for de Chemant by Josiah Wedgwood, but its high firing shrinkage was to lead to considerable difficulties for imitators in their attempts to control dimensional stability and hence obtain a good fit in the mouth. The eventual demise of all-porcelain dentures was hastened by their brittleness and sometimes lurid colouring, but at the close of the 18th century they were very much in vogue, and no self-respecting dentist, particularly in the capital, would dare not offer to provide them – nor would a dentist whose ambitions aspired to practising there.

Lesec's advertisement in the *Newcastle Chronicle* shows a delicate balance between salesmanship and professional responsibility, with a healthy awareness of economic factors:

ADAMANTINE TEETH.

> MR LESEC, Surgeon Dentist, begs Leave to announce to the Public, that he has, with much Labour and Difficulty, brought to Perfection, a Composition for Artificial Teeth, equal in strength to Adamant. The advantages of such an Invention can only be adequately appreciated by those who have felt the Inconvenience from the Use of Artificial Teeth of other Substances; for, however well such Pieces may be fitted both as to Shape and Colour, it is an offensiveness in the Mouth which the greatest Attention and Delicacy are not entirely capable of overcoming. To those therefore who can judge from Experience he submits his discovery, not doubting but they will influence their Friends who may require such Aid — From the great Difficulty of the Process in making them, and their Durability when made Mr Lesec is obliged to charge double the Price of those made of any other Substance; it will therefore be optional for those who honor him with their Favors, either to have them of the one or the other, as he still continues to make Artificial Teeth in the Manner his Friends are already accustomed to.....

The extent to which these new teeth were adopted in Newcastle is unknown, as also is Lesec's provision of them in either the north or London. Yet his concentration of effort towards a profitable livelihood would seem to have been supported by the provision of responsible treatment and an astute mind. Newcastle was probably well served by him in the few years he was active there.

******

If John Lesec had been the first full-time resident dentist in Newcastle, an important stage in the development of dental practice in a provincial town, he might not have held this distinction had Charles Edward Whitlock not been quite so stage-struck.

The name of Whitlock is not unknown to local historians or to students of the theatre because of his activities as actor and then actor-manager of the new Theatre Royal until he was bought out in 1791, but they seem generally unaware of (or have chosen to ignore) his parallel activities as a dentist. It has been suggested that Charles may have been the son of Michael Whitlock, an operator for the teeth with a particular reputation for his artificial teeth and confident at transplantation, who alternated between Durham and Newcastle at weekly intervals in the autumn of 1760,[9] but this relationship remains to be proven. Nevertheless it would offer a reasonable explanation for Charles's acquisition of dental skills, which remained important to him throughout his life, not merely because they would have enabled some extra income if the theatre takings were leaner than hoped for.

The headquarters of drama in Newcastle from 1747 until 1787 had been the Turk's Head Long Room, known as the theatre in the Bigg Market, although such dramatic representations as had been the rule were really illegal under prevailing law, and admission to them was obtained only under subterfuge. An example of this occurred in Worcester in 1770, when Sarah Kemble (later Mrs Siddons) acted with her future husband; the entrance to the 'concert' was free, but the audience had to purchase packets of tooth-powder at 2s, 1s, and 6d each respectively.[10]

If this same subterfuge was adopted in Newcastle, then the availability of tooth-powder would have been enhanced in 1774, when Charles Whitlock joined the company of comedians, then managed by Austin and Heatton. Yet his advertisement in the *Newcastle Journal* shows that he took his dentistry as seriously as his acting:

February 10, 1774

WHITLOCK, Dentist,

Begs Leave to acquaint the LADIES *and* GENTLEMEN *of Newcastle*,

THAT he performs evey Operation necessary for beautifying and preserving the TEETH and GUMS.

He scales and cleans the blackest Teeth, restoring them to their natural Complexion, and the Mouth to its wonted Sweetness, without Pain.

Makes and fixes artificial Teeth in so exact a Manner as not to be discernable from the natural ones.

Such Teeth as project, so as to deform the Mouth, he regulates, &c.

Those Ladies and Gentlemen who please to honour him with their Commands, (during the Stay of the Comedians) are requested to favour him with them, at Mrs Gale's, in Newgate-street.

Where may be had, his Tincture for the Scurvy in the Gums; and his Paste or Powder for cleaning and preserving the Teeth.

In 1778 Whitlock took over from Heatton, so with Joseph Austin as co-lessee, he ran a circuit consisting of Newcastle, Sheffield, Lancaster, Chester, Warrington and Preston (and including Manchester for two seasons), which occasioned the performers travelling over 1100 miles each year, at a time when road travel was still not without its difficulties. Thus he could be in Newcastle only for part of the year, in the winter season, which generally ran from January until late March or April. In 1785, he married Elizabeth Kemble at York (after which she joined the company), with the effect that he became the brother-in-law of both John and Stephen Kemble and Mrs Siddons. Elizabeth, not handsome but more vivacious than sister Sarah, must have taken after her brother and another of her sisters in size – Stephen was later able to play Falstaff without padding, and Frances Ann was said to be as 'big as a horse' – and she also had something of the Kemble manner and voice; whilst the Newcastle press were generally polite about the performances of the company's leading lady, later Irish critics were to remark that her voice was more noticeable for its strength than its sweetness.

The managers appointed to the new Theatre Royal, which opened in Mosley Street on 21 Jan 1788 with great celebrations, were Austin and Whitlock, who were able to draw on their existing experience at the theatre in the Bigg Market, but Austin retired at the end of the first season, to be replaced by Joseph Munden. Despite his managerial responsibilities, Whitlock, who was less flexible and benevolent than Austin, still wanted to act, but his roles tended to be the 'second leads', characters such as Bassanio, Cassio, Horatio, etc. Quite where he fitted his dentistry into all these exertions is unclear, but at the start of each season a polite reminder appeared in the local press, as it did at Chester:[11]

> C.WHITLOCK, DENTIST, respectfully informs the Ladies, Gentlemen, and Public, that he continues to perform operations on the teeth, and shall be happy to receive their commands at Mr. Bulmer's, No.2, Northumberland place. He has just made a fresh parcel of very fine tooth-powder, which he recommends; and has brought from London a quantity of tooth-brushes of superior quality.

It has been ironically observed that the drawing powers of Mrs Whitlock were perhaps greater than those of her husband. This is now somewhat difficult to substantiate, although the leading actor George Frederick Cooke (when very drunk) once referred to him as 'that tooth-drawing reptile'.[12] Nevertheless it is clear that Lesec's arrival on the scene was in no way jeopardized by Whitlock's established presence.

In September 1790, the theatre's committee was informed that Whitlock had bought out Munden, but he in his turn was bought out by his brother-in-law Stephen Kemble a mere six months later, receiving payment of £1000 for his properties. Despite this, he returned to the area the following year (1792), thanking his Newcastle patients for their past favours, announcing that he would be paying his annual visit to Durham towards the end of April, and purposing that he would pay his respects to Newcastle, as a dentist, in the course of the next year. His return was a little earlier than planned, since it was in the December that he announced he would be at Mrs Turner's, in Mosley Street, though for a fortnight only, but this advertisement reveals an increasing emphasis on dentistry once his management of the Theatre Royal had been concluded, and Stephen Kemble was attracting the London stars to appear on this northern stage.[13] No longer was he offering just the basic clinical techniques, but

> he continues to perform all Operations on the TEETH, supplies real and artificial Teeth on Gold or Ivory Sockets, Gold Screws, &c.&c.

After this, his advertisements in the Newcastle press cease, until a notice in August 1793 informed readers that Mrs Whitlock and her husband were among the last emigrations to America in the theatric line. Their successful sojourn there lasted about ten years, albeit punctuated by a premature obituary in April 1799, for which the *Newcastle Chronicle* had to make public apology some weeks later. Although they made a comfortable independence there, with Charles Whitlock including some of Washington's own family among his patients, Mrs. Whitlock re-appeared at Drury Lane in 1807. Yet Newcastle must have maintained an attraction for them, for they had returned north by 1811, where, according to William Macready, 'they were highly respected and mingled in the best society of the place', despite her love of acting being so great as to blind her to her disqualifications.[14] Nevertheless she continued to act, but not Charles, who was firmly described in the 1811 trade directory as 'dentist', in company with Charles Wawn and J Summers. The clinical call had remained.

******

With Lesec and Whitlock having departed the town, so that the only dental expertise available was from the surgeon Frederick Horn, the field was open to the short-term visitors, but these seem to have been surprisingly few and far between. Judging from their advertisements, their skills covered the spectrum from those of the highly-trained London men, through the less reputable and those practising a combination of trades, to the opportunist of very doubtful pedigree, and their stay in Newcastle or its neighbourhood was rarely more than a few weeks.

Of the highly-trained men, Mr Matson was a characteristic example of the London-based dentist who was extending his practice by provincial forays once the roads had improved, but since his arrival in Newcastle was in March 1791, when both Lesec and Whitlock were active, he may have felt that local demand was not such as to make any return worthwhile. This was in fact William Matson, who has been recorded as practising near Holborn Bars in 1794 and then in 1802 at Kirby St, Hatton Garden, in partnership with Alexander Rowland (although the latter, with his son, appears to have abandoned dentistry for the macassar oil business by 1809). If his claims that he had received instruction from Mr Berdmore are true (unlike those of Robert Wooffendale), then his skills may well have matched the prolixity of his prose. Thomas Berdmore (1740-1785) had been attached to the Racquet Court practice in Fleet Street, originally established in 1702 by John Watts (later master of the Company of Barber-Surgeons), and of high reputation, since its principals had included another master of the Barbers' Company (Samuel Rutter) and a royal Operator for the Teeth (William Green). Berdmore himself succeeded Green in his court appointment at the age of 26, and was author of *A Treatise on the Disorders and Deformities of the Teeth and Gums* (1768), which, although one of the earliest books on practical dentistry in English, yet lacks the stature of those written in France by Fauchard and Bourdet.

Matson's advertisements included a reference to filling decayed teeth, although he did not specify whether he used gold or lead foil for this purpose as Berdmore had recommended, and he also prided himself on his replacements:[15]

> fixing in real and artificial ones, from a single Tooth to a whole Set, at 5s. each, on a Construction entirely new, without tying; they remain quite firm and fixed, putting the Wearer to no kind of Trouble or Inconvenience, and perform all the Functions proper to the Teeth with the greatest Facility and Pleasure, and likewise prevent that fetid forbidding Smell proceeding from Foulness.

This charge of 5s per replacement tooth was well below the usual London prices, which ranged then from 10s 6d to an exorbitant 5gns, but no comparison is possible with the fees of either Lesec or Whitlock, since these were not publicised. Matson's charges for his Imperial Tooth-Powder at 2s 6d per box, however, do correspond quite well with Lesec's at 2s 9d; as the latter figure occurs in many advertisements for other proprietary dentifrices, this must have been regarded as the accepted rate.

Matson attended Durham for just two days at the end of March 1791 before returning to Newcastle, where his press notices continued until 4 June. This 3-month visit was far longer however than the mere fortnight or so by the son of the Chevalier Bartholomew Ruspini, one notice of his presence in the town being merely tucked into the middle of a long advertisement for some of his father's many preparations, *viz*: the balsamic styptic, *A Treatise on the Teeth* (the 8th edition of which was just due to be published), dentifrice-powder and tincture, elixir for the toothache, and tooth-brushes.[16] Both father and son were Dentists to the Prince of Wales – readers were rarely allowed to forget this – but James Bladen Ruspini's visit to Newcastle in the autumn of 1797 was patently little more than part of a national sales-campaign.

The remaining London man to pay a brief visit to the town, in 1799, was Crawcour, 'Surgeon Dentist, from the Strand', who also offered a wide range of treatments, including filling up decayed teeth with gold, silver or leaf lead.[17] The Crawcours, of Polish origin, have remained a difficult family to elucidate since they nearly always advertised merely as 'Mr' or 'Messrs'. One at least was visiting cities and towns in the north of England early in the 1780s

– there had been a Mr Crawcour in Newcastle in 1783 – but it is not clear whether this was the same man as the 1799 visitor, although the latter is probably the same as the surgeon-dentist at No.439 Strand, London, in 1805, and who was at No.46 two years later when promoting his own preparation of 'Genuine Russian Tooth-Powder'.[18] Nor is it clear whether this 1799 Crawcour was of the generation preceeding the five dentist brothers (Barnett, Moses, David, Israel and Abraham), whose sons, too, followed the same occupation, or whether he was actually one of the brothers.

The Crawcour name has become associated with charlatanism because of their widespread use of their *Mineral Succedaneum* (an amalgam of mercury and coarse filings from French silver coins), which they claimed equalled gold as a filling material but cost considerably less. Their clinical technique was such that these fillings were inserted over the decay, using far too much free mercury which was frequently swallowed, with resultant excessive salivation as well as periapical abscesses and much pain; the subsequent 'Amalgam War' took nearly a century to settle before more refined preparations finally became acceptable alternatives to gold. The *Mineral Succedaneum* was still to be developed in 1799, but a pattern had already been set of extensive advertising and flying visits around the country, so that the perpetrator was well away from the scene by the time his angry patients had realised the failure of the glamorous promises. Typically, the Newcastle stay was short, as 'he must proceed on his journey to Carlisle', though he had also managed a very brief visit to Morpeth within this time. Superficially, this advertisement looks as reputable as those of Matson and Lesec, and the treatment offered may indeed have been professionally responsible, but the present-day historian approaches the name of Crawcour with much caution; such hindsight might have been appreciated by many in the early 19th century.

Two other short-stay visitors combined their dentistry with another trade or interest, a not uncommon practice amongst the less skilled in order to ensure a reasonable and steady income. E Braham, 'Late from Berlin, the Capital of Prussia' but having just departed from Whitby in October 1793, was a peripatetic individual whose chiropody was clearly predominant over his dentistry. Despite describing himself as 'Corn Operator and Dentist', his Newcastle advertisements are pedally orientated, with his oral treatment confined merely to curing the toothache in a minute's time, 'be the Pain ever so Violent', applying a 'Curious Liquid that removes all rheumatic Complaints in the GUMS', and fixing teeth from one to a whole set 'in a Manner not discernable from natural Ones'.[19] Although this combination of trades may seem curious to some modern eyes, they both deal with the hard tissues of the body, of reasonably easy access if equally odiferous. The toothdrawers of earlier centuries had not infrequently combined these activities (although phlebotomy was the more usually associated) in their efforts to gain a reasonable living, and such duality was to persist well into the 19th century.

Mr MS Leve, on the other hand, amplified his income by promising to cure all venereal complaints in the easiest and most expeditious manner. On his brief visit in March 1795, when he claimed to be 'Surgeon and Dentist to the Royal Family in Copenhagen' – an assertion which may be true, but has yet to be substantiated – he nevertheless offered a wide range of dental skills, including extracting, filling hollow teeth, curing the scurvy, scaling, cleaning and whitening the teeth, replacing missing units, restoring decayed gums and fastening loose teeth.[20] Leve's actual skills were probably less than his claims since he disappears without trace, as also does the opportunist Sergeant Summers, of the Cumberland Militia, who described himself in May 1799 as 'Dentist', seemingly on the strength of a secret given him by a celebrated German dentist on his death-bed, for kindness shewn him by the proprietor. This was a 'VALUABLE SECRET for extracting TEETH, whether broken in the Gums, or in any State, without the Assistance of any Instrument, and without the least Pain'; in addition to this he felt competent to clean and replace teeth and to cure the scurvy in the gums, at the Barrack Tavern in Sunderland.[21] This smacks strongly of the charlatanism that was still prevalent in dentistry, particularly in more rural areas, but the possibility cannot be entirely excluded that the advertisement was no more than a hoax, perpetrated after a night's heavy drinking.

At the opening of the 19th century, not only was provincial dentistry expanding rapidly, but Newcastle was poised for its imminent commercial and economic growth, and associated population expansion. As a result, the scope of dental services in the new town was easily able to develop still further. The skills and prestige of later men such as Charles Newby Wawn and Richard Downing (erstwhile partner, and brother-in-law, of the great Joseph Fox, in London) should not however lead to undue over-shadowing of their professional predecessors. The people of Newcastle were already aware of what could be offered by the modern dentistry of the era, in terms of range of operative treatments and skill allied to professional care. Demand for such treatment, to which later dentists might respond (and some clearly did so, with enthusiasm), had been created by an awareness and appreciation of the activities of the earlier reputable practitioners. The dental services in Newcastle in the 1790s had prepared the way forward.

References

1. *Whitehead's Newcastle and Gateshead Directory*, 1790.
2. Miller FJW. The Newcastle Dispensary 1777-1976. *Archaeol Aeliana* Ser 5 1990; *XVIII*: 177-195.
3. *Newcastle Weekly Courant*, 1 Feb 1723/4; *Newcastle Journal*, 7 Apr 1739.
4. Boyes J. Newcastle – A study in local dental history. *Archaeol Aeliana* Ser 4 1958; *XXXVI*: 147-163.
5. *Newcastle Courant*, 29 July 1786.

6. *Newcastle Advertiser*, 17 July 1790. Identical advertisements by Lesec in the *Chronicle* and *Courant* on this and subsequent occasions.
7. *Newcastle Advertiser*, 12 March 1791.
8. *Newcastle Advertiser*, 15 Nov 1794.
9. Boyes J. Medicine and dentistry in Newcastle upon Tyne in the eighteenth century. *Proc Roy Soc Med* 1957; *50*: 229-235.
10. Oswald H. *The Theatres Royal in Newcastle upon Tyne.* Newcastle upon Tyne: Northumberland Press Ltd, 1936:4-5.
11. Eg *Newcastle Chronicle*, 27 Feb 1790 and 19 Feb 1791.
12. Cited by Hare A. *George Frederick Cooke: The Actor and the Man*. Bath: Pitman Press, for the Soc for Theatre Research, 1980:53.
13. *Newcastle Chronicle*, 8 Dec 1792.
14. Pollock Sir F (ed). *Macready's Reminiscences, and Selections from his Diaries and Letters*. London: Macmillan & Co, 1875:53.
15. *Newcastle Chronicle*, 28 May 1791.
16. *Newcastle Advertiser*, 23 & 30 Sept 1797.
17. *Newcastle Courant*, 3 Aug 1799.
18. Campbell JM. *Dentistry Then and Now*. Privately printed, 1981:265-8.
19. *Newcastle Advertiser*, 12 Oct 1793.
20. *Newcastle Chronicle*, 14 March 1795.
21. *Newcastle Chronicle*, 11 May 1799.

Chapter 7

DR JOHN CLARK: THE FORGOTTEN PHYSICIAN 1744-1805

FJW Miller

Introduction: the puzzling memorial

In 1775 John Clark, then 31 years of age, came to Newcastle from Kelso to practise as a physician. He does not seem to have had any previous connection with the town or introduction to any physician or surgeon, and he arrived shortly after another physician, a Dr Wilson, had left for London. Clark therefore had to make his own way but was to remain in Newcastle until his death in April 1805 at the age of 61 years.

In November of the same year Dr JR Fenwick of Durham, who had previously practised in Newcastle and, between 1786 and 1791, had been on the staffs of the Infirmary and Dispensary, delivered a memorial address to the Literary and Philosophical Society. That Society had been founded some twelve years earlier with Clark as a Vice-President.[1] Fenwick's address entitled 'A Sketch of the Professional Life and Character of John Clark M.D.' was then published early in 1806.[2]

Fenwick begins 'A man who lived so honourably to himself, and so usefully for others, should not be allowed to sink into the grave unnoticed' but then, rather strangely, goes on 'and that although his life was marked by no singular events, though I cannot offer to your consideration those splendid qualities which command admiration, you will yet take an interest in tracing the progress of a man most deserving of praise in private life, and whose writings have improved the important art which he exercised'. That, surely, is a strange introduction to the memorial address of a man who had been a physician in the town for thirty years. Indeed it hints of a major difference between his private and professional lives and that the latter was hardly deserving of praise. That statement and others throughout the paper leave the reader wondering what Dr Fenwick really thought about Dr Clark whose friendship he professed. Printed as an appendix is a short letter from Dr John Ramsay, another physician to the Infirmary, written on 1 September 1805 at the request of Dr Fenwick.[3] It is full of praise for Clark's clinical skill and care for his patients and is 'that testimony ... which twelve years' intimacy has afforded me.' Dr Ramsay's praise was unstinted.

Following those communications and a short note in Mackenzie's *History of Newcastle*, the next references to Clark and his work I have been able to find appear in GH Hume's *History of the Infirmary* and in Sir WE Hume's short account of the Infirmary written for the bicentenary celebrations in 1951.[4,5,6] They all refer to his work during the extension of the Infirmary 50 years after its foundation and the events concerning the accommodation for patients with 'Fever' which resulted in local controversy. The details of that crisis will be considered later, but perhaps some explanation of Dr Fenwick's guarded statement about the lack of 'qualities which command admiration' may be found when GH Hume, writing of Clark, says 'He seems to have had a lifelong struggle with ill-health, but in spite of ill-health, to have been a man of indomitable energy and unquenchable interest in his profession. Of somewhat rough manners and hasty temper, he possessed the intellectual force which compels confidence ... such a man is equally successful in winning friends and in making enemies'.[7] Nearly 50 years later Sir WE Hume (the son of GH) names the three outstanding personalities at the Infirmary at the end of the 18th Century as John Rotherham and John Hall (physicians) and William Ingham (surgeon) – he did not include John Clark though he does acknowledge his work in the extension and reorganisation of the Infirmary.[8] Clark, therefore, is hardly remembered in the medical lore of Newcastle and Tyneside except perhaps as a hard working but ill tempered Scot. Yet he founded the Newcastle Dispensary which served the town for nearly two centuries and played a major role in the first extension and reorganisation of the Infirmary. An examination of the man and the local medical situation of his time would therefore seem reasonable. We must begin by looking at his origins and the first half of his life.

Origins and early days

Clark was born in May 1744 at Graden, a farmstead in the parish of Roxburgh about equidistant between Town Yetholm and Kelso.

He was the first of seven sons born to William Clark and there were also three daughters, but we do not know if he was the eldest child. No details of his home life are known and there are no Clarks at Graden now, but his first school was at Linton about three miles from home. Then, when he was eleven, he was placed in the Grammar School at Kelso and seems to have attended for five years. There is much one would like to know about this period. Did he travel each day, and if so how, or did he stay with someone in Kelso as a boarder on a weekly or longer basis? There was a large family and one wonders how the others were educated.

Whatever the arrangements, he must have made good progress, for in 1760 he entered the University at Edinburgh to be educated for the Church. But his interests took another direction and he changed to medicine, the teaching of which was taking a great part in the glow of the Scottish Enlightenment.[9] Soon, however, he experienced a set back in health, difficult to explain or understand, which seems to have affected him at intervals all his later life. Fenwick relates that Clark suffered an accident when a slate, falling from a roof, struck him on the head. That injury was followed by severe headaches, general nervous complaints and a disordered state of the organs of digestion from which he suffered throughout his life.[10] He had, in fact, been away from his country home for less than a year, and could not have been more than 17 years of age. We have no details of how or where he lived, or his financial situation as the son of a country farmer with a large family. It is also difficult to associate the headaches, general nervous complaints and abdominal symptoms: were they attacks of severe migraine, had he a peptic ulcer, or had he attacks of partial intestinal obstruction possibly as a result of bovine tuberculosis in earlier childhood?

There seems little doubt that his final illness some 40 years later was intestinal obstruction followed by peritonitis, but that might well have been due to quite a different cause. Throughout those 40 years there do not seem to have been any signs of neurological damage or disease and he certainly led a hard and busy life. Yet, whatever the origin of his symptoms while at University, they were enough to make him return home without finishing the course of lectures which would have enabled him to obtain the degree of Doctor of Medicine. It is possible, however, that he returned because he simply failed to cope with the city life of the time. Whatever the reason, he went home in 1761, yet before the end of the same year had become apprenticed to a Mr Watson, a former Naval surgeon, practising in Kelso. There he remained the full five years of his apprenticeship and must have learned much of the practical art of the medicine of the day. We have no evidence that he suffered from ill-health during that period and in the autumn of 1766 he returned to Edinburgh to complete his lectures. Fenwick says that, on this occasion, he soon attracted the interest of Dr John Gregory, the Professor of the Practice of Physic (1766-1773); but the abdominal symptoms soon recurred and resisted all Dr Gregory's attempts to help, until finally he recommended that Mr Clark should 'try the effects of a warm climate'.[11]

That was not easy advice to follow. Fenwick mentions the Clark family's large size and straightened circumstances and that it was necessary for John to support himself. He therefore sought and, with the help of friends, obtained a post as a surgeon's mate on a ship of the East India Company. The pay would be small, but he would have some opportunity for private trading. So, at the age of 24, he again left home and travelled south, but before joining his ship, attended a course of William Hunter's lectures in London, enabled to do so without payment of the usual fee. Fenwick gives no hint, but one wonders if he had an introduction from John Gregory explaining his situation.

Voyages East 1768-1772

The East Indiaman the *Talbot*, c650 tons, Captain Sir Charles Hudson, left England on the 22 March 1768 with 108 crew and 132 passengers and military recruits. The passage to India took five months. They sailed down the West Coast of Africa and rounded the Cape to Madagascar. By then fever and scurvy had appeared and in his journal Clark enthusiastically describes the welcome sight of 'rice, India corn, sugar cane, sweet-potatoes, melons, pumpkins, and oranges'. But he also records that in the wet season, November to March, 'the atmosphere is dark, gloomy and much rain falls'. After a stay of ten days they sailed on and by 25 August dropped anchor at 'Culpee in the river of Bengal'. Travellers to those parts will not be surprised to learn that 'within two weeks many of our people, officers and passengers as well as common seamen, were attacked with sickness, often a vomiting but always a purging of gall'; and he goes on to describe the weather in September as intolerably hot, sultry and suffocating with fogs and dews at night. By the end of that month there were 'few or no hands on board of our ship capable of doing duty'.[12] During October the weather improved with refreshing breezes but attacks and outbreaks of diarrhoea continued.

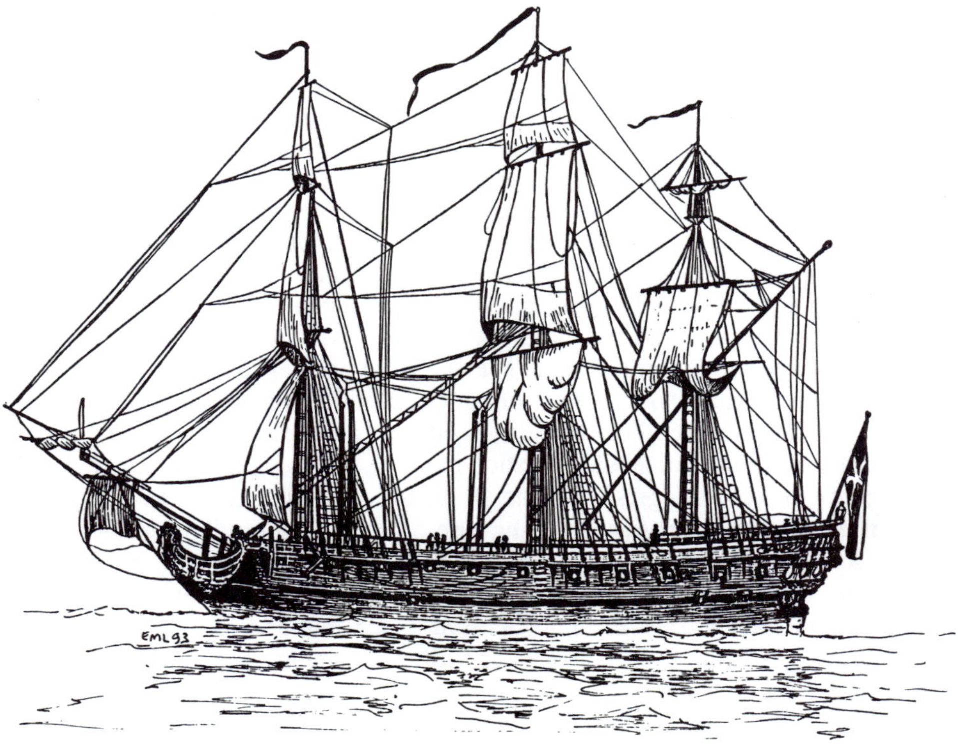

Figure 1. An East Indiaman of about 1750: redrawn by E Lazenby from Culver HB *The Book of Old Ships*; New York: Garden City, 1935.

By January and through February the weather was 'serene, dry and temperate, with agreeable breezes' and on the 22nd March after a stay of six months and just a year after leaving England they began the return voyage. Clark does not give, as he did on the outward voyage, the number of crew or passengers nor does he record whether they had lost any of the original crew, but he does go on to say 'at this time almost all our people were able to do duty; however, several of them, who had suffered much in the sickly season, had not regained their usual strength and vigour' – and then shows his concern and foresight for the possibility of prevention which later was to be so conspicuously displayed in Newcastle, for he continues '... but when it is considered on what poor diet seamen are obliged to live, at Bengal, their slow recovery from diseases will be easily accounted for ... the only vegetables which seamen are allowed in abundance are yams and rice ... During the last two months ... in Bengal about twenty of our people had the venereal disease ... for the most part ... in the form of ulcers [or] warts ... on the penis ... only two had a virulent gonorrhoea ... the disease was only to be cured by mercury'.[13]

In July they met bad weather – 'one violent hard gale continually succeeding another ... obliged us ... to lie to ... as the ship became leaky ... it was necessary to keep the pumps almost constantly at work'. During June and July many of the crew had scurvy and the officers were not totally exempt, so that by the middle of July 'it was unanimously agreed to bear away for Madagascar, as being the nearest and best port for refreshment, and the only means of preserving the lives of our seamen; and of course the ship and cargo'. Their plight was indeed desperate. Leaving Bengal, the crew, officers and all, consisted of 87 people. By then 33 of the 'best' hands were confined below deck and those able to work 'were so much enfeebled, that the duty of the ship required the assistance of the passengers and their servants'. They lay at Madagascar all the month of August – 'as soon as we arrived ... the sick were supplied with oranges in abundance, and vegetable soups ... we had the good fortune to lose none of our people'.[14] Leaving Madagascar in the first week of September, by mid October they anchored off St Helena. There Clark was very critical of a situation in which with adequate fertile land 'the gentlemen [passengers] who can afford to live on shore, meet with proper refreshments ... yet this is not the case of the common sailors' ... for whom no vegetables could be obtained 'but at an exorbitant charge ... the soldiers who reside on this island are subject to the same disease' (scurvy). After two weeks they sailed again but met with variable winds and calms and there was a return of scurvy before they made Scilly on 5 January 1770 and 'on the 16th we arrived in the Downs, which put an end to our tedious and disagreeable voyage'.[14] During the voyage 13 people had died, 10 of the ship's crew and 3 recruits, and they had been away from March 1768 to January 1770.

In all the detailed and thoughtful accounts of the voyage Clark says nothing of himself or his health. It cannot have been an easy experience, yet after spending the summer and autumn of 1770 in Roxburghshire, presumably at his home at Graden, he was prepared to undertake a second voyage in the same vessel with the same captain.

The *Talbot* again left the Downs on 16 February 1771 with a company of 107 crew, 16 passengers and 70 military recruits. On this second voyage Clark kept a daily record of latitude, longitude, temperature, direction of wind and comments on weather. He also described sporadic illness, largely with intestinal symptoms, and after only two weeks at sea 'a black boy, a native of India, died of a consumption', who, when they sailed 'was reduced to that stage of the disease, from which none recover'.[15] As they approached the Equator, many people complained of prickly heat but fortunately scurvy did not appear and they reached Johanna, chief of the Comera Islands, without major trouble. There they took on water, provisions and fruit, sailed again in three days, and on 25 July, after five months, reached Madras. The ship's company were soon hard at work thoughout the day and as early as the second day after arrival many were seized with sickness and purging and one young man appears to have died from heatstroke. Clark does not seem to have seen the man at the beginning of his illness for he says his 'assistant' was first called as Clark himself was away from the ship.

After one month, on 25 August, they sailed for Macao with a crew sick with fever and dysentery. Many of the men who still did duty looked 'pale and wan'. The voyage was slow and it was 19th October before they reached harbour where intestinal troubles continued and one man died from tetanus. Five months later, on 7 March 1772 the return began via Java and the Cape of Good Hope which they rounded on 4th June without any scurvy and made for St Helena 'but had no vegetables' so that by August scurvy was again apparent. Yet when this second voyage ended on 1st September and they had been away from England for 18 months they had lost only one person on the outward and three persons on the return voyages. As in the first voyage Clark says nothing about himself or his health in a direct way and one feels he was a competent and concerned ship's doctor.

He did not go to sea again but was not idle, for in his book on 'Fevers' there are records of visits made to patients during 1772 and part of the following year, whilst he was working near his home at Graden.[31]

But he also had copious notes and records of his travels made, as he says, during the 'tediousness of many a vacant hour at sea'. These notes were transformed into *Observations on the Diseases which prevail in Long Voyages to Hot Countries.*[12-15] Quickly finished and published, the book was dedicated to the Court of Directors of the East India Company. Clark then seems to have spent the winter of 1772 in London seeing his work through the publishers and the first edition appeared in 1773. (A second edition followed in 1792 and a third in 1809). For the book and dedication Clark received one hundred guineas from the Company.

His thoughts must then have turned to his future. He had not completed his courses of lectures at Edinburgh and could not be recognised as a Doctor of Medicine at that University but he did apply to, and receive from St Andrews the required Doctorate, given, probably, on the strength of his published work.

That Diploma allowed him to enter practice as a physician and in the same year settle in Kelso which, at that time, had a population of about 4,000, was a market town, and not far from his birthplace. He must have known the town well, for he had finished his apprenticeship there only four years earlier. But it soon proved too small for his ambition and in 1775 he moved to Newcastle where he would live and work for the rest of his life.

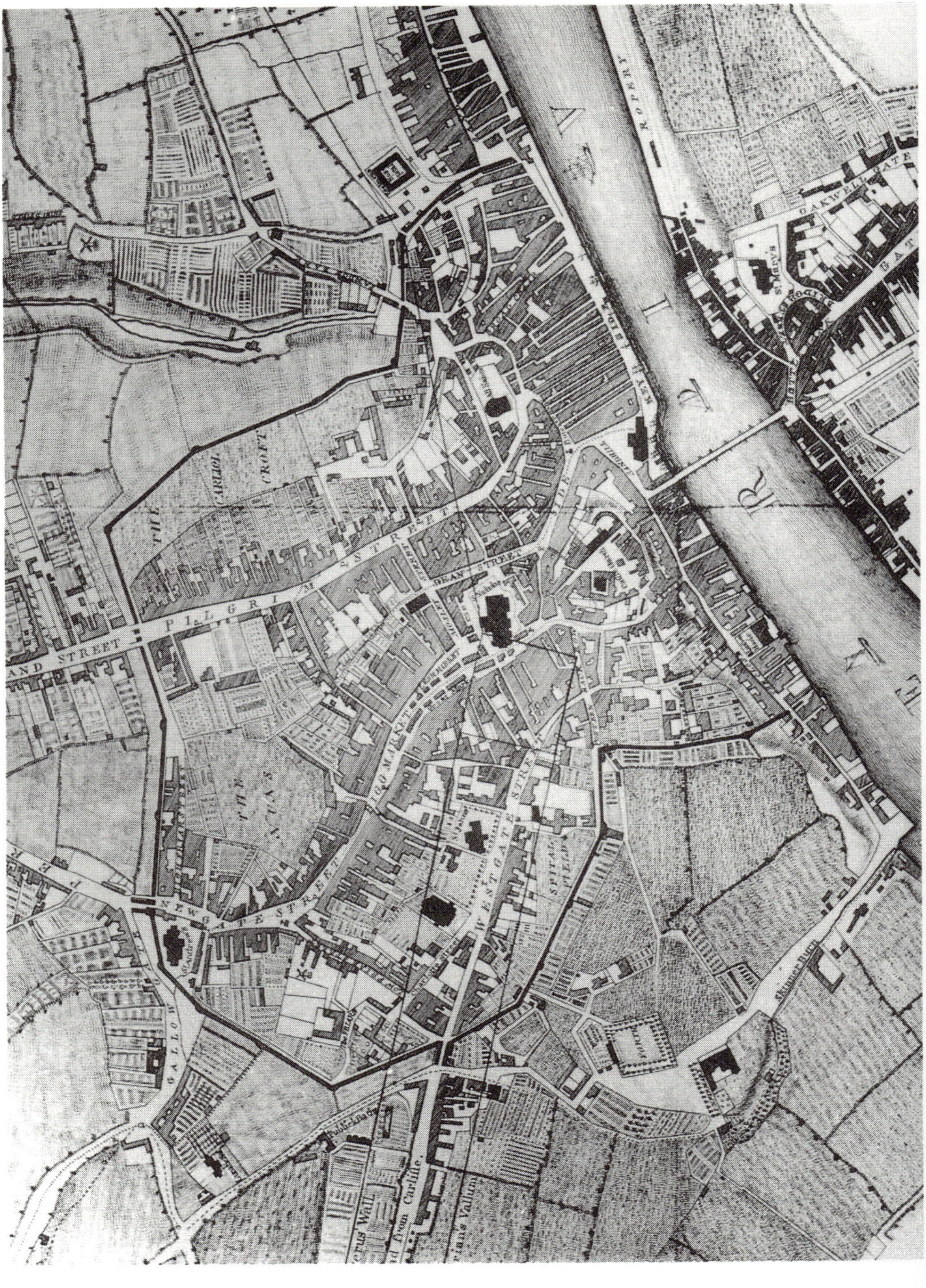
PILGRIM STREET
NEWGATE STREET
OAKWELL GATE
ROPERY

Newcastle and its doctors in 1775

The New Castle was then nearly seven hundred years old. The town and its 25,000 inhabitants, largely confined within its medieval walls, was the largest between York and Edinburgh. One bridge, crossing the Tyne where the Romans first built in Hadrian's time, brought the traveller to the Sandhill near the Guildhall and the commercial centre. From there three routes diverged. The steep 'Side' passed St Nicholas Church to the Bigg Market, St Andrew's Church and to the New Gate; East and North the way led to All Saints Church and Pilgrim Street and Gate; West lay through the Castle Garth to St John's, Westgate Street, the West Gate and the Hill beyond. The Quay formed the north bank of the river on land reclaimed slowly over past centuries. From the Quay running north was a mass of narrow 'chares' whose high, crowded houses were the homes of poor families and where infective illnesses flourished.

Throughout medieval times the town had been a base for both defence and offence against the Scots and also a local commercial and market centre for the north bank of the Tyne. It still supplied London with coal carried by sea in large fleets of collier brigs. About this time the manufacture of glass, the beginning of iron and chemical works were heralding the industrial growth of the next 150 years. Yet only thirty years had passed since cannon had been mounted against the possibility of attack by Charles Stuart and his Highlanders and one wonders about the popularity of a Border accent.

The city guild of Barber Surgeons dating from 1442 regulated apprenticeships, entry to and the practice of its members as surgeons.[16] There were also a small number of physicians who had doctorates of medicine from Scottish or continental universities. They practised internal medicine and acted as consultants to the surgeons. But essentially all were in competitive practice. Apothecaries, also qualified by apprenticeship, prepared, stocked and sold medicaments but were not allowed to prescribe or give advice to customers. However, the boundaries between the groups often seemed indistinct and financial and social tensions were usually present.

The medieval monasteries and nunneries had long since been suppressed. Each of the four parishes in the town had responsibilities for its own Poor Law relief and each maintained a Poor House. Despite the sea trade with the Thames and London there is little doubt that at this time Newcastle and its people had strong local sentiments and inter-relationships based on local families and their traditions. Its 'outlets' were towards the sea and seafaring, and the lure of London rather than movement to other parts of the country.

Figure 2 (opposite). Newcastle in 1788. Beilby Plan.
The Bridge reached Sandhill, whence Pilgrim Street, Bigg Market and Newgate Street, and Westgate Street ran to their gates in the Edwardian Walls. The Infirmary lies outside the walls near the south-west corner of the Forth.

In 1751 the local population joined in the national movement which created the voluntary hospitals. In January of that year a proposition to found an Infirmary for Newcastle, Northumberland and Durham was first brought before the public in the *Newcastle Courant* when a letter signed only with the initials 'BK', but thought to be written by a young surgeon, Richard Lambert, urged that Newcastle should follow the example of other places and provide a hospital to care for the Sick and Lame Poor. The emphasis was particularly on the care of victims of injury and accident and those requiring surgery, who could not be looked after in their own houses, or pay for the treatment. The appeal also touched civic pride and the response, both personal and municipal, was immediate. Subscription lists were opened, in three months staff had been appointed and temporary accommodation was in use in Gallowgate. By October 1753 the first patients were admitted to the newly completed Infirmary building on the Forth outside the city wall.[17]

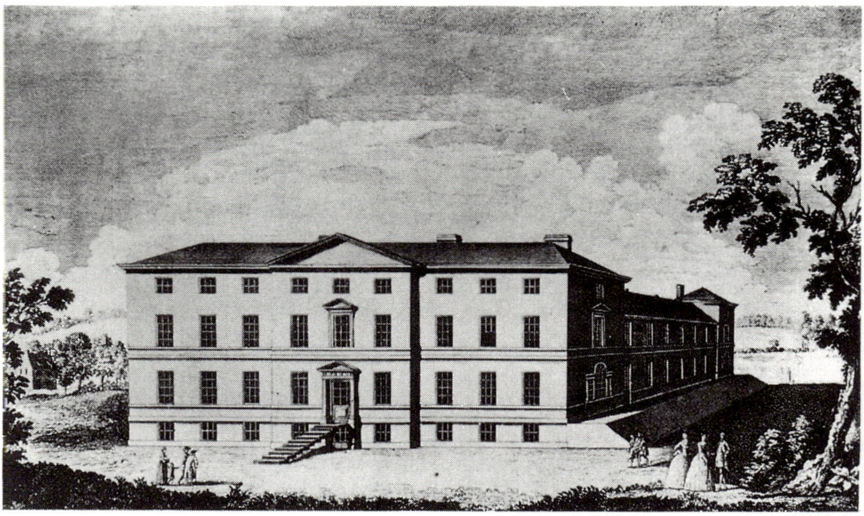

Figure 3. The Infirmary on the Forth, 1753-1906.

Clark comes to Newcastle

Clark arrived in Newcastle in 1775 as Dr A Wilson, an Edinburgh graduate, left for London. He is said to have had 'but little business' although he had been on the Infirmary staff for 3 years and probably in the town since 1758. His successor on the staff was Dr Pemberton and the next vacancy at the Infirmary did not occur until 1786 on the death of Dr Rotherham.

Clark's move from the smaller town of Kelso to Newcastle was certainly an attempt to break into a bigger and more lucrative field of practice. It was both bold and risky. Wilson seems to have given up the struggle although he may have been in Newcastle for nearly 20 years. Clark was a lowland Scot from a farming community without any introductions or social links. Novocastrians had no reason to welcome people from North of the border which for so long had been a source of trouble. In other growing towns such as Manchester and Liverpool Scottish physicians were hardly welcomed.[18] But Clark did begin practice and Fenwick says that he 'advanced but slowly against so powerful an opposition'. He was, and would be for some years, the only physician not on the staff of the Infirmary. It is unlikely that he had financial support from his own family, but he may have acquired some capital by trade during his voyages or by marriage.

We do not know the date or place of his first marriage or the financial situation of his wife, but Mackenzie states Mary Clark was a widow and that they had two sons, both of whom died in infancy.[19] Mrs Clark died in May 1781.

The first General Directory for Newcastle issued in 1778 records that five physicians were in practice and all, including Dr Clark, lived in Pilgrim Street which led north to the Pilgrim Gate and was considered socially desirable.[20] Only one surgeon of the ten in practice lived in the same street and he, Mr John Anderson, became a close colleague of Clark during the foundation of the Dispensary and afterwards. Little is known of Clark's home life except from Fenwick who says he was 'an affectionate husband and father, a warm and steady friend, an indulgent master, a man of unbounded benevolence, equally inaccessible to suspicion and incapable of practising deceit', but he also says 'Dr Clark was rather hasty in his temper; a fault which is so often connected with great and generous qualities that it generally meets with too much indulgence in society'.[21]

Two years after the death of Mary, Clark married Susannah Heath in the Chapel of St Andrews on the first of May 1783. The first child of that marriage was born on 5 June of the next year and baptised in the Unitarian Chapel in Hanover Square where John Clark's name is included in the Register of the Minister and those who regularly assembled in that Chapel. Thereafter the births and baptisms of six sons and one daughter were recorded at intervals to 2 September 1802.[22]

Susannah survived her husband and was with him during his last prolonged illness. Of the family, William the third son, became Professor of Anatomy at Cambridge.[23]

Foundation of the Dispensary 1777

Dr Fenwick's phraseology in his address is not always easy to understand or assess but he indicates that the opposition and difficulties which Clark had encountered on building a practice amongst those able to pay fees had made him 'in his zeal for the improvement of his profession offer his services to the poor'.[24] It is not, however, clear when or how he began to do so. There is little doubt that he was in touch with and aware of the works of physicians outside Newcastle. The Unitarian Minister at Hanover Street,

William Turner, had come to Newcastle from the Warrington Academy where both John Aikin and William Percival had been educated; Aikin's book *Thoughts on Hospitals* and the work of Percival and his group in Manchester would be known to him.[25] In London Lettsom had been one of the leaders in the establishment of the Dispensary service since 1770 – a service which did not simply dispense medicines but would make home visits to sick persons confined to bed many of whom could not be admitted to hospital. That movement expanded rapidly in London. Outside London the Edinburgh Dispensary in 1776 was the first to be established[26] and Clark would certainly have known of these developments and similar plans for Liverpool and Manchester.[27,28] Clark was not a man to miss an opportunity and in April 1777 a few private gentlemen met together under the chairmanship of the Mayor, Mr John Carr, and agreed to the opening of a Dispensary linked to the names of John Clark and Mr John Anderson who, as we have seen, lived near Clark in Pilgrim Street. Clark was certainly the major influence at that meeting and pushed matters ahead, printing the proceedings and appealing for financial support. Particular care had been taken to avoid the impression that the new project should appear to be in opposition to the Infirmary 'whose practice is confined chiefly to surgery and to the relief of chronic diseases. Its gates, from unavoidable necessity, are shut against the poor labouring under Fevers, pleurisy, sore throats and all other internal inflammations, cholera, colic, dysentery, smallpox and measles and, in short all the acute disorders of adults and children – the practice must be confined to the diseases which are not admitted to the Infirmary'.[29] Those reassurances were indeed very necessary, for the Infirmary staff resented what they regarded as possible competition and only two of the Infirmary physicians and one surgeon, J Anderson (not on the Infirmary Staff), became active members of the Dispensary when work began. After the April meeting subscription lists were opened and regulations were drafted. There was to be a General Court of Governors meeting four times a year, when each Governor would have a vote (an annual subscription of £2 or more brought that right, or a donation of £20 brought Life Governorship). Subscribers of lesser amounts did not have the right to vote. Admission to assistance was by presentation of a dispensary letter obtained from a Governor, subscriber or their agent.

A second meeting of subscribers was held on 29th September 1777 to confirm the Regulations and, despite the fact that the available capital was only £143, a decision was taken to begin work immediately.[30] The proceeedings of this meeting were also published and laid down principles of operation which remained essentially the same until 1948. The central figure in the work of the Dispensary was the Apothecary (later the Resident Medical Officer) who was the only resident member of staff. A person wishing to be 'admitted' into care obtained a Dispensary letter and sent to the Dispensary before 10 am if they required to be visited at home, or attended with the letter for help and advice as an out patient. Any patient was accepted except maternity work for which a separate hospital had been founded in 1760. Thus the Dispensary cared for a wide range of people and all types of illness in very variable environments. Those who worked in the Dispensary must always have been conscious of the relationship between housing, social conditions, nutrition and the prevalence and severity of illness.

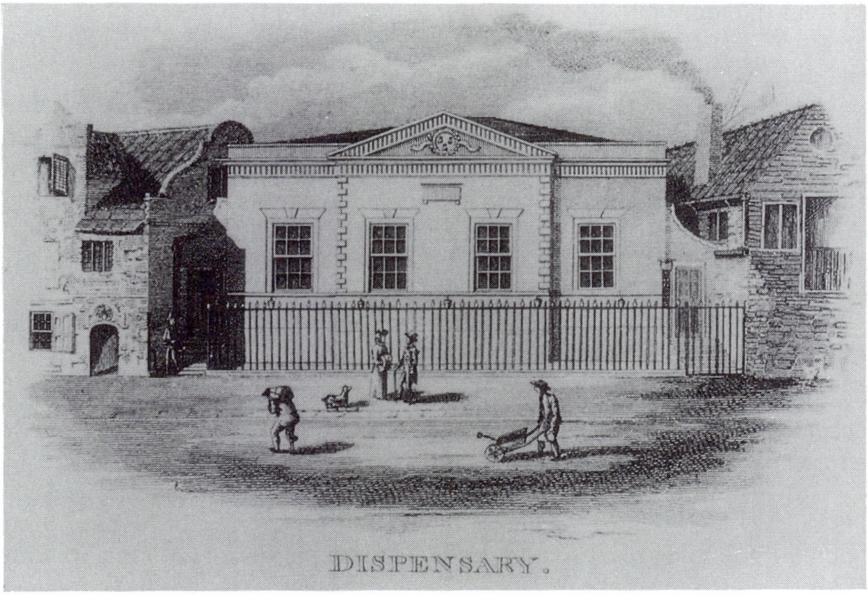

Figure 4. The Dispensary, Low Friar Chare, 1790-1838.

After four years operating from an 'entry' off the foot of the 'Side' new accommodation was found near the Queen's Head Hotel in Pilgrim Street and work continued there until 1790. Each year the annual report, unsigned but bearing the stamp of Clark's personality reported an increase in the number of patients. Clark himself did much home visiting and kept full and careful notes of the people, children and adults, he attended. He was particularly concerned with illnesses associated with 'Fever' and with the different types of fever, 'relapsing', 'intermittent' and 'continuous'. In his voyages East he had become familiar with the effect of the Peruvian bark (quinine) upon patients with repeated attacks of relapsing fever, many of which must have been due to malaria. This impressed him so much that, unfortunately, he thought the 'bark' was the cure for all fevers – and that all fevers had the same cause. Throughout the first two years of the Dispensary he collected clinical records and, in 1780, published *Observations on Fevers especially those of the Continuous type and on the Scarlet Fever attended with Ulcerated Sore-Throat.*[31]

In 1785 the Duke of Northumberland consented to be Patron and the Annual Report proudly contained the names of five Presidents and four Vice

Presidents, all giving evidence of greater support and of Clark's growing influence in the area.

He was not content to care only for sick patients. In 1786 another publication described detailed proposals for a general inoculation against smallpox which was so frequently a danger and cause of death, blindness and scarring.[32] That publication was followed by another in 1790 also published without signature but, like that of 1786, bearing every sign of Clark's authorship.[33] That report restated the rules and organization of the Dispensary and detailed its work since 1777.

It also marked the third move of the Dispensary to much more suitable premises in Low Friar Chare not far from the White Cross in Newgate Street. The Dispensary was now firmly established and, although it moved again in 1838 and 1926, continued to work and serve the people of Newcastle on the same broad lines until 1948 and the beginning of the National Health Service. Clark deserves to be remembered, if for nothing else, as its founder and for his early place in the history of the Dispensary movement.[34]

Clark's clinical practice

Eleven years after Clark's arrival in Newcastle, in 1786, a vacancy occurred in the staff of the Infirmary when Dr Rotherham retired and shortly afterwards died.

By that time Clark must have been well established in practice and the Dispensary was steadily becoming recognised for service to the poor ill at home or attending as out patients. He had also published both the account of his voyages and his experience of 'Fevers' in Newcastle and, at the request of Dr Dugud Leslie of Durham, an account of an outbreak of Influenza in that city during 1782 to which he had added the story of a similar outbreak in Newcastle later the same year.[35] We have seen he was also a regular Member of the Unitarian Congregation. It is not surprising therefore after eleven years of active work and growing influence he should be a candidate for the Infirmary vacancy. The other candidate, Dr John Fenwick, we know as the author of the valedictory address. A member of a local family, his father had practised in Morpeth but it is uncertain when John began to practise in Newcastle. His name did not appear in the Newcastle Directory of 1778 but he had worked at the Dispensary since 1784 and in that capacity Clark and he were colleagues.

The election was made at a Special Court of Governors held on 12th April 1787. Meetings to make honorary appointments were advertised in the local press and were regarded as important. Only Governors were entitled to attend and to vote, and canvassing and lobbying were the usual customs. Unfortunately, the minutes of that meeting are quite inadequate but no fewer than 155 Governors attended and voted. Such an attendance was far greater than at an ordinary Quarterly Court, indicating the interest aroused and the degree of canvassing when an appointment was at stake. No record is given of the proceedings or the persons who proposed the candidates.

There is merely a list of the names of those who attended, and beside the name of each is the letter 'ff' or 'C' indicating how the person voted. Ninety names were marked 'ff' and 65 marked 'C' and the four members of the Infirmary staff who voted all supported Fenwick.[36]

The minutes of both Quarterly Courts and of the Weekly Committee at this time are very sparse and may well be a sign that the general work of the hospital and local interest had deteriorated.

Private practice, however, must have continued and Clark must have had plenty to do. Patients could approach him directly or he could be called into consultation by either another physician or a surgeon. He probably continued to do his share of visiting of Dispensary patients but at no time in its history do the Annual Reports detail the number of home visits made by individual doctors.

Clark, we know, kept full notes of the people and children he visited from the Dispensary in its early days and Fenwick in his address became almost lyrical about Clark's conduct of a consultation and of his care for his patients saying 'Doctor Clark was formed to excel in the profession he exercised ... no man was ever more thoroughly attached to his profession ... to it he sacrificed not only ... pleasures but likewise society ... He also listened with benevolence to the diffuse and occasionally irrelevant details which severe suffering will draw at times from even the most resigned and sensible persons ... knowledge of facts which will materially assist him in forming his opinion ... His instructions were distinguished by their perspicuity ... nothing which could be useful was omitted. He listened to the opinions of others with attention and, in delivering his own, always adduced the reasons on which it was founded ... His manner, on such occasions was singularly happy ... Extensive as his practical knowledge was, it was not more conspicuous than the judgement and discrimination with which he applied it ... In the same proportion as he was patient and cautious in forming his opinion, was his practice vigorous and decisive'.[37]

Fenwick next praises Clark's writings as the best guide then existing for those who 'practise physic in hot climates' and goes on to commend his use of mercury, as calomel, in both acute and chronic rheumatism and also as a treatment for dysentery and 'some states of Remittent Fever, when local affections of the abdominal viscera attend the disease, he considers it, combined with opium, to be the best remedy which can be had recourse to'. These and other usages sound very strange today but they seem to have met with approval at that time and physicians were certainly expected to act with potent remedies.

Election to the Infirmary May 15th 1788

Clark had failed when opposed by Fenwick, but only a year later in April 1788 another vacancy was caused by the death of Dr Brown the Senior Physician who, in 1760, had succeeded Dr Henry Askew when he left after only one year in office.

On this occasion there was no opposition. At a Special Court on 15 May, Thomas Charles Bigge of Benton House, named John Clark to succeed Dr Brown. The name of his supporter is not legible. Clark was then elected unanimously by the twenty five Governors present.[38] Obviously the situation was very different from the previous year and it looks as if the absence of competition for the appointment had been well known. At that time there seems to have been only one other doctor in the town practising as a physician but not on the Infirmary staff.

So, thirteen years after his arrival in Newcastle and eleven years after the foundation of the Dispensary, Dr Clark became a member of the staff of the Infirmary. It would be necessary for him to attend regularly for the examination of patients presenting with letters from subscribers and presumably to make regular visits to the wards to see his own patients though as yet there was no separation of 'medical' and 'surgical' patients. The appointment would certainly have increased yet further his standing in the town.

For the immediate future, however, one gets the impression that he was still very much more concerned with the growing work of the Dispensary. In addition to his regular attendances we have seen he was almost certainly the principal organiser of the scheme for a 'General Inoculation' in Newcastle and the author of the pamphlet setting out the 'Proposal' for that scheme.[39] The hope that such a scheme could be introduced in Newcastle had been raised first in 1779 only two years after the Dispensary opened but abandoned for lack of funds. But in 1786 it was revived because 'especially amongst the poor, Inoculation had made little or no progress'. Since 1779 general inoculations of the poor had been held in Chester, Leeds and Liverpool. In Newcastle patients were to be inoculated in their own homes and supplied with medicines from the Dispensary. Women who could not afford time from work to look after their children would be paid 5s for one child and up to 10s for four or more. Subscriptions were requested, a committee would be formed and the 'consent and Patronage of the Magistrates, the Clergy and the principal inhabitants be obtained'. There followed an estimate that 153 lives a year might be saved. In the first inoculation some 208 childen were treated and 'everyone passed through the disease with utmost safety'.[39]

But he planned to go further and as early as 1793 had hoped that it might be possible to form a Board of Health with a House of Recovery and means of 'cleansing' both the persons and the clothes etc of those suffering from infectious fevers. That plan could not then be financed but it was not forgotten and remained an ambition and hope for Clark and his colleagues.

The numbers of patients cared for at the Dispensary were slowly but steadily increasing and in 1788 for the first time exceeded a thousand (1057). In that year also the names of three new physicians, Drs Moorhouse, Milne and Young, joined the four, Hall, Pemberton, Fenwick and Clark also at the Infirmary. Thus, all the physicians practising in the town joined in helping at the Dispensary. Mr John Anderson, the only surgeon who attended, was able to visit a patient at home when required.

The report of 1790, issued about the time of the move to Low Friar Chare, carries a detailed table of the causes which had brought nearly 11 000 patients to seek help and reveals that acute infections, mostly respiratory and intestinal, were by far the most frequent reasons for 'admission'.[33] Some 860 patients were thought to have tuberculosis (156 had already died); 232 had had smallpox with 59 deaths; scarlet fever 203 cases and 26 deaths.[33] Clark thought of prevention as well as cure and records the inoculation of 1056 children in the preceding four years; 852 were under three years of age and three deaths were recorded. Natural infection was thought to carry a mortality of one in six cases, so he was able to argue lives had been saved.

After the account of work done the 'rules and orders' governing the conduct of the Dispensary were set out in detail for all to read and understand. Altogether it is a clear and concise document which emphasises the Prevention of Contagion and draws attention to a hand-bill on the subject given to every Dispensary patient. Thus from its beginning the idea of prevention and control of infective disease was prominent. An 'Inoculating Department' was to be established and would have its own committee of fifteen Governors of the Dispensary with an equal number of subscribers. It would organise the spring and autumn inoculations which were to be done by surgeons at the homes of the children 'and the Physicians would give their assistance when necessary'. Sixteen surgeons, probably all except two of those in practice at that time, are listed, the only time the surgeons as a body appear as assisting in the work of the Dispensary.[33]

In 1801 the inoculations of children gave place to vaccination as Jenner's work became recognised and by that time nearly 3000 patients had been seen and the work of the visiting physicians had been supplemented by home visits made by Mr James Wilkie the Apothecary and Mr Murray, a surgeon, employed part time for that purpose. Affairs continued in that way at the Dispensary, but as we shall see, Clark became more and more caught up in the complex situation at the Infirmary and remained so until his death in April 1805. Strangely, the annual report of the Dispensary for that year does not carry any mention of Clark's work during the 28 years since its first opening in 1777. His name simply vanishes from the list of physicians.

The Infirmary 1788-1801

When Clark became a member of the Infirmary staff in April 1788 Dr Hall was senior physician and would remain so for another five years. He was the son of a local surgeon, enjoyed an extensive practice and had served on the Dispensary with Clark since its foundation. With partners he established a private asylum and also public baths in the area now known as Bath Lane just outside the Town Wall as it swept south to the West Gate. In 1788 he was serving a second term as President of the recently formed Philosophical and Medical Society.[40] He had also, many years earlier, in 1766 opened a private mental home at Belle View near the Leazes. The next senior, Dr Pemberton, also from a local family and, like Clark, a member of the congregation of Hanover Square Chapel, had been appointed to the Infirmary when Wilson left in 1775. He was also physician to the Lying-In Hospital then situated in Rosemary Lane near St John's Church. He remained on the Infirmary staff until 1800. Dr John Fenwick, appointed only a year earlier than Clark, was in active practice in the city but was to resign and move to Durham in 1791. Whilst in Newcastle he, like Hall, served as a physician at the Dispensary and remained a friend, being with Clark during his last prolonged illness in 1804-5.

The four surgeons had all been appointed earlier, A Abbs (1773), Wm Ingham (1778), H Mewburn (1782) and R Keenlyside, son of W Keenlyside, (1784) would all serve to the end of the century, Mewburn retiring in 1799 to be succeeded by F Horn. Ingham, certainly the most powerful locally, seemed to have considerable influence on both Keenlyside, and later on Horn. He was also widely known for his professional skills and his training of apprentices. All the surgeons seemed very conscious that the Infirmary had been initiated by a surgeon and its prime purpose was to treat accidents and provide surgical care for patients who could not be looked after at home. There seemed always to be an undercurrent of tension between physicians and surgeons.

The responsibility for the Infirmary in terms of finance, general management, the appointment of staff and indeed the admission and discharge of patients rested with the Governors. A Quarterly Court to discuss and vote on matters of policy was held four times each year. Special Governors Courts could be called whenever required, notice having been given by advertisement in the Newcastle papers.

Day to day affairs and detailed management were in the hands of a Weekly Committee responsible for the patients' adherence to the Rules, for the admission of new patients (except accidents) and discharge of others. That committee was appointed at each Quarterly meeting as a panel of 12 Governors from each of Newcastle, Northumberland and Durham. All the 36 were eligible to attend, but few did, and there did not seem to be any set quorum. Medical and surgical staff who were Governors were also able to attend.

At each meeting the Apothecary and Matron presented their reports and raised any complaints from or about patients. The Apothecary then reported on patients to be discharged and on those who had been in hospital for more than two months with the advice of their doctors regarding further treatment. Major decisions needing an early answer required a special meeting of the Governors.

The minutes of each meeting are written in ink and vary greatly in legibility and fullness and generally deteriorate as time goes on. The duration of meetings was never indicated. In the early years they were signed by the Chairman. Only occasionally were financial details given. Presumably they were in the hands of the Treasurer who kept his own accounts and settled bills, etc. The Chairman was chosen at each meeting from the members present so there was little continuity of management.

In his history of the Infirmary on the Forth GH Hume records that he scrutinised the committee minutes to the end of the 18th century and comments upon the misbehaviour of patients on the one hand, and nurses and servants on the other; about complaints from the patients regarding food and drink. He records the low wages and the rising cost of food, particularly after 1793 and the renewal of the long continued war with France.[5] These conditions also affected the readiness of subscribers to pay their annual contributions and there was recurrent general anxiety about finance. But there were also other considerations urging change.

The Infirmary at Newcastle had been founded and opened at almost the same time as the hospitals in Manchester and in Liverpool. All these institutions had similar difficulties but those in Liverpool and Manchester could be said to arise more quickly than those of Newcastle because both towns were growing much faster. In all three places the hospital premises had been built rapidly and enthusiastically but with little knowledge and no experience of the difficulties of organisation, design and the dangers for the individual patient inherent in the situation. Certainly, in Newcastle and probably in the other two towns, the moving figures had been surgeons whose patients required operative care but whose dwellings could not provide the essential conditions required; industrial accidents and street accidents were common and increasing; bladder stones were frequent, leg ulcers also. Apart from surgical situations the population as a whole was visited regularly by epidemics of respiratory and alimentary infections, acute rheumatism and carditis. Scarlet fever, smallpox, measles and whooping cough were all childhood hazards whilst tuberculosis in various forms affected patients of all ages. Diphtheria had not been separated from other forms of acute tonsillitis, or typhoid from typhus. Although it was recognised that disease could spread from person to person in the community, there was no knowledge of the many different ways that happened and no concept of bacteriology. Spread was most often thought to be caused by 'contagion' or 'miasmas', by contact with patients' clothes, or by changes in the air and attention was focussed on ventilation and the removal of objectionable smells.

Pressure for admission to hospital led to overcrowding and the system of letters of recommendation gave the subscriber some power of selection of patients. Ill patients often came from distances in primitive transport. These types of difficulties arose in the hospitals of all three towns and all were under pressure from overcrowding and the presence of 'hospital infection', when in 1771 the small book *Thoughts on Hospitals* was published in London.[25] The author, John Aikin was only 24 years of age and was still serving an apprenticeship to the famous and formidable surgeon and accoucheur Charles White in Manchester. Dedicated to John Haygarth the physician at Chester, with it was printed a letter from the more senior Thomas

Percival, also of Manchester. That publication was full of practical common sense regarding the design of hospitals, the consideration of the selection of patients likely to benefit, 'those with external injury in a sound body', the 'difficulties which applied to wounds made by surgeons', 'a hospital should be a place designed for the cure of the sick and not an alms house for the support of the indigent and decrepit'. Percival's 'Letter' supported Aikin's thesis and emphasised 'Air, Diet and medicine are the three great agents in preventing and correcting putrefaction and contagion in hospitals'. That book had great influence for many years to come.[25]

In all three growing towns local politics and interests were often in conflict and many of the early hospital physicians were in fact members of Dissenting congregations known to each other and almost certainly in regular correspondence. John Aikin, the author, was the son of John Aikin, the Principal of the Dissenting Academy in Warrington founded in 1757. He had been educated there before his first apprenticeship as an apothecary and his medical studies in Edinburgh. In Manchester he met again with Thomas Percival who had also been educated at Warrington – indeed in 1757 he had been the first student enrolled in the Academy. Both were Unitarians as was George Bell, appointed when Percival resigned as physician to the hospital in Manchester. In Liverpool, James Currie was also a Dissenter. Percival was also one of the chief founders of the Literary and Philosophical Society in Manchester. Here also were connections with Newcastle and we know that William Turner, also educated in Warrington, came to Newcastle in 1783 as minister to the Unitarian congregation in Hanover Square where John Clark, his wife Susan and family were members. Thus, there was certainly a network of like-minded men between the towns.

In Manchester local politics were confounded by increasing pressure on the hospital and in the 1780s and later that problem was met by the formation of an outdoor service conducted by hospital staff able and willing to do home visiting and later still by the opening of accommodation for fever patients in a building near the hospital but physically separate from it.[28] By that time in Newcastle the Dispensary with its home visiting service was striving to meet the same need. Apart from the fact that some physicians gave service to both institutions, in Newcastle the Infirmary and Dispensary remained separate, while demands on the Infirmary for all types of help increased steadily and overcrowding was a constant problem. Financial support, which did come in response to particular appeals, was not sustained in the intervals.

Writing in 1827 Mackenzie said 'This Institution continued to produce the most beneficial effects; but, at length many of the original statutes for its regulation fell into disuse; while others from great improvements in the management of hospitals became unavoidably defective'.[41]

There had long been difficulties over the admission of 'fever' cases (an omnibus term for many infections) and Hume, himself a surgeon, says 'it was at length decided in 1774 by the Governors that no fever cases should be admitted'.[5] That did not remove the difficulties concerning febrile patients who came from a distance. Hume also regrets that the Reports of the period do not give any indication of the volume or type of work done or the results obtained. There is no evidence that hospital notes were kept and there was no separation of patients into 'medical' or 'surgical' wards.

The 1801 extension and reorganisation

To try to understand something of the atmosphere and functioning of the Infirmary at that time I have followed Hume's example and scrutinised the Minutes to 1805. They are kept in chronological order, those of the Court and Weekly Committee following each other in the same volume.

The Chairman was appointed each week from the Governors present. Comments from the weekly visitors are quite rare. The Matron or the Apothecary occasionally complained of the conduct of patients, particularly of men who left the hospital without leave and sometimes returned late, showing evidence of drink; of the behaviour of nurses taking gifts from patients, allowing bread to be taken from the hospital or food to be brought in. Patients complained about the food, especially the bread and beer. The names of those patients admitted or discharged were recorded at each meeting but no indication is given of their illnesses or condition.

The staff appointed in April 1751 had moved with the hospital to the Forth in 1753. There were then four Physicians and two Surgeons; an Apothecary and Matron who were residents and initially only two nurses. Matron had power both to engage and dismiss nurses but these events and their changing numbers are not recorded.

In December 1753 Mr Gibson the Apothecary resigned and W Keenlyside was appointed in his place.

From the early months there were complaints that the chimneys smoked, that noise was a problem and that the 'offices became nauseous and offensive to all persons who go nigh them'.

In 1758 Dr Cooper, one of the first physicians, died following a fall from his horse and Henry Askew, the son of the powerful Adam Askew, was elected to the vacancy but he resigned within a year.

In January 1760 Mr Samuel Hallowell the senior and respected surgeon also resigned as did Mr W Keenlyside the Apothecary. A month later at a Special Court both Henry Gibson and W Keenlyside offered themselves as candidates for the vacancy and at a Special Court on 14 February 1760 with 120 Governors present, Keenlyside was elected by a large majority and John Dent was appointed Apothecary without opposition.

Weekly committee meetings were poorly attended, usually by only 3-5 Governors, one or two surgeons, usually Hallowell and Lambert, and only occasionally a physician. But in February 1760, when an appointment was to be made, there was a large attendance of Governors — the result of canvassing for and by the candidates. At the same meeting there was a letter from several members of the Surgeons' Company of the Town asking that the

Rules be changed to increase the number of surgeons. The next Court held on 3 April 1760 was stormy but by a narrow vote (31 to 29) the number of surgeons was increased to four to equal that of the physicians. Henry Gibson, the former Apothecary, was appointed without opposition and then John Rayne was elected from 9 other candidates. Both Keenlyside and Gibson were to give long sevice and were regularly present at both Courts and at weekly meetings. Over the years the surgeons attended the meetings much more regularly than the physicians and certainly give the impresson of acting much more as a group.

Over the years also, more and more people sought admission, until in May 1799, at a Special Court, the Chairman proposed a motion that the Infirmary be considered full when there were 80 patients in the House. This was opposed vigorously by both Dr Clark and Mr Keenlyside and the former moved that the Apothecary should, every Thursday, make out a list of patients with the time of admission, the nature of their complaints and the name of their physician or surgeon. There is no evidence that this was done and problems seem to have continued.

In March 1800 Mr Mewburn resigned after 17 years' service and in April was succeeded by Mr F Horn, proposed by Mr Gibson whose apprentice he had been before serving in the Royal Navy and returning to practise in Newcastle. The April meeting saw an unusually large attendance and a sudden move to increase the number of surgeons to six was defeated by 134 to 76 votes. The proposal which was quite unexpected gave rise to a resolution that no proposition respecting an alteration in staff should be proceeded upon without previous agreement at a quarterly meeting. But it was certainly an indication of pressure from the surgeons.

Throughout the year 1800 committee attendances were small and in August, Matron (Miss Jackson) entered in the House Visitors book 'From non-attendance of the Committee (I) have been under the necessity of taking upon myself to apply to another Baker instead of Mr Harrison who has of late supplied the House with bread very unsuitable both in respect of quantity and quality – signed Mary Jackson'. She was then empowered to purchase bread until arrangements could be made, but it reveals a most unsatisfactory situation.

At the October Court Dr Steavenson was elected in place of Dr Pemberton who had resigned and thus, after 13 years, John Clark became senior physician. There seems by then to have been a general wish to revise the Statutes and Rules laid down in 1751 and when a Mr Walton placed his suggestions before the Governors the meeting resolved that a Special Court should be held on 6 November to consider the matter.

Despite advertisement in the papers, insufficient Governors attended that Court and as Dr Clark had suggested various important changes in Statutes and Rules a Committee of Governors was appointed to 'take all the statutes and rules into their consideration and frame such a code for the future conduct of the Charity as should appear to be made necessary or expedient by change of circumstances' (Minutes 6 November 1800). There were eleven members of the Committee and such of the Physicians and Surgeons who were Governors. The committee was to request advice and assistance from all other members of the Honorary Staff and report at latest by April 1801. It did so on 26 March. The April Quarterly Court then ordered that the new version of the Rules be printed and a copy sent to each Governor before a Special Court on 25 June. The result was a formidable document of 48 pages comprising 22 Statutes followed by 120 rules for patients, for Treasurer, Honorary Medical Staff, for Apothecary and Matron, nurses and servants, for the Library, and for the Professional conduct of Physicians and Surgeons. Finally there was an appendix containing forms of letters and a Table of Diet. No copy remains with the minutes, but one is in my possession.[42]

The question of alteration and extension of the Infirmary was first raised and discussed at the House Committee on 4 June. Only four members were present including John Clark and Mr Ingham and it was agreed that the question should be added to an advertisement for the Special Court on 25 June.

A week later on 11 June Clark circulated to every Governor, in a printed pamphlet of some 15 pages, the results of his study of the works of Percival, Aikin and the Committee of the Royal Society of Medicine in Paris and of Physicians in Glasgow, Woolwich, Liverpool, Northampton, Leeds and Manchester. He compared results and suggested improvements required in Newcastle and argued strongly for separation of patients and arrangement, according to diseases, into suitable wards.[43] That he was able to respond so quickly is evidence of long preparation.

At the Special Court on 25 June under the Chairmanship of Sir Matthew White Ridley the old code of laws was repealed and the new code confirmed.[44] Three committees were then formed, one to superintend the printing of the new code, the second to act as the new House Committee and the third to consider and report upon the required alterations and improvements. The membership of the second and third committees was the same and in each committee the presence of three members would form a quorum.

The third committee, Thomas Bigge the Chairman, reported on 21 July, and presented the report to a Special Court on 6 August 1801, making proposals for improving the ventilation, altering the wards, and building an extension which would accommodate 34 patients, making, with 50 in the old building, a total of 84 beds. 'But as the Infirmary would still be very imperfect your Committee propose to set apart, together with a distinct wash house for cleaning and purifying the patients' clothes, two rooms capable of containing six beds each, for infectious diseases of accidental occurrence to which patients may be removed to prevent the contagion from spreading through the whole house'.[44] Attached to the report was a plan and elevation of the new building and there the 'house for fever' is described as having 6 beds on each of three floors. At each level there was to be a door communicating with the main hospital. This was described as an important improvement in the house for fever, but there is no indication of an authorisation of the departure from the text of the Bigge Report.[45] There is therefore a discrepancy from the beginning. Nevertheless, at the next Court on 6 August the report was approved and a decision taken to solicit subscriptions immediately. The Duke of Northumberland opened the list with a draft of £500 and by 3rd October £2857 15s had been given. (Dr Clark and Mr Ingham each gave £21.)

On 11 October Dr Clark issued a second edition of his June letter to Governors with an appendix and asked his medical friends to suggest 'any useful internal improvement which may still be adopted in the execution of the Building'.[46] In it he describes the fever house in considerable detail with 16 beds for patients and 2 beds for nurses. Again the description in the text does not quite correspond with that in the appendix, but the text still uses the phrase 'infectious fevers of accidental origin'.

At the House Committee on 29 October Dr Clark requested and it was agreed that a register be kept of all accidents received during the year, but there is no evidence this was done. Work on the extension proceeded though not without difficulty with tradesmen.

During all that time John Clark, of course, was still very active in the work of the Dispensary which had been established for more than twenty years. He had always been in touch with many physicians in other cities and influenced by their writings and knew by experience the toll constantly exacted by acute and chronic infections. In line with that concern, in November 1801 he established a new Committee 'for increasing the usefulness of the Dispensary'.[47] It consisted of 17 members including Clark. Four members (Lloyd Wm, Lawton S, Headlam TE, and Revd D Prosser) were also members of the Infirmary committees responsible for the extension and John Anderson and Thomas Leighton were practising surgeons, all being Governors of the Infirmary. Meeting on 27 January 1802 that committee resolved to 'inquire into the causes which produce, preserve, and propagate the contagion of fever in Newcastle and Gateshead ... that they digest a plan to eradicate the contagion ... and that they point out the most likely means of raising a fund to carry the plan into execution'.[47] A report of 30 pages was printed and copies sent to the Mayor and Magistrates, the Clergy and Gentlemen composing the Vestries and also made available to the public. A forceful document, it describes the spread of 'fevers' particularly from the 'narrow lanes and courts such as those of Pandon, on the Quay, in the Castle Garth, Long Stairs, Sandgate and Pipewell Gate'.

It then goes on to recommend that a Board of Health be instituted and that a House of Recovery be provided for the reception of those persons labouring under fever. Control of the arrangement would be from the Dispensary whose physicians would care for the patients and whence medicines would be supplied. There were also to be provisions for cleansing of 'bed-clothes and apparel'. Finally, 'an inspector to visit houses where people have fever', should be appointed by the Committee at a moderate salary. The Dispensary committee could not 'raise a fund adequate for the purpose' and suggested that money should come from charitable sources and from the parochial rates.

The report ends with three short Appendices reprinted from previous writings, the first on the spread of Contagious Fevers in Newcastle written by Dr Ramsay in October 1793, the second by Dr Clark a month later when he had first proposed that a Society of Health (similar to those at Chester, Bury and Lancaster) should be established in Newcastle and that Society should provide a House of Reception. The third and last appendix was the 'Instructions and Rules' to be observed by patients of the Dispensary – these had been printed in 1791 and since then given to all Dispensary patients.[47] Thus the Committee restated old concerns and ambitions. That report, circulated in Newcastle from 14 May 1802, was sent to all Governors of the Infirmary and Dispensary and must have been read together with the edition of the 'Plan for the Internal Improvement and Extension of the Infirmary at Newcastle' issued by Dr Clark in October 1801. As already explained, it contained proposals for the 'fever wing' which did not quite correspond with those in Dr Clark's original publication, the number of beds it would contain was unchanged at 16 but in the appendix two were to be kept for nurses, thus reducing the patients' accommodation to 14 beds, and omitting the description of fevers 'of accidental occurrence'.[48]

The publication of that report from the Dispensary with the suggestion of a Board of Health and House of Recovery undoubtedly caused alarm in those opposed to the admission to the Infirmary of patients with 'Fevers'. Evidence of that concern was soon apparent for at the Weekly Committee on 29 April 1802 it was agreed that 'Dr Clark be requested to consult with the gentlemen of the Faculty ... the propriety of allowing the Fever Wards of the New Building to be appropriated to the purposes of an Institution for the prevention of Contagious Fevers and to report their joint opinion to this Committee'. The minutes do not say who made the proposal. There is no evidence that any such consultation took place but the pace of events quickened and on 27 May at the Weekly Committee it was agreed that a further Special Court should be held on Thursday 24 June at 10.30 am to take into consideration a 'Proposition for rendering the Fever house of the hospital more generally useful, the additional expense thereby incurred not to be defrayed by the funds of the Infirmary'.

This was a climax and a crisis. If the proposition were accepted it would mean that 'Fever' cases would be admitted from the community to the fever beds and the expense be borne by the parishes or other charity and would also, in effect, bring the Dispensary into association with the Infirmary. It was, of course, a challenge from those who agreed with Dr Clark and the work of the Dispensary. Just one week later at the House Committee on 3 June came a further resolution that the 'Physicians and Surgeons be requested to send to the Secretary, sealed up, on or before Wednesday 23 June, their opinion on the following point – whether there will be danger to the patients in the other parts of the Infirmary from a general admission of Fever patients to the Fever House, either upon the supposition that the only communication between the two buildings remains open for the convenience of admitting patients from the old House by means of a double door or is walled up'. The attendance of the Faculty at the meeting was particularly requested.

There must have been considerable local excitement for 105 persons are listed as attending. Staff had submitted opinions (Dr Wood had already published his) and they were read and 'debated'. Finally, the following Resolution was moved by Sir JE Swinburne and seconded by T Bigge Esq.

'That the Fever House of the Infirmary be opened for the General Reception of persons labouring under contagious fevers and that a Committee be appointed for doing this in the manner most beneficial to the public but without expense to the Infirmary'. Mr Bigge had been chairman of the committee appointed the previous year and both he and Sir John Swinburne were strong supporters of Clark. But it was not to be, the resolution was soundly defeated by 78 votes to 21.

The medical staff, who all voted, were equally divided, Clark and Ramsay, physicians, and Keenlyside and Abbs, surgeons, were for the resolution; Steavenson and Wood, physicians, and Ingham and Horn, surgeons, were against it.

Throughout this time there had been considerable anxiety about the finances as the work of extension and alteration slowly progressed. This seemed to be reflected in the handwriting of the minutes which become almost illegible, several sections appear to be in different hands, and none are signed, indicating a period of doubt and confusion. At another Special Court on 19 August, after inspection of the accounts, a full statement was deferred until the October Court 'when it is hoped the Building Committee will be enabled to present an accurate summary of the accounts'. Dr Clark does not seem to have attended during this time, but he had not accepted defeat.

The opinions of the Medical Staff submitted to the Special Court of 24 June are not recorded in the minutes of that Court, but six weeks later on 16 August 1802 Dr Clark circulated to all Governors a substantial *Collection of Papers relating to Fever Wards in Newcastle and other Infirmaries*.[48] After a preface of 44 pages he criticised 'old Infirmaries, many extremely defective', and advocated 'annexing to them fever houses which have incontestably been proved to be of infinite more service to the poor and to all ranks of society than every other department of these charitable Institutions'. This was hardly the language to mollify any opposition. The Collection begins with a plan of the Infirmary and the proposed extension and recounts in detail the proposals for the fever wards which, when the garret was floored, made room for 20 fever patients instead of twelve – here said Dr Clark, opposition began. Clark also restates his belief that infection in 'Fevers' spread by 'contagion' from patients or their clothes, but not through the air at any distance. That, in fact, is the real point of difference between the adversaries. 'Fevers' had not been differentiated other than smallpox, measles and scarlet fever and there was little knowledge of methods of spread and none of causal organisms. 'Contagion' seemed to mean spread through air, particularly in crowded and ill- ventilated rooms, but also it was believed by some that it could operate at considerable distances. The protagonists simply were at cross purposes, arguing with more feeling than knowledge.

The *Collection* also contains his earlier correspondence with 24 physicians all over the country asking their opinion upon Fever Wards and the arrangement he proposed. His letter and their replies he now published in detail, claiming support for his views. The answers, however, vary considerably and probably not all his correspondents had fully appreciated the situation in Newcastle. They occupy 120 pages of the *Collection of Papers* and are followed by reprints of other letters sent to the Court of 24 June – letters from 'A Governor', from Dr Wood, from 'A Governor of the Infirmary', from Mr Ingham who denied he had ever heard a hint that any part of the new building was to be used as a fever house for the reception of patients in general. In it he states 'I will maintain there are other ways of communicating the contagion of fever besides proximity to the infected'.

There were further letters both for and against the fever unit and a second communication from Mr Ingham on 20 June, just before the meeting on the 24th. In it he says he did not concur at any time with the establishment of a fever house for the reception of patients in general, but would support the establishment of a fever house in a proper situation. In view of the final outcome, this is very significant. All that collection of 239 pages was presumably printed and circulated at Dr Clark's personal expense.[48] But it was only a beginning. Three days later on 17 August, Dr Fenwick published a letter supporting Dr Clark's views.[49] In 36 pages he argued the advantages of an 'attached' fever house but then said that 'if it be not granted' it was the duty of those in opposition to bring forward a plan for a separate Fever House.

In September came a broadside from Frederick Horn. Not only did he argue strongly for a House of Recovery 'at a proper distance' but he documented the growth of the proposed Fever Wards at the Infirmary from two rooms each of six beds for infectious diseases of accidental occurrence to a unit of 20 beds occupying the garrett also, and the growth of the idea of a Board of Health. That, with a great deal of self justification, required a preface of 20 pages and a reply of 88 pages.[50]

All these publications must certainly have fuelled considerable local controversy and matters needed to be brought to a head. That step was taken at the Weekly Meeting on 23 September when Mr Stokoe the Architect was directed to give an account of the sum expended beyond the estimate and the alterations 'which have occasioned such excess'. The Secretary was also directed to call a meeting 'to determine the propriety and expediency of opening for general reception the Fever House annexed to the Infirmary and also, if judged necessary, to rescind such part of the 15th rule for the Governance of the Charity as may be supposed to apply to the admissability of contagious fevers' – Clark's opponents had mounted their offensive.

Although I cannot find any reference in the Minutes, Dr Clark, after the meeting of 24 June, had appealed to the Bishop of Durham as Grand Visitor, who had then requested a meeting of a Special Court for 12 October. At that meeting the Bishop was in the Chair and no fewer than 240 Governors were present so that proceedings were adjourned to the nearby Assembly Rooms. Hume says that after protracted debate, a compromise was reached but the minutes simply state that the following resolution was moved from the chair and unanimously adopted:[51]

> It appearing to this Court that the measure of opening for general acception the Fever Wards of the Infirmary is disapproved by many of the respectable inhabitants of Newcastle (although it is the opinion of very many of the most eminent physicians that such fever wards may be opened for general acceptance with perfect safety — an opinion confirmed by the uniform experience of every Hospital in which such wards have been established) — and that a proposition has been made to establish a House for the general reception of Fevers detached from any inhabited building — Resolved that in the event that such a separate House of Reception together with the funds for its support be not approved by the Grand Visitor on the 31st day of October 1803 he be then empowered to order the Fever House annexed to the Infirmary to be opened for the general reception of Fever Patients.

It was then resolved that the proceedings be advertised twice.

The names of Governors attending this meeting are not given and there is no indication that Clark was amongst those present. Those who opposed Clark and his supporters had indeed won the day and patients with 'contagious' fevers would not in future be admitted to the Infirmary.

It is difficult to think that the Court had not been 'packed' and the long resolution hardly seems spontaneous. Furthermore there must have been the expectation that funds to build a 'House of Recovery' within a year were, or would become available despite the fact that the alteration and extension of the Infirmary was proving much more expensive than originally estimated.

The final phase

Clark by then was both ill and disappointed. Yet he would not remain silent, and, in December 1802, he published a 'second part' of the *Collection of Papers intended to Promote an Institution for the cure and prevention of Fevers*.[52] They were offered as a complement to the Collection published in August. Some had already appeared in print. The first 36 pages are 'Remarks on Mr Horn's letter to the Governors of the Infirmary'. This is followed by correspondence which Dr Clark had undertaken with physicians in many centres. Next is a reprinting of the letter from JR Fenwick in answer to Mr Horn's Pamphlet (13 pages). Clark then prints further letters 'Relative to the economy, safety and necessity of opening the Fever-House annexed to the

Infirmary'. Next he reprints the Requisition to the Lord Bishop asking for a Special Court. That request carried the names of 122 Governors, (2 staff members).

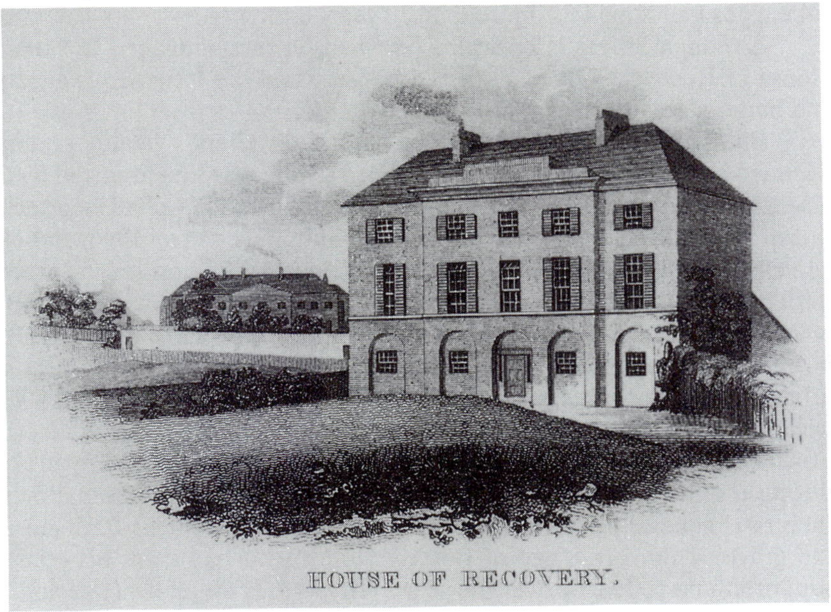

Figure 5. The House of Recovery, Wardens Close, 1804.

It is followed by a proposal for a House of Recovery dated 28 September 1802 which states that 'At a Common Council held yesterday, the Mayor of Newcastle be authorised to subscribe such a sum as may appear to him necessary towards establishing a house for the general reception of contagious fevers, detached from any inhabited building – signed by 88 Governors (including four staff members) who offered support and help towards the establishment of a House of Recovery. It was dated 28 September, only seven days after the Requisition to the Bishop.

Somehow the resolution adopted at the Special Court on 12 October had grown from those two conflicting views.

Clark wrote a further 100 pages on 'Summary remarks on the means of exterminating Typhous Fever, The Scarlet Fever and the Smallpox in Cities; in Towns; in Country Villages; in Boarding Schools and in Private Families'.[52]

It was Clark's last effort. He did not often attend meetings while the alterations to the Infirmary went slowly on and financial worries increased. But he did not resign from the Infirmary.

The provision of a Fever Hospital did proceed; the Corporation gave a site in Wardens Close just outside the Town Wall. Subscriptions were raised and the hospital opened in 1804. In 1805 the Infirmary minutes record that patients with 'accidental Fevers' were removed from the Infirmary to the

House of Recovery and at the costs to relatives or overseers of the Parish. The patients were looked after and medicines supplied from the Dispensary but there was no attempt to form a Board of Health as Clark and his colleagues had hoped for more than 10 years earlier.

Although Hume is critical, Clark had, in fact, managed to obtain a House of Recovery linked to the Dispensary and the Infirmary was larger and better suited to its purpose than previously.[53]

But Fenwick says that from this time on Clark's health gradually declined and 'in the last week of October 1804 he was first attacked by that disease which was destined to close it'.[54] He seems to have had an attack of intestinal obstruction which was relieved, but followed in mid-November by a second and more severe attack. Yet he endeavoured to continue in practice until the end of 1804. In January 1805 he left for Cheltenham and then Bath where his attacks of obstruction continued and became more severe. At Bath he met and spent much time with Dr Currie of Liverpool who also was affected by his last illness. Of similar outlook, they were firm friends. Fenwick, who had also travelled to Bath and was often present at the meetings of Clark and Currie, writes very sensitively of the time.[54] But early in April during another attack Clark developed signs of peritoneal inflammation and then fatal general peritonitis. He was buried at Weston near Bath close to the grave of the Mr Bigge of Benton House who had been his constant supporter and colleague over the years. He was only 60 years of age and had spent half his life in Newcastle.

The Infirmary minutes for April 1805 simply record his death without any expression of thanks for his services or of sympathy for his family. The report of the Dispensary for that year makes no reference to his death – his name simply disappears. Yet by Clark's efforts the Infirmary had been re-organised, and the Dispensary founded and established so that it continued to serve the community until 1948.

Epilogue

Clark lived before the beginning of knowledge of bacteriology, but he thought in terms of prevention and limitation of spread of disease in the community as well as its treatment in the individual. He understood the need for organisation, and design in hospitals, the importance of record keeping and numerical information. His origins were humble in a world where social standing and acceptance were important. As a lowland Scot educated near home, he entered a town where clannishness was strong. He needed to be tough to make his way whatever the superficial politenesses, and medical practice was competitive. As one of many Scots coming to the towns of the North, he certainly earned a reputation for brusqueness and plain speaking. Yet, in just two years he had been the greatest influence in the foundation of the Dispensary – and that against considerable opposition from the staff of the Infirmary. When at last he was elected a physician to the Infirmary there seems always to have been tension between physicians and surgeons with the latter very conscious that the Infirmary had a surgical emphasis from the beginning and very anxious that there should always be room for their own patients so often 'emergencies' as a result of accidents. The physicians and surgeons were both trying to cope with different situations without either the technical knowledge or basic resources to do so. Both were the prisoners of their time. Yet looking back after nearly two centuries one cannot but be sad that Clark pushed his case too hard and suffered in so far as his real achievement in establishing the Dispensary was never sufficiently recognised or remembered. Paradoxically, in the 1802 settlement he obtained the House of Recovery he had wanted ten years earlier and its care devolved upon the staff of the Dispensary as he had wished. Seventy years later it became part of the Municipal Health Department after Dr HE Armstrong, the first Medical Officer of Health, moved into that position from the Dispensary where he was Resident Medical Officer. John Clark deserves to be remembered.

In an interleaved collection of papers published at this time and used by someone associated with the Infirmary during the early years of the 19th Century there is a handwritten anonymous poem of some nine verses. Its old oxidised words reveal something of what one Governor, and perhaps many others, thought of the behaviour of the adversaries at the time. The first and second verses run:

The Devil amongst the Doctors

1. Doctor Clark, Doctor Clark
You should now cease to bark
By squabbling you never can win it:
And you'd no right at all,
When once sent to the wall
Thus fiercely again to begin it.

2. And you Mr Ingham
Can ne'er indeed bring 'em
To join you by furiously fighting;
And believe me 'tis true
Tho' I say it of you,
That you damn your own cause by your writing.

(Anon)

Acknowledgements

In the preparation of this paper I have received much help and encouragement and wish to thank particularly the Staffs of the Tyne and Wear Archives, the Robinson Library of the University of Newcastle upon Tyne and the Library of the Literary and Philosophical Society of Newcastle upon Tyne.

The author also wishes to thank the Wellcome Trust for support during the later stages of the preparation of this paper.

Figures 2, 3 and 4 are taken from illustrations in *Description and historical account of the town and county of newcastle upon tyne and its vicinity*, Mackenzie E, 1827.

The figures have been prepared by the Audio-Visual Department, University of Newcastle upon Tyne.

Efficient secretarial help was cheerfully given by Mrs Cora Wheeler.

References

1. Watson RS. *History of the Literary and Philosophical Society of Newcastle upon Tyne 1795-1896.* London: Walter Scott, 1897:46.
2. Fenwick JR. *Sketch of the Professional Life and Character of John Clark MD.* Newcastle upon Tyne: S Hodgson, 1806:67.
3. Ramsay J. *Letter printed with the address of JR Fenwick.* (Ref 2)
4. Mackenzie E. *Description and Historical Account of the Town and County of Newcastle upon Tyne and its Vicinity.* Newcastle upon Tyne: Mackenzie and Dent, 1827:105.
5. Hume GH. *History of the Newcastle Infirmary. Newcastle upon Tyne.* Newcastle upon Tyne: Andrew Reid, 1906.
6. Hume Sir WE. *The Infirmary, Newcastle upon Tyne 1751-1951.* Newcastle upon Tyne: Andrew Reid, 1951:24-6.
7. Hume GH. *op cit*:33-6.
8. Hume Sir WE. *op cit*:18.
9. Risse GB. *Hospital Life in Enlightenment Scotland.* Cambridge University Press, 1986:7-25.
10. Fenwick JR. *op cit* ref 2:3-4.
11. *ibid*:4.
12. Clark J. *Observations on Diseases which prevail in Long Voyages to hot Climates.* London: Murray, 1792:15.
13. *ibid*:18-9.
14. *ibid*:22-9.
15. *ibid*:31-2.
16. Pybus FC. The Company of Barber Surgeons and Tallow Chandlers of Newcastle upon Tyne. *Newcastle Med J* 1928; *9*:147-63.
17. Miller FJW. The Infirmary on the Forth 1753-1906 *Archaeologia Aeliana* 1986; Fifth Series, *14*:143-65.
18. Pickstone JV, Butler SVF. The Politics of Medicine in Manchester 1788-1792: Hospital Reform and Public Health Services in the Early Industrial City. *Med Hist* 1984; *28*:227-49.
19. Mackenzie E. *op cit* ref 4:504.
20. Whithead W. *Newcastle Directory for 1778.* Newcastle upon Tyne: Thomas Angus, 1778.
21. Fenwick JR. *op cit* ref 2:43-4.
22. Church of the Divine Unity, Hanover Square, Newcastle upon Tyne, *Register of births and baptisms 1779-1844.* Tyne and Wear Archives Service, TWAS:1787/9.
23. *Dictionary of National Biography. 10*:403.
24. Fenwick JR. *op cit* ref 2:8-9.
25. Aikin J. *Thoughts on Hospitals (with a letter to the author by Thomas Percival).* London: Johnson, 1771:82.

26. Comrie JD. *History of Scottish Medicine to 1860.* London: Bailliere Tindal & Cox, 1927:131.

27. Loudon ISL. The Origins and Growth of the Dispensary Movement in England. *Bull Hist Med* 1981; *55*:322-42.

28. Pickstone JV, Butler SVF. The Politics of Medicine in Manchester 1788-1792: Hospital Reform and Public Health Services in the Early Industrial City. *Med Hist* 1984; *28*:227-49.

29. Anon. 1 *A Plan for Instituting a Public Dispensary.* Newcastle upon Tyne: Saint, 1777.

30. Anon. 2 *An Account of the Newcastle Dispensary for the Relief of the Poor instituted 1777 published by Order of the Governors.* Newcastle upon Tyne: Saint, 1778.

31. Clark J. *Observations on Fevers especially those of the Continuous type and on the Scarlet Fever attended with Ulcerated Sore-Throat as it appeared at Newcastle upon Tyne in the year 1778.* London: Cadell, 1780.

32. Anon. 3 *Proposals for Promoting General Inoculation in Newcastle.* Newcastle upon Tyne: S Hodgson, 1786.

33. Anon. 4 *The History and Statutes of the Newcastle Dispensary.* Newcastle upon Tyne: Hall & Elliott, 1790.

34. Miller FJW. The Newcastle Dispensary 1777-1976. *Archaelogia Aeliana* 1990; Fifth Series, *18*:177-95.

35. Leslie PD. *An account of the Epidemic of Continued Fever commonly called Influenza as it appeared in the City and Environs of Durham in the month of June 1782.* London: Crowder, 1784.

36. Infirmary Minutes. *Special Court of Governors 12 April 1787.* Tyne and Wear Archives Service, TWAS HO/RVI/2/9.

37. Fenwick JR. *op cit* ref 2:45-50.

38. Infirmary Minutes. *Quarterly Court, 15th May 1788.* Tyne and Wear Archive Service, TWAS HO/RVI/2/9.

39. Anon. 3 *Proposals for Promoting General Inoculation in Newcastle.* Newcastle upon Tyne: S Hodgson, 1786.

40. Hume WE. The Medical Societies of Newcastle upon Tyne. *Newc Med J* 1958; *25*:163-226.

41. Mackenzie E. *op cit* ref 4:503.

42. Anon. 5 *A code of Statues and Rules for the Government of the Infirmary.* Newcastle upon Tyne: Walker, 1801.

43. Clark J. *Letter sent to all Governors 11th June 1801 reprinted in 'A Collection of Papers relative to the safety and importance of annexing Fever Wards to the Newcastle and other Infirmaries'.* Newcastle upon Tyne: S Hodgson, 1802:206-21.

44. Clark J. *A Code of Statutes and Rules for the Government of the Infirmary, – and of the Plan lately adopted for its Internal Improvement and Extension.* Newcastle upon Tyne: Walker, 1801.

45. Clark J. *A Collection of Papers intended to promote an Institution for the Cure and Prevention of Infectious Fevers ... together with the communications of the most eminent physicians ... annexing Fever Wards to the Newcastle and other Infirmaries. Part Second.* Newcastle upon Tyne: S Hodgson, 1802:62.

46. Clark J. *An Account of the Plan for the Internal Improvement and extension of the Infirmary at Newcastle, October 11th, 1801.* Newcastle upon Tyne: Walker, 1801:52.

47. Anon. 7 *Dispensary Committee. Proceedings for Promoting an Institution for the Cure and Prevention of Contagious Fevers in Newcastle and Gateshead.* Newcastle upon Tyne: S Hodgson, 1802:26-8.

48. Clark J. *A Collection of Papers intended to promote an Institution for the Cure and Prevention of Infectious Fevers in Newcastle and other populous Towns.* Newcastle upon Tyne: S Hodgson, 1802:239.

49. Fenwick JR. *State of the Question relating to the Proposal of annexing Fever Wards to the Newcastle Infirmary Addressed to the Governors.* Newcastle upon Tyne: S Hodgson, 1802:36.

50. Horn F. *A Letter to the Governors of the Infirmary at Newcastle occasioned by the late Publications of Drs Clark and Fenwick. Preface 20 pages.* Newcastle upon Tyne: Brown, 1802:88.

51. Hume GH. *op cit* ref 7:34.

52. Clark J. *op cit* ref 45:230.

53. Hume GH. *op cit* ref 7:36.

54. Fenwick JR. *op cit* ref 2:30.

I have made extensive use of the Minutes of the Court of Governors and the Weekly Committee of the Newcastle Infirmary which are held in the Tyne and Wear Archives in Blandford Street, Newcastle upon Tyne, NE1 4JA under the following reference numbers.

TWAS	HO/RVI/2/1	29 May 1751 - 25 April 1754
TWAS	HO/RVI/2/2	8 Oct 1753 - 10 Jan 1760
TWAS	HO/RVI/2/3	31 Jan 1760 - 13 Dec 1764
TWAS	HO/RVI/2/6	6 April 1769 - 30 March 1775
TWAS	HO/RVI/2/7	6 April 1775 - 6 June 1783
TWAS	HO/RVI/2/8	3 July 1783 - 28 March 1786
TWAS	HO/RVI/2/9	6 April 1786 - 12 Aug 1790
TWAS	HO/RVI/2/10	18 Dec 1794 - 12 April 1798
TWAS	HO/RVI/2/11	19 April 1798 - 21 May 1801
TWAS	HO/RVI/2/13	8 Nov 1804 - 30 March 1809

Chapter 8

THE LIFE AND WORK OF WILLIAM HEWSON, HAEMATOLOGIST AND IMMUNOLOGIST

Nicholas Wilford.

Introduction

William Hewson was one of the most accomplished anatomists of the 18th century. Born in Hexham and trained there and in Newcastle, he went to London and became a pupil and later a colleague of the brothers John and William Hunter. He made remarkable discoveries in his tragically short career. This account of his life is a modified version of an essay successfully submitted in 1991 for the William Hume Essay Prize.

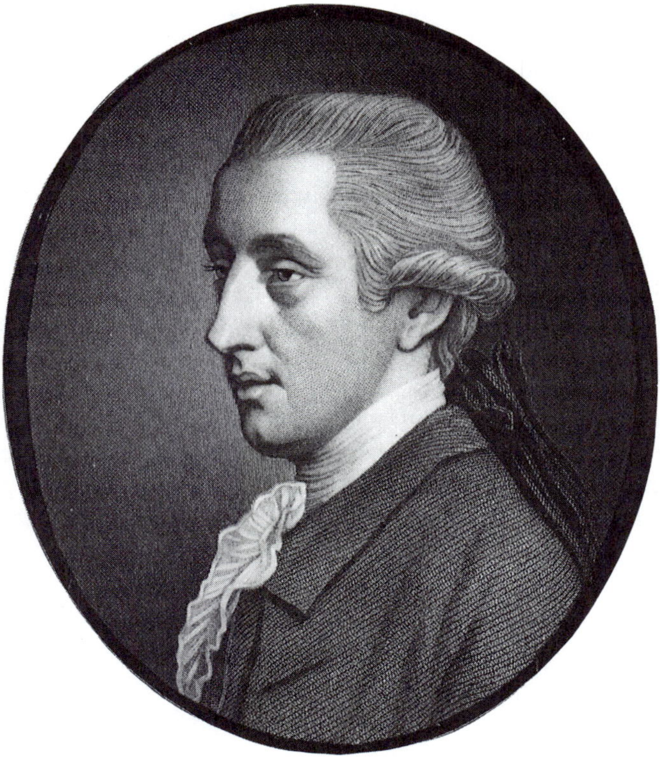

Figure 1. William Hewson

> I forget whether I ever acknowledged the receipt of the prints of Mr Hewson. I have one of them framed in my study. I think it is very like.
>
> ***Benjamin Franklin***

The early years

William Hewatson (he adopted the form Hewson many years later in London) was born on 14 Nov 1739 at Hexham, where his father had a practice as a surgeon and apothecary. William's mother was of the prominent local family Heron and was born in the town. Hexham in the early 18th century was 'not very populous'; Hutchinson in about 1743 had computed its inhabitants at 2000 souls.[1] However the town had some important manufacturing industries (including the making of leather, gloves and hats) and workers in these industries, and in the extensive local farming community, would have been in need of a surgeon and the drugs of an apothecary.[2]

William was one of 11 children. From an early age he stood out among them in talent and aptitude, and was sent to the Royal Free Grammar School in Hexham, which was at the time in the charge of Rev Abraham Brown, a curate from nearby Whitley and a famous teacher. William found no difficulty in gaining very good results in all subjects.[2] When he left school his father decided to give him a training in his own profession, and William was soon sufficiently knowledgeable of the work of an apothecary to be of assistance in the preparation and dispensing of drugs and was considered responsible enough to visit his father's patients.

After a few years he was apprenticed to his father's friend in Newcastle-upon-Tyne, the eminent surgeon Mr Richard Lambert. Here William soon developed a detailed knowledge of human anatomy. Mr Lambert had recently formed a medical charity in a house in Gallowgate, which was later to become the Newcastle Infirmary.[2] By the time William joined Lambert the Infirmary, with additions and improvements, was receiving patients and was well established, providing a stimulating environment both for study and practice.

When Hewatson's apprenticeship came to an end he moved to London to further his knowledge and to gain experience. Mr Lambert's reputation was nationally known and William therefore found little difficulty in being admitted to Guy's and St Thomas' where he attended the lectures of Dr Colin Mackenzie (midwifery), Dr Hugh Smith (physic) and Dr William Hunter (anatomy).[2]

The Hunters, William and his brother John, soon considered Hewatson to be sufficiently skilled and reponsible that during the Seven Years War when John Hunter was away, Hewatson was left in charge of both pupils and patients,[3] and thereby 'he gained money when most students in surgery are spending it'.[4]

It was at this time that William began to write his name 'Hewson'. Mackenzie suggests that the Londoners' 'habits of abbreviation' pronounced it so, and William therefore began to spell his name in order to suit their pronunciation,[5] but perhaps the Northumberland accent had something to do with their misinterpretation.

William Hunter thought so highly of him that he suggested that if Hewson were to study for a year in Edinburgh he would take him into partnership on his return. So Hewson travelled north, carrying letters of recommendation from both Hunter and the great Sir John Pringle (of military medicine and sanitation fame, and a well known member of the Royal Society).

During his academic session at the University of Edinburgh he studied under Professors Alexander Monro *secundus*, Cullen and Gregory, before returning to London in 1762. Monro is thought to have been a particular influence on Hewson, as indeed he was on the study and science of anatomy throughout the country. But Hewson was intelligent enough to form his own opinions on many of the disputed questions, and his relative disrespect for learning anatomy by careful note-taking at lectures may have aggravated the later disagreements with his former teacher.

The following year, at the tender age of 24, he became a partner and joint lecturer in anatomy with Hunter in Litchfield Street. During the summer of 1765 he studied in France, Flanders and Holland before returning for the autumn anatomy lectures.Though his professional rise was rapid and demanding, William continued to make frequent visits to Hexham, after his father died in 1767, to visit his family and to ensure they lived sufficiently well.[6]

The treatment of pneumothorax

In 1767 Hewson suggested that air in the pleural cavity (which he described as emphysema, but now known as pneumothorax) was responsible for the 'difficulty in breathing, and shortness of breath, tightness in the chest and the sense of suffocation' sometimes seen after fractures of the ribs. Since these symptoms were similar to those of hydrops pectoris (pleural effusion) and empyema he suggested that a similar method of treatment might be of benefit, and as a result Hewson's first published work was on 'The Operation of Paracentesis Thoracis, proposed for Air in the Chest, with some remarks on the Emphysema and on Wounds of the Lungs in general'. This was read by William Hunter to the Society of Physicians in 1767, published in their *Medical Observations and Enquiries*,[7] and reprinted by the Sydenham Society in 1846.[8] A controversy soon arose however between Hewson and his renowned former lecturer, Professor Monro, regarding the origin of these ideas. Monro declared that he 'had made that observation' in his lectures in 1761 and earlier. After various bitter communications Hewson conceded thus:

> About the middle of last Summer I was told by a gentleman from Edinburgh of your manner of treating me, at which time I was a little surprised, as I was not conscious of having given you the least cause of complaint. But having since learned from other gentlemen who attended your lectures before the time of publishing that paper (and who at my request, consulted their notes) that you had mentioned it, I cannot now doubt that you had made the observation before me. At the same time I must assure you, that to suppose I knew it at the time of publishing that paper was doing me an injustice.[6]

The Lymphatic System

It was his next series of investigations however which brought him distinction, but also into another bitter controversy with Monro, regarding the priority of the discovery of the lymphatic system. In 1768 Hewson spent some time at Brighton, where he carried out experiments on monkfish in order to establish whether a lymphatic system existed in fish. He had already used small live fish from London markets but had no success with these or with larger dead ones. After many failures, both with skate and cod, he was 'at last so fortunate to discover the lacteals and get a pipe into one of those vessels on the mesentery of each of these fish; and injecting by this pipe, I found where the larger vessels lay; after which there was but little difficulty in tracing the whole system.' These celebrated findings are now acknowledged as the first known descriptions of the lymphatic system in fish.

The results of Hewson's investigations with fish and also with 'amphibia' (a term which then applied to turtles) were read by William Hunter to the Fellows of the Royal Society, and in the Society's Journal Book is the following entry:[9]

> Mr Hewson's descriptions were greatly illustrated by the exhibition of a series of preparations taken from turtles and divers fishes, wherein these vessels were injected and shown to the naked eye in their rise, progress, communications and insertions, to the great satisfaction of the Society. Thanks were returned to Dr Hunter and Mr Hewson for these very ingenious communications.

Hewson's findings were important. The Hunters had suggested that lymphatics have an absorptive role, but until then no lacteals or lymphatics had been identified in fish. The subsequent recognition by Magendie that the blood vessels also have an absorptive function obviously showed the Hunters' conclusions regarding the lymphatic system to be at that time premature though, as we now know, correct.

In 1770 Hewson was elected a Fellow of the Royal Society (his proposers including Sir John Pringle, William Hunter and Benjamin Franklin, the American philosopher) and he was later awarded Sir Godfrey Copley's Gold Medal 'for his papers on the lymphatic system in birds, amphibious animals and fishes'. These achievements were completed at the age of 31. William Hunter, 20 years his senior, had become a Fellow only three years previously and was never awarded the Copley Medal.

At this time, Hewson's dispute with Monro was mainly concerned with the discovery of the lymphatic system in birds and turtles. Monro wrote to the Royal Society claiming priority for these discoveries and later published a pamphlet (1770) repeating the claim. Hewson's reply, in an appendix to his *Experimental Inquiries* Part 1,(8) conceded the point, discussed earlier, about the operation of paracentesis, but with reference to the lymphatic system he successfully vindicated his priority. In addition, some years previously John Hunter had made observations on the 'absorbent' vessels of birds and reptiles, and the following passage from Hunter's *Essays and Observations* reveals that Hewson was aware of them:

> In the beginning of the winter 1764-5, I got a crocodile which had been in a 'show' for several years in London before it died. It was .... perhaps, the largest ever seen in this country, ... and was about five feet long when it died. I sent to Mr Hewson, and before I opened it, I read over to him my former descriptions of the dissections of this animal, relative to the 'absorbing system', both of some of the larger lymphatics and of the lacteals, with a view to see how far these descriptions would agree with the appearances in the animal now before us, and on comparing them they exactly corresponded. This was the crocodile from which Mr. Hewson took his observation of the colour of the chyle. The intention of my showing this crocodile, and also reading my former dissections to Mr Hewson was, that he might see that I had a tolerable description of this system in the Amphibia; because I found him busy in the pursuit of this system in various animals, and hinting himself to be the discoverer of it even in birds, and to convince him that this description must have been written some considerable time before, in all probability before my going abroad. As crocodiles are seldom to be had in this country, I could hardly have dissected two crocodiles, besides this, between May 1763 (the time I returned from Portugal), or the autumn 1763, when the turtle was dissected, and the beginning of the winter 1764-5. Mr Hewson at the time appeared satisfied, or at least made no remarks.[10]

The Monro-Hewson controversy was said by a medical journalist of the 1820s to have:

> excited more interest than the subject of the discovery; for, instead of its being followed up by the investigations of succeeding anatomists into the anatomical disposition of the absorbent system in other animals than those in which its presence had been ascertained and described by Monro and Hewson, so entirely did the interest cease and the matter fall into abeyance, that a physiologist of the present day has raised a question whether there was any truth in the discovery at all.

The physiologist in question was Magendie. Though some of Hewson's initial theories and conclusions were incorrect, he was able to demonstrate clearly the absorbent function of lymphatic vessels, that lacteals and lymphatics interconnect to form one system, that this system has an extensive distribution and that the fluid in this system can coagulate. Hewson identified that the red lines leading from wounds are a result of lymphatic inflammation and he described the metastatic nature of cancer when passing between various groups of lymph nodes.

Marriage and professional discord

In 1768 Hewson first met Miss Mary Stevenson, whom he was later to marry on 10 July 1770 (honeymooning in Hexham). Mary (usually known as Polly) was the daughter of the lady with whom Dr Franklin resided during his 15 years in London, and Franklin was so fond of Polly that he could hardly have been more pleased if his own son had married her.

In 1769 Hewson left the apartment in Windmill Street allotted to him by Hunter ever since the anatomical school had opened, and moved to nearby Broad Street in order to remain near the lecture theatres. He continued to teach with Hunter and take his share of the profits for two further years. Hunter then announced that, since Hewson now had a family (his first son had been born some months previously) and was no longer living under the same roof, he would not be able adequately to carry out his duties, and the partnership was dissolved. Obviously Hewson was surprised and saddened, and later angry when he learnt that he would not be allowed to take away the preparations that he himself had made. Evidently there had been an agreement that any preparations Hewson made during the partnership would remain in his own possession if it were ever dissolved. William Hunter saw things a little differently and made his views clear as follows:

> Dr. Hunter expects Mr. Hewson should go on with his Business as usual during the Remainder of the Term they are to continue together; and during that time should make Preparations, at Dr. Hunter's Expence, such as the Dr. should direct to be made, and others, so that those directed are not neglected or omitted: That all the Preparations are to be the Doctor's sole Property, and at his absolute Disposal, so that if he afterwards should give any of them to any Person (which he would not be understood to promise) such Gift is to be considered as the sole Effect of his Goodwill.[11]

It seems that the Hunters were famous for their short tempers, and both their intransigence to argument and their often very unreserved language were well known. Benjamin Franklin was called in to act as a mediator between Hewson and Hunter and among his papers is a list of William Hunter's petty, but amusing complaints regarding Hewson's conduct; these include:[12]

> That he gave Leave to go to Blenheim once, but not repeatedly, not for an Absence of 10 days from Business, which was the more inconvenient as Dr. H. was then indisposed with a Lax....
>
> That Mr. H. would have used a Body of Dr. Hunter's Purchasing to make a Skeleton, who it could not be expected should purchase Bodies for him for such purposes.
>
> That he had employ'd a Man to pick Bones out of the Tubs and fit up a Skeleton for him, without Leave of Dr. H. which ought not to have been done till the Lectures were over.
>
> That Mr. H.'s Behaviour to Dr. H. was extreamly rude, and that he had said, *he was a Fool to expect that Dr. H. would act like a Gentleman.*

Franklin was able to secure a partial reconciliation, though Hewson did not receive all of his preparations. It is interesting that Hunter used Franklin's help in order that some of the preparations could be returned without loss of face. Franklin writes thus:[13]

> Some time last Summer, after your Parting, you wrote me a Note, which I cannot at present find, but I think the Purport of it was, that you had some Preparations which you could spare, and were dispos'd to give me, desiring I would call and look at them; I did so, and accepted them. I apprehended it to be your Supposition in giving them to me, that as I had no Use for them, I should probably give them to Mr. Hewson, which I immediately did.

It is thought that neither Hunter nor Hewson bore any long term animosity towards each other and some of Hunter's later writings are full of praise for Hewson's achievements.

The specimens which were returned were to make an important contribution to Hewson's own school of anatomy. He established a demonstration theatre and classes in Craven St, Strand and built a large adjoining house for his family. He set to work at once to prepare a series of specimens to illustrate his teaching, many of them similar to those he had made for William Hunter's museum. Among the Hunterian manuscripts preserved in the library of the University of Glasgow is one giving descriptions of about 60 injected specimens. These cannot now be traced but it seems likely that they would have formed a very interesting collection. Some of them were of whole bodies with a two colour injection:

> The head and trunk of a lad about 16 injected red by the arteries and yellow by the veins, the heart also injected and in situ. The trunks of the great veins and the whole vena portarum are the objects aimed at. Cava superior, the two subclavians and two jugulars are well seen, so is the cava inferior but vena portarum is particularly well injected and dissected — a beautiful preparation.

It was not just the elder Hunter however who is recorded as objecting to Hewson's conduct; John Hunter recorded his own impressions of Hewson's work:

> First he published what was not his own, second he published what was not his own, third he published what was not his own, fourth he published what is disputed or denied and fifth he published nonsense.[14]

Regarding this charge of plagiarism, it has already been noted that Hewson's papers on the 'absorbents' in birds, reptiles and fish had been presented to the Royal Society by John Hunter's brother William in 1768 and 1769. If there had been any suspicion at that time of incorrect procedure, then one would have thought that the Hunters would have revealed it, particularly John, who was never shy of controversy. Benjamin Rush in his *Travels Through Life* left this record: 'It was while I was dissecting a body by his side that Dr. Hewson succeeded in an experiment which proved the existence of lymphatic vessels in Fishes.'[15] John Hunter's discovery of lymphatic vessels in the necks of birds had always been adequately acknowledged by Hewson, although Hunter remained suspicious that Hewson would attempt to steal some undue credit.

Blood morphology, haematopoiesis and coagulation

Before he began to teach his anatomy course Hewson gave an inaugural lecture to the leading scientists of London, on 'The Spleen and Thymus'.[16] He spoke of the lymphocyte-distributing function of the thymus, the reason for its gradual atrophy in early adolescent life and perhaps even previewed Burnet's concept of 'first' and 'second' level lymphocytes, all these ideas being suggested many years before they became more firmly recognised. He examined the fluid of the lymphatics and the thymus and noted the 'pale globules' in the blood, thus describing the lymphocytes common to all these fluids.[17]

In addition to his observations regarding the lymphatic systems in a number of animals and his findings that the absorptive function of the lacteals was 'on the extremities of the villi', Hewson's *Experimental Inquiries* document some other very important findings, particularly concerning blood cell formation and morphology. Although Leeuwenhoek and others had seen that the red cells of amphibia were flat and elliptical they had still believed that human and quadruped red blood cells were globular. Magnus Falconar, who completed and published the third part of *Experimental Inquiries* after Hewson's death, thought that this misconception was rather amazing, but attributed it to the great concentration of corpuscles in human and mammalian blood which would make the shape of individual cells difficult to determine. However, he found that when human red cells were diluted with serum so that individual cells could be distinguished, the discoid nature of the cells became apparent. Some had previously suggested that red cells were annular; the careful observations of Hewson and Falconar showed this not to be so. They did, however, make several errors in observation and therefore in the resultant theories; they failed to realise that the red cells were biconcave and that the dark spot seen at their centre was only an optical expression of this fact.

In the third experiment, the effects on blood cells of what we now call osmosis were investigated. An animal's requirement for serum salts, in order to keep blood cells flat, was recognised in what was possibly one of the earliest examples of the concept of physiological saline.[6]

The fifth experiment was devoted to a theoretical discussion of blood cell formation and thymic function. Hewson had suggested that one role for the lymphatic system might be in blood cell formation in addition to its suggested role in the absorption of nutrients. He tied a ligature around a thymus *in vivo* and many lymphatic ducts became visible. Microscopic examination of their contents revealed a fluid which was identical to that in the lymphatic glands; it contained:

..a great number of small, white, solid particles, exactly resembling in size and shape the central particles found in the vesicles in the blood, or such as are found in the fluid of the lymphatic glands.[17]

Hewson concluded that the lymphatics are probably the excretory ducts of the thymus and suggested that the microscopic cells are common to both the circulatory and the lymphatic systems.[18] When he incised the thymus a 'white thick fluid' oozed out, exactly as it did from the lymph nodes, and when this fluid was diluted with serum and Glauber's solution it contained:

..small particles precisely corresponding with those found in the lymphatic vessels passing from the thymus, and with those found in the fluid of the lymphatic glands.[19]

Hewson thus identified the lymphocyte as a common component of certain body fluids and concluded that:

One use of the thymus is to secrete from the blood a fluid, containing numberless small particles, similar to those found in the lymphatic glands; and that the lymphatic vessels arising from the thymus convey this secreted fluid through the thoracic duct into the blood vessels, and thus become the excretory ducts to this gland.[19]

He suggested that the structure and uses of the thymus are 'similar to those of the lymphatic glands, to which it may be considered as an appendage'.[19]

On opening a lymphatic vessel close to a lymphatic gland both 'solid particles' (lymphocytes) and 'solid particles within vesicles' (red blood cells) were identified. Hewson and Falconar thought that the particles within the vesicles were the same as those which were not surrounded, and that in the latter either the vesicle was a secretion from the particle or that lymphatic vessels are able to form 'vesicles' from lymphatic fluid. They thought that the vessel, in addition to supplying the vesicle was also able to give the corpuscle its red colour, as up to this point the central particle was white. Obviously Hewson mistook lymphocytes as being the dark particles identical with those seen at the centre of the red cell, and he and Falconar failed to realise that the red cells seen in the lymphatics occurred there by accident in the preparation of the specimen. As a result of these misconceptions, they postulated the erroneous theory that red cells were formed in the lymph glands, thymus and spleen, where they were built up from a central 'solid particle' and a red 'vesicular' portion derived from the walls of the lymphatic vessels. These errors can generally be attributed to the inadequacies of simple microscopes and to the fact that the cells were observed without prior staining. That Hewson and Falconar observed as much as they did, is a remarkable tribute to their own powers of observation and to the skill of the craftsmen who made their lenses.[6]

Hewson also drew attention to the 'curious circumstance of the thymus being largest in the earlier periods of life, and becoming gradually less as the animal advances towards maturity' and the fact that this is a constant occurrence in the human subject. From this he logically concluded that:[20]

> The thymus is necessary to perform an office requisite in the foetus-state, and in the early part of life ...[and] ..that it may act as an auxilliary to the lymphatic system, for the purpose of forming more of the central particles of the blood than could have been made by the lymphatic glands alone during that time, when nature needs them most...

Thus Hewson thought that the thymus was large in the fetus, because the need for blood was greater in fetal life than the lymphatic glands could supply. As the animal grew larger and the lymphatic system more extensive, it would be able to produce the amount of blood required without help from the thymus. It was also suggested that the thymus gland is placed in the chest because the space it occupies there is not required during fetal life. After birth, when respiration commences, the growth of the lungs demands that the cavity of the chest be enlarged. This was said to occur partly by the absorption of the thymus but mainly by the growth of the structures constituting the chest wall.[21]

The spleen also was thought to 'secrete blood'. This was suggested since it was observed that if the spleen was diseased the body gradually wasted. Also it had been proved that 'solid particles' were made by the lymphatic glands and thymus and were conveyed into the circulation by the thoracic duct. It was suggested that these were carried to the spleen where once again they could acquire their 'vesicle' to become fully formed red blood cells.[22] In retrospect many of Hewson's conclusions were clearly making a major mistake in confusing red cells with lymphocytes, this theory however was a vast improvement on the previously suggested synthetic role for the lungs and blood vessels. As Hewson said,

> ... since [these particles] are so complicated in their structure, it is improbable they should be made by mechanical agitation in the lungs or blood vessels, as has been suspected, but probably have some organs set apart for their formation.[6]

Coagulation

Hewson's experiments on the coagulation mechanism showed that 'coagulable lymph' (which we now recognise as fibrinogen) was responsible for clotting. He found that freezing blood would suspend coagulation, and that this could be restored by thawing. After delaying coagulation with cold temperatures or neutral salts, Hewson was able to separate off a coagulable plasma containing a factor which could be precipitated at a little over 50°C. This factor, 'coagulable lymph', he identified as being responsible for clotting.[23]

Success and tragedy

Hewson's first course of lectures was so popular that more than half of William Hunter's pupils from Windmill Street attended. As Lettsom's biography of Hewson recorded, 'The theatre in which he delivered his lectures and expounded his doctrines was crowded with men of science, as well as with pupils, to listen to a youth grown sage by experimental researches'.[4] Though heavily occupied with lecturing he had not abandoned his other skills and as a surgeon had gained one of the most lucrative practices in London. After 18 months his practice in midwifery and surgery had enlarged to such a degree, and his anatomical lectures were so successful, that his future seemed assured. On 18 April 1774 he sustained a cut in the dissection theatre, resulting in a severe fever. By the 23rd some temporary improvement was noted prior to a rapid worsening and he died on 1 May, in his 35th year.[24] He was buried at the church of St Martin-in-the-Fields, though the exact site of his grave is now unknown. Among the church's Notices of Burials is recorded 'May 6 1774, William Hewson, a man.' Benjamin Franklin wrote:[25]

> He died last Sunday Morning of a Fever which baffled the Skill of our best Physicians. He was an excellent young Man, ingenious, industrious, useful and belov'd by all that knew him... He was just established in a profitable growing Business, with the best Prospects of bringing up his young Family advantageously. They were a happy couple! All their Schemes of Life are now overthrown!

Hewson left two sons and a daughter, the second son being born three months after Hewson's death. Mrs Hewson remained an affectionate friend of Dr Benjamin Franklin and following his advice she emigrated to America and brought up the children firstly in Philadelphia and then in Bristol, Pennsylvania, until her death in 1795. William Hewson Jr died in Vera Cruz in 1802 and Dr Thomas Tickell Hewson died in 1848. Thomas had received his early education in England before he emigrated with his mother to Philadelphia. He graduated in Arts at the University of Pennsylvania in 1789, before studying medicine under Dr John Foulke. He then returned to England to serve as a house surgeon at St Bartholomew's Hospital, later going to Edinburgh for further study. He returned to practise in Philadelphia in 1800, and in 1822 organised a private medical school where he taught anatomy and practice.[26] Subsequently he became President of the College of Physicians of Philadelphia. Thomas Tickell Hewson's eighth son was Dr Addinell Hewson (1828-89), the first to use electricity to detect the translucency of tissues in fractures.[6] Addinell Hewson's eldest son, Dr Addinell Hewson Jr, became Professor of Anatomy in two American medical schools, and in turn his son Dr William Hewson became a physician practising in Philadelphia. Thus every one of six successive generations of the Hewatson/Hewson family was represented in the medical profession.

Grandfather Hewatson had not lived long enough to witness his son's rapid rise in London; he had died in 1767. Many of William Hewson's siblings died prematurely. As a consequence by the turn of the century the name Hewatson had disappeared from Hexham.[2]

At the time of his death Hewson was busy preparing the third volume of his *Experimental Inquiries*, which was completed and edited by Marcus Falconar. On his death bed Hewson chose this 20-year old as his successor at the Craven Street school. He had been one of John Hunter's pupils at St George's Hospital in 1771. Falconar ensured that the school went from strength to strength and retained its already fine reputation; but he too died young, in 1777, and the museum of the Craven Street school was sold.[27]

In addition to having exceptional skill both professionally and academically, and notwithstanding his temporary disagreements with Monro and the Hunters, Hewson was socially well liked; he was kind, and lively in conversation. His personal friends included Sir John Pringle, Dr Halle (Professor of Physic at the University of Leiden) and Dr Simmons who, quoting the words of Hewson's widow, wrote that 'a better son and husband or a fonder father than Mr. Hewson never existed'.[28]

Respecting Hewson's position in medical literature and science, Gulliver admiringly suggests in his preface[8] that Hewson's work on blood was a model of experiments which were nicely devised, well executed and clearly reported.

Hewson's investigations of the thymus introduced a rational method of research into this important area of physiology and his theories regarding 'solid, dark particles' (which we now recognise as lymphocytes) and his observations regarding their common presence in blood, thymus, lymph nodes and thoracic duct, were pioneering ones, made with what we would consider to be relatively primitive equipment. Some of his deductions have only now, over 200 years later, gained widespread recognition.

Hewson's work has received high praise. His contribution to our understanding of the lymphatic circulation has been compared with that of Harvey in connection with the circulation of the blood. Some rather uncertain evidence suggests that Edward Jenner had such respect for Hewson's work that he and John Hunter purchased between them many of Hewson's preparations of the lymphatic system, although Hunter opens an incompletely-dated letter to Jenner with the remark 'I could not buy a single preparation for you, they all went so dear'.[29]

Indeed the scope of Hewson's experiments in such a brief career seems remarkable. He investigated most of the major haematological topics and should perhaps be regarded as the Father of Haematology. In addition, I would suggest that his discovery of some of the essential components of the immune system should secure for him the equivalent rank in the rapidly developing science of Immunology.

Appendix

Bibliography of William Hewson (from Gulliver[8])

The operation of Paracentesis Thoracis, proposed for Air in the Chest; with some Remarks on the Emphysema, and on Wounds of the Lungs in general. *Med Observat Inquiries* 1767; *3*:372-96.

An Account of the Lymphatic System in Birds. *Phil Trans* 1768; *58*:217-26.

An account of the Lymphatic System in Amphibious Animals. *Phil Trans* 1769; *59*:198-203.

An Account of the Lymphatic System in Fish. *Phil Trans* 1769; *59*:204-215.

Experiments on the Blood, with some Remarks on its Morbid Appearances. *Phil Trans* 1770; *60*:368-83.

On the Degree of Heat which Coagulates the Lymph, and the Serum of the Blood; with an Inquiry into the Causes of the inflammatory Crust, or Size, as it is called. *Phil Trans* 1770; *60*:384-97.

Further Remarks on the Properties of the Coagulable Lymph, on the Stopping of Haemorrhages, and on the Effects of Cold upon the Blood. *Phil Trans* 1770; *60*:398-413.

On the Figure and Composition of the Red Particles of the Blood, commonly called the Red Globules. *Phil Trans* 1773; *63*:303-23.

An Experimental Inquiry into the Properties of the Blood, with some Remarks on its Morbid Appearances; and an Appendix, relating to the Discovery of the Lymphatic System in Birds, Fish, and the Animals called Amphibious. London: T Cadell, 1771.

Experimental Inquiries, Part the Second, containing a Description of the Lymphatic System in the Human Subject, and in other Animals. Together with Observations on the Lymph, and the Changes which it undergoes in some Diseases. London: J Johnson, 1774.

Falconar M. *Experimental Inquiries, Part the Third, containing a Description of the Red Particles of the Blood in the Human Subject and in other Animals; with an Account of the Structure and Offices of the Lymphatic Glands, of the Thymus Gland, and of the Spleen; being the remaining part of the Observations and Experiments of the late Mr. William Hewson, FRS and Teacher of Anatomy*. London: T Longman, 1777.

A Letter from the late Mr. William Hewson FRS to Dr. John Haygarth. *Med Phil Commentaries* 1775; *3*:87-93.

References

1. Hutchinson W. *A view of Northumberland, with an excursion to the Abbey of Mailross in Scotland.* Newcastle: T Saint, 1778:105.
2. Welford R. *Men of Mark 'twixt Tyne and Tweed,* Vol 2; London: Walter Scott, 1895.
3. Hinds AB. *A History of Northumberland*, Vol 3 – Hexhamshire, part 1. Newcastle-Upon-Tyne: A Reid, Sons and Co, 1896: 304.
4. Lettsom JC. Biography of William Hewson. *Trans Med Soc* 1810; *1*:51-63.
5. Mackenzie E. *A descriptive and historical account of the town and county of Newcastle upon Tyne.* Newcastle upon Tyne: Mackenzie and Dent, 1827; I: 63 footnote.
6. Bailey GH. William Hewson, F.R.S. *Annals Med Hist* 1923; *5*:209-224.

7. *Medical Observations and Enquiries by a Society of Physicians in London*, London: William Johnston, 1768; III: 372- 396.

8. Gulliver G. *The Works of William Hewson F.R.S.* London: Sydenham Society, 1846.

9. Hewson W. *Journal Book of the Royal Society of Physicians. 27*: 241-244.

10. Hunter J. *Essays and Observations on Natural History, Anatomy, Physiology, Psychology, and Geology.* London: J Van Voorst, 1861; 2: 334-5.

11. Wilcox WB (ed). *The Papers of Benjamin Franklin.* 29 vols. New Haven and London: Yale Univ Press, 1959-92; 18: 211.

12. *ibid* 18: 192-3.

13. 30 Oct 1772; *idem* 19: 353.

14. Owen RS. *Owen Correspondence.* British Museum (Natural History); 15: 470.

15. Corner GW (ed). *The Autobiography of Benjamin Rush.* Princeton: Univ Press, 1948: 52-53.

16. Pettigrew TJ. *Memoirs of the Life and Writings of the late John Coakley Lettsom.* 3 vols. London, 1817; I: 143-144.

17. Gulliver *op cit* note 8, 259.

18. *ibid*, 258-260.

19. *ibid*, 260.

20. *ibid*, 263, 279.

21. *ibid*, 280.

22. *ibid*, 282-6.

23. *ibid*, 15.

24. *Dict Nat Biog.* 9: 763-764.

25. Willcox WB. *op cit* note 11, 5 May 1774; 21: 208-9.

26. Packard FR. *History of Medicine in the United States.* 2 vols. New York and London: Hafner, 1963 (reprint); II: 999-1000.

27. Dobson J. *John Hunter.* Edinburgh and London: E&S Livingstone, 1969: 202-3.

28. See Mary Hewson's letter of 30 Aug 1782 in Gulliver *op cit* note 8, xv.

29. Dobson, *op cit* note 27, 203-4.

Chapter 9

JOHN HEYSHAM MD

W P Honeyman

John Heysham was born on 22 November 1753 at Lancaster where his father was a ship owner. He attended the local Quaker school at Yealand near Burton in Westmoreland, this being run by Messrs Jenkinson, where he received his basic classical education.[1] There is no history of medical men in the Heysham family but he took the decision to embark on this career at the age of 16 and became apprenticed for five years to Mr Parkinson, a surgeon at Burton. Under his indentures, he had to learn the 'art and mystery' of an apothecary with the preparation and compounding of drugs; his surgical experience included bleeding, cupping and tooth drawing and he studied anatomy and the course of diseases in the human body, as well as gaining experience in veterinary problems. The Vicar of Burton, Rev Dr Hutton, tutored him in the classics as well as in mathematics.

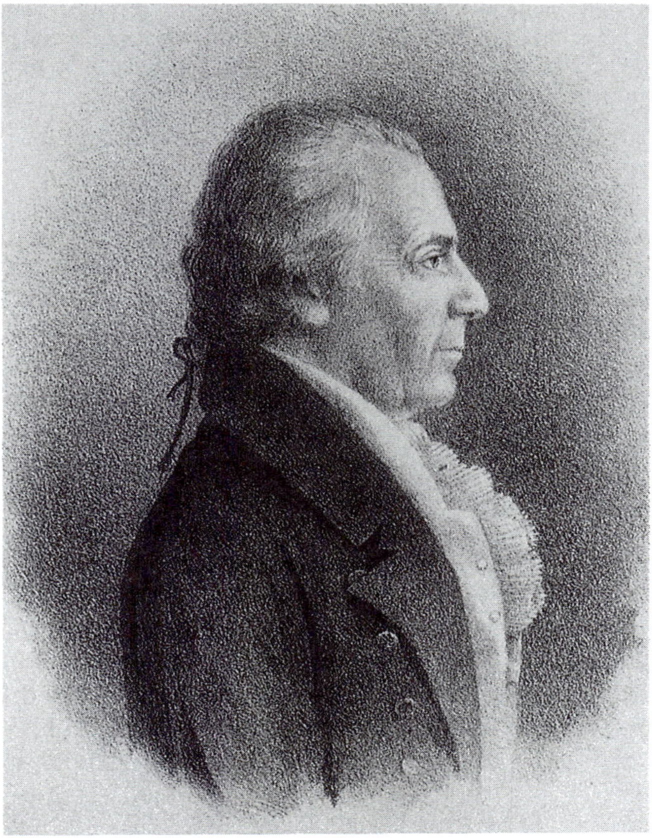

Figure 1. John Heysham

Having inherited his father's handsome personality and habits of perseverance and not a little of his mother's thrift, he was well equipped for the next stage of his training. Lancaster is 170 miles from Edinburgh and, there being no coaches, he made the journey on horse back passing through Kendal, Penrith and Carlisle; it was perhaps this early view of Carlisle, a walled city by the river, that was to attract him back for his medical career.

For three years in Edinburgh, he studied under Monro, Cullen and Black, gaining his doctorate in medicine in June 1777.[2] His thesis, *De Rabie Canina* was an historical review of hydrophobia and its treatment, manifest as an 'aversion and horror at liquids, exciting a painful convulsion of the pharynx occurring at an indetermined period, after the canine virus has been received into the system'. He deduced:

> first that, this virus is unquestionably present in the saliva, secondly that in its nature and effects, it differs from all other contagions with which we are yet acquainted. Thirdly that its properties are very foreign from those of putridity. Fourthly, that it cannot be so united with air as in that manner to give the infection to the human system. Fifthly, that it is so far of a fixed nature that the saliva is capable of giving the infection after the thinner parts have been evaporated by exposure to the open air. And, lastly, that amputation of the member bit or complete extirpation of the part, are the only certain prophylactic yet discovered, by which we are able to counteract the influence of this poison.

He then described the remedy prepared by William Hill of Ormskirk, Lancashire:

> Powder and chalk, half an ounce; armenian bole, three drachms; allum, ten grains; powder of elecampene root, one drachm; oil of anise, six drops. Such a dose to be taken every morning, repeated to the sixth time...... and with regard to its efficacy, this has now been so thoroughly established by experience, that there can be no room to doubt it.

However, John Fothergill, reporting on a case of a hydrophobia in 1774, when a 40-year-old man and his servant maid were both bitten by a cat and had been given the Ormskirk medicine, commented that 'it is with some repugnance we point out that the inefficacy of a medicine, which in this country has established a reputation as its being an infallible preservative.' Heysham would not have been aware of these comments by this physician, 40 years his senior, as they were published in *Medical Observations & Inquiries* in 1779.[3]

This thesis gives an early indication of the care and thoroughness in any investigation or problem Heysham was to meet throughout his life.

After graduating Heysham spent a year in Holland and London to further his medical knowledge and then came to Carlisle in 1778, where he rented rooms in St Cuthbert's Lane in the centre of the city, close to the Cathedral.

Carlisle, originally founded as a Roman Fort in AD 78, was the site of much warring and eventually became a walled city set in the Eden Valley with the rivers Caldew and Petteril to the West and East. It was only after the Jacobite Risings of 1715 and 1745 that Carlisle began to develop with properties being built outside these city gates. Manufacture of linen, woollen and cotton cloth started: the development of the 'military road' to Newcastle opened up trade with the north-east of England and the Newcastle company of Scott, Lamb & Co started a calico printing business in 1761 in Carlisle.[4] In 1763, the population of the city was 4158 in 1059 families. With the development of the textile factories, Scottish and Irish families came seeking employment; the rapid increase in the number of inhabitants seeking accommodation caused gross overcrowding in the limited number of houses in the Lanes area abutting the Eastern wall of the city. Heysham's awareness of the problems of these families in unsuitable accommodation caused him to take an early interest in the statistics relating to population and disease in Carlisle. *Observations of the Bills of Mortality in Carlisle for the year 1779* was the first of nine annual reports that he wrote.[5] In these Heysham recorded the deaths occurring in the population with details of ages and the causative diseases. General comments were made on the weather, including an earthquake in 1786. Epidemics were recorded, also selected cases of medical interest with full clinical details, discussion and management.

1779: Thirty-nine persons (including 31 children under 5 years) died in Carlisle in an epidemic of 'Scarlet Fever and Sore Throat', which lasted for six months; as it was an uncommon disease and not perfectly understood, Heysham discussed this at length, differentiating between scarlatina and scarlet fever, and deducing that it was a contagious disorder, due to 'a peculiar kind of poison, of a volatile nature, readily mixed with air.' Treatment was detailed:

> of all remedies made use of in this Epidemic, none was of more real advantage than bleeding, which was sometimes repeated three of four times; so great was its efficacy, that I believe not one patient died, who lost a sufficient quantity of blood early in the disease.

Tartar Emetic and Saline Mixture were routinely advised and 'a gargle of red wine and water was useful in washing off any mucous slough.'

There was an epidemic of smallpox in the last six months of the year when out of 300 cases, 90 died, including 86 under the age of 5 years. It worried Heysham that although in the same period several hundred were inoculated in the neighbourhood of Carlisle, not one of them died; had the 300 cases been inoculated, only six fatal cases might have been expected instead of the actual 90 deaths.

> Yet so great is the prejudice against the salutary practice of inoculation amongst the vulgar, that few, very few, can be prevailed upon either by promises, rewards or intreaties to submit to the operation. No wonder that in rude, ignorant and barbarous times, superstition hurried men into the grossest absurdities; when in a polished and enlightened age, in an age too, when the experience of full twenty years has clearly demonstrated the utility of inoculation, we see the bulk of mankind

> ready to sacrifice their children and all that is dear to them, to a foolish prejudice.

At this time, inoculation was still as introduced into England by Lady Montagu in 1717, using a thread soaked in material from a smallpox pustule. It was not until a further 21 years had elapsed that vaccination from cowpox was introduced in Carlisle.

> In February, a poor girl either for some real, or imaginary complaint, was advised by an acquaintance as ignorant as herself, to take a large quantity of steel filings, which had been procured from a White Smith, or Watch Maker.

After being in severe abdominal pain for two days, she died: she had denied knowing of any cause for illness but after her death, steel filings were found in her room: she had been seen to take three teaspoonfuls mixed with treacle. Analysis of the filings showed contamination with lead and copper to be present.

> Let the death of this unfortunate woman be a caution to others: and let Watch Makers and White Smiths be careful to whom they sell steel filings, especially till they are separated from every impurity by the loadstone or some other method.

1780: The 'chincough' or whooping cough was fatal to 10 children under the age of 5, who had not had any medical attention. Measles accounted for a further 33 deaths in children (25 under the age of 5).

'A very remarkable case of Dysphagia Spasmodica, and Epileptic Fits,............' was that of Jane Stockbridge, 41 years old with a history of fits dating back over 12 years, and dysphagia for 7 years. Seen by Heysham on 7 January 1780, a surgeon was called in on the next day: after initial difficulty from the stricture, a bougie was passed into her stomach; this precipitated a violent epileptic fit lasting for 30 minutes. Medication was then started as pills of Cuprum Ammoniacum half gramme in a paste of bread, taking one and half to two tablets morning and night: after eight months her fits ceased and therapy was discontinued: in June 1781, she was free from all complaints.[6]

1781: In this year there was a severe epidemic of Typhus Carcerum. It started in a house, in which lived six very poor families in cramped and squalid conditions; because of the window tax, the stagnation of air 'rendered still more noxiously the filth and uncleanliness of the people.' One of the patients was a weaver who, when recovered, returned to his work spreading the disease until eventually the whole city was affected: out of 500 cases, 48 died. Heysham published *An Account of the Jail Fever or Typhus Carcerum as it appeared at Carlisle in the year 1781*.[7] This work detailed the circumstances of the outbreak, the diagnosis and course of the illness; the main interest was in the change of treatment advocated, namely up to two and a half bottles of port wine daily and Peruvian bark, in double the dose usually prescribed.

Smallpox continued to take its toll of the children, 19 dying. Consumption accounted for a further 26 deaths. 'One fell a victim to the venereal disease, or rather to the want of the common necessaries of life.' A 17-year-old girl, because of a 'disappointment in love', took a teaspoon of arsenic: seen by Heysham, she was given Tartar Emetic and next day she was bled 8-10 oz. Details of her condition and treatment are given but she died five days after taking the arsenic: examination of her stomach revealed ulceration, the size of a crown piece in the pre-pyloric area.

> To conclude this melancholy subject, I think it is a duty incumbent on all surgeons, apothecaries and others who retail arsenic, never to trust the care of so deadly a poison to an apprentice whose unsuspecting youth may be easily imposed upon by the specious pretences of the desperate, profligate and base.

1782: Jail fever and smallpox continued to take their toll, the latter causing 30 deaths. An outbreak of Catarrhus Contagiosus or influenza soon became widespread but only one death ensued, a 64-year-old with pre-existing lung disease.

Until this year, Heysham had carried out his medical practice from his rooms in St Cuthbert's Lane. He was now finding these to be inadequate and, realising that the medical needs of the poorer members of society were increasing, he sought help from Dean Percy. The Chapter was prepared to grant him the use of a room within the Cathedral precinct for the formation of a Carlisle Dispensary.[8] A committee of eminent persons was appointed and subscriptions were sought to defray the expenses of running the Dispensary; John Heysham was appointed as the first physician, and William Graham a surgeon, both giving their services gratuitously. The Carlisle Dispensary opened on 1 July 1782 but within four months Mr Graham died, being attended by Heysham.

> On Thursday evening 10 October 1782 I was called in a great hurry to Mr Graham, a surgeon aged 46 years, a gentleman of a robust, strong and somewhat corpulent habit of body, who had lived freely and had been accustomed to considerable exercise and fatigue. I found the house overwhelmed in the deepest distress, and as soon as I entered his room he told me with considerable emotion and haste that he was on the point of death; that he breathed with great difficulty, and that he was affected with a violent pain under the sternum extending from the cartilago ensiformis to the clavicles and from thence to his arms and wrists. His face was covered with a clammy sweat and his hands were cold. His pulse was exceedingly weak, intermittent, and beat only about 26 strokes a minute. I was informed by some of the family that immediately before my arrival he had himself opened a vein in his arm and had lost about a pound of blood. I gave him 30 drops tinc thebain in a cup of peppermint water which he vomited in the space of two minutes. Dr Carlisle soon afterwards came in, and he took half an ounce of a mixture of equal parts elix guiac vol and tinct valerian vol and died in less than 15 minutes from the time I saw him and about an hour and

> a quarter after he was first seized with the complaint. He was perfectly sensible and spoke within a minute or two of his death. He had eaten his dinner in good health and had assisted in getting in some oats into his barn, with which he was somewhat heated.
>
> What is remarkable, another gentleman in the neighbourhood of Carlisle was on the same day suddenly seized with a violent pain in his breast and arms and died in a very short time. He was likewise somewhat corpulent and had lived freely.
>
> What was the nature of the affection of which these two gentleman died, for their symptoms were nearly similar? I confess my ignorance, never having seen or remember to have read any case of a like nature. Dissection perhaps might have elucidated the matter.

In the same year, two cases of Heysham's were to lead to severe differences of opinion with Graham's replacement as surgeon, John Hodgson. Ann Liddle, aged 60, was a baker, managing a public oven: she was accustomed to taking large quantities of snuff. For eight years she had suffered from severe pain 'on the right side of her face and head: she imagines it begins in her cheek and thence extends all over that side of her head.' Never clear of pain, it was worse in the colder weather and most moderate in hot weather. Treated initially with up to 60 drops of laudanum, no relief was obtained by day or night: Heysham then tried Fothergill's treatment for similar symptoms and for three months, she took extract of hemlock morning and night, but without benefit. After a further three months, she was suffering constant pain with frequent severe spasms, originating 'in the cheek bone near to the antrum maxillare.' Heysham decided that the antrum should be drained, calling in the surgeon John Hodgson for the procedure to be carried out on the next day, April 24: 'there was not the least discharge of matter or any other appearance of disease in the part.' Decoct Peruvian bark and elix aloes were injected into the antrum daily, the orifice being kept open by a small piece of gentian root: over the next three weeks, three dead insects were discharged. This was not the end of her problem for her symptoms continued: Heysham reviewed her case comparing it with Fothergill's sixteen cases of facial pain.[9] Detailed notes over the years reported no change in her symptoms despite frequent consultations with Heysham: 'August 28, 1789, not having seen her for a considerable time, I called upon her today, and was sorry to find no abatement of her pain, or any prospect of death soon putting a period to her misery.'

Also in 1782, Heysham was called in to see Hugh Sutherland, aged 65 years, with an acute retention of urine.

> I sent for Mr Hodgson, who I had just before left at the Blue Bell, and that there might be no delay, I went to his shop to get the necessary instruments ready: he had none, but we borrowed a couple Catheters of Mr Creighton. In his first attempt to introduce the catheter, I saw he was extremely awkward and gave him some instructions, which however, he was too self sufficient to pursue: in short, after a trial of twenty

> minutes or more, during which he put the poor man through a great deal of torture and bought away nothing but blood, he then .... gave the matter up.

A second surgeon, Mr Joseph Blain, was able to pass a catheter without difficulty and with immediate relief to the patient.

The surgical management of these two cases of Ann Liddle and Hugh Sutherland led to an acrimonious dispute between Heysham and Hodgson in which serious allegations over professional judgement, competency and confidentiality were made by each party. A 15-page pamphlet by Hodgson *A State of Facts.....* was answered by Heysham in a 25-page statement *More Facts or a Reply to a Pamphlet entitled a State of Facts...*[10,11] As these cases referred to patients accepted for treatment by the Carlisle Dispensary, the Surgeon and Physician had to state their cases at length in front of the Committee of Management; as a result a new appointment of Surgeon was made.

1783: Smallpox again caused deaths — 19, of which 17 were under 5; a general campaign of inoculation in Carlisle was carried out by the Surgeons in the City.

Heysham details the treatment of three girls suffering from St Vitus's Dance cured by Cuprum Ammoniacum: 'My patient who is about 8 years of age gradually increased the dose to nine Pills in the day, which contained five grains and a half of the Cuprum.'

1784:

> The Diabetes is a rather curious affection, and tho' it has long been noticed by medical writers, yet the causes of it, whether remote or proximate, have not been ascertained; nor have the experiments either of empirics or regular physicians discovered any remedy which can be depended on for its cure.

This case was in a woman aged 33 years with onset a year previously, following childbirth. Heysham 'evaporated five pounds of her urine and obtained from it seven ounces avoirdupois of a sweet substance of the colour and consistence of toffy.' Initial treatment taken four times daily was an 'electuary of bark, alum and most astringent gums washed down with wine and water acidulated with elixir of vitriol, or alum water.' No benefit ensued nor from a tincture of cantharides in daily doses of up to 640 drops. She died ten months later.

Also reported is 'a Case of Hydrocephalus Internus or Dropsy of the Brain, which terminated fatally.' Aged 8 3/4 years, he had had a fit: on making a diagnosis, Heysham's treatment was 'in the space of about 53 hours, half an ounce and two scruples and a half of strong mercurial ointment, were carefully rubbed into his thighs and legs, and four grains of calomel were given internally, the latter chiefly with an intention of producing a stool.'

1785: Percivall Pott's treatise, *Remarks on that kind of Palsy of the lower limbs, which is frequently found to accompany a curvature of the spine and its treatment* had been noted by Heysham and he reported on this case, the first to be cured of this condition in Carlisle.[12] George Robinson, aged 18 was only able 'with the assistance of two sticks, with great difficulty to hobble over a smooth floor.' To the tumour of his dorsal spine, a large caustic was applied on each side: two large eschars were formed to which three kidney beans were applied to continue the discharge. Within seven months, he was able to walk the ten miles from his home to Carlisle and in a further four months returned to his work as a weaver: he was dismissed 'cured, with directions to keep the issues open some time longer.'

1786: An epidemic of measles, not seen for six years, was traced as spreading from Northumberland: six or seven hundred cases developed in Carlisle, 28 deaths being in children; nine also died from chincough.

1787: 'An Account of a Female Child which was born at Carlisle, at the full time, alive and which lived five days and twenty hours, without the smallest appearance of a brain.' Heysham had been called to this case one hour after the delivery of 26-year-old Mary Clarke's sixth child, a girl; he attended until the death of the child and was present when two surgical colleagues carried out a detailed postmortem examination. From the findings,

> I think the following obvious inferences may be drawn...... that the living principle, the nerves of the trunk and extremities, sensation, and motion, may exist independent of, and that the natural vital, and animal functions, may be performed without the brain. And as the external organs of sense viz. the eyes, the nose, the tongue, and the ears, all seemed perfect may we not therefore suppose, that the optic, the olfactory, the gustatory and the auditory nerves may exist independent of, and unconnected with either the brain, or the spinal marrow? I content myself with little more than describing this extraordinary case, and leave to others, to deduce from it, such conclusions as the appearances observed, may be thought to warrant.

He compared this case with those of Dr Monro, two of which were illustrated, '...... I think we may infer from his silence, ... that they were really born dead'.[13]

At the end of 1787, no further Bills of Mortality were produced nor reports of cases published, but Heysham continued as Physician to the Dispensary as well as in his practice in Carlisle.

Over the years, Heysham had taken a particular interest in smallpox and had been very active both at the Carlisle Dispensary and in his private practice in taking every opportunity in advocating inoculation in childhood as a prime means of reducing the high mortality from this disease, particularly in the first five years of life. It was in the year 1800 that Dr Robert J Thornton came to the North of England to promote the use of inoculation with cowpox. 'I was equally anxious to establish the cowpox at Carlisle......and Dr Heysham an eminent physician of that City, proposed setting an example by having his own child, only six weeks old inoculated.'[14] Letters from Heysham to Thornton in October to December 1800 record that three attempts with charged lancets failed. The unusual step was then taken, for a villager near Penrith to take on horseback, his 5-year-old daughter with her 'pustule in a proper state.' On her arrival after the journey of 26 miles, Heysham was then able to inoculate directly nine patients at once and more next day.

The successful inoculation with smallpox of his daughter was recorded in a letter from Heysham to Thornton, five years later when the situation in Carlisle and other towns in Cumberland were reviewed in letters published in *Vaccinae Vindiciae* in 1806.[15]

> I have the pleasure to inform you that ever since you introduced the cowpox into Carlisle, which was in the Autumn of 1800, vaccination has been regularly practised by all the medical gentlemen here with the best effects. I think that I may venture to say, that all the children of the opulent, the greatest part of the middling ranks and a very considerable number of the inferior classes of society have been vaccinated. Since that time the smallpox has occasionally occurred but has never raged as an epidemic, and the mortality from that disease has been comparatively small indeed.
>
> My little girl who was vaccinated soon after she was born, from the patient you were so kind as to send from Lowther, was inoculated on 20 November 1804 in both arms with smallpox matter. Both arms inflamed to a very considerable degree and the inflammation did not completely subside till the 7th December: but neither disease or eruptions succeeded. She went to school, ate and slept well all the time. Several other children by way of experiment have also been inoculated with smallpox matter but I have not heard of one who received the infection.

On 4th May 1789, John Heysham married Elizabeth Mary Coulthard, only daughter and heiress of a rich tanner. They moved into a three-storey house opposite to his previous lodgings in St Cuthbert's Lane. His wife died 14 years later, during which time a son had died in infancy, with four sons and three daughters surviving.

The study of nature was a life-long interest of Heysham's: as a youth in Lancashire he had roamed the countryside, following the birds and animals in their haunts. These activities continued in Cumberland. In 1788 he was elected an Associate of the Linnaean Society but it was not until 1794 that his only recorded work, 'A Catalogue of Cumberland Animals' was published as an addendum to Hutchinson's *History of Cumberland*.[16] In this detailed list of animals, birds and insects are recorded many of his interesting experiences and observations; he followed a female peregrine on the crags near the Twice Brewed Inn on the Roman Wall, eventually shooting it after it had been five hours on the wing.

Rev Macpherson in his *Fauna of Lakeland* (1892) makes frequent references to Dr Heysham's detailed findings, including 'Dr Heysham devoted nearly three columns to the Hen Harrier and his account of the birds which nested at Newtown, near Carlisle, is infinitely the finest piece of writing that his pen has bequeathed to us.'[17] He observed swifts nesting in the Cathedral near to his house, comparing dates of their arrival and departure with local meteorological records: his servants when mowing a field of grass, found a nest of 12 young corncrakes: he 'killed a female merlin on her nest on Rockcliffe-Moss....... that was in the evening, I left a trap at the nest and went the next morning and found the male taken.'

The fine collection of birds which he collected over the years was housed in the Deanery of Carlisle in the care of his friend, Dean Milner and on the latter's death, it passed to Dr Thomas Barnes at the House of Recovery.

It was from the compilation of population statistics in *Observations on the Bills of Mortality in Carlisle 1779-1787* that Dr Heysham became known far beyond the walled City of Carlisle.[5] A census in July 1763 had recorded that within the city and its suburbs there were 1059 families with 4158 inhabitants. In January 1780 Heysham had a further census carried out under his own inspection when the figures showed that in 891 houses, there were now 1605 families and 6299 inhabitants: the increase was attributed to the recent opening of four calico printing works in which 800 workers were employed. The detailed information in this first year comprises not only a census of families and their houses, but also a statistical analysis of the ages of the population, their deaths, the diseases from which they succumbed and the months in which they died. As in other censuses, errors arose from the ascertainment of the number of births solely from baptismal rolls, many of the births to Dissenters not being on a birth register. The diseases were identified by Cullen's *Synopsis Nosologica Methodica*, third edition.

Though the Bills of Mortality covered only the years 1779-1787 for the inhabitants of Carlisle, Heysham's researches were spread much further afield. Wales of Christs' Hospital, London had a correspondence with him in 1781/82 asking that Parish Registers in the County of Cumberland be consulted to obtain the numbers baptised and buried in each parish for 10 year periods 1688-1697, 1741-1750 and 1771-1780. Unfortunately no complete records were obtained for various reasons.[18] Nevertheless extracts from parts of these figures are to be found in Hutchinson's History of Cumberland: 'they were collected by a Physician of eminence in 1781.'[19]

Heysham's Bills of Mortality (1779-87) were brought to the attention of the insurance world through Joseph Milne, Actuary to the Sun Life Assurance Company: the correspondence is recorded verbatim in the Appendix to Dr Henry Lonsdale's *Life of John Heysham MD* 1870.[1] Much further research for each year to 1813, of births and deaths, movements of soldiers and their families, recession in the factories etc was needed to bring the statistics up to date. The final Table was published by Milne in 1815 'showing the Expectation of Life at every age, according to the Law of Mortality at Carlisle.'[20]

The First Annual Report of the Registrar General by Lister for the year 1839 showed how the figures for an annuitant's expectation of life varied on comparing the tables of Milne, founded on mortality observed in Carlisle, with those by Price in Nottingham: calculations by Milne forecast that out of 100 000 persons aged 25, 51 335 would be expected to survive until the age of 65 years, whereas Price's figure was 34 286 surviving.[21] Dr Henry Barnes, Physician to the Cumberland Infirmary, in his President's Address at the 64th Annual Meeting of the British Medical Association in Carlisle in 1896, drew attention to this discrepancy.[22] He referred to the earlier Northampton Table, drawn up by Dr Price, a Unitarian Minister, from accounts kept in the town's records, during the 46 years 1735-1780 of the ages at death of 4689 persons buried in the parish of All Saints. In Northampton the population was apparently static due to the non-inclusion of some births, *ie* those of Baptists; in the rest of the country, including Carlisle, there was a general increase. The Government had used the Northampton Table for calculation of annuities; they found that mortality was one-third less than the Table predicted; payments were accordingly higher, resulting in a loss to the Treasury of two million pounds. The accuracy of the Carlisle Tables was soon recognised and they were adopted by life assurance companies in this country as well as in America. In the fifth report of the Registrar General (1843) Dr Farr stated:

> I avail myself of this opportunity to pay my humble tribute to the fairness of the Carlisle Tables; to Dr Heysham, who collected the facts with so much care; and to Mr Milne, who cast these facts so judiciously to the purposes of life insurance.

Dr Henry Lonsdale, born in Carlisle and a Physician at the Cumberland Infirmary for 22 years, spent much of his time in writing biographies of local worthies. His *Life of John Heysham MD* (1870) gives many details of the life of this physician, helped in accuracy by the fact that a member of Heysham's family was alive at the time it was written. It includes some details of his social life. Heysham was friendly with several of the big landowners in the area and from them he acquired natural history specimens and had the opportunity of furthering his interests in this subject: holidays were spent 'naturalising and shooting.' Heysham lived near the Cathedral and the Dean was included in his circle of close friends. More notorious was his habit of dining with friends at each others' houses in the winter months, when they would sit down and dine at 3 pm rising from the table at about 10 pm during which time, each would have downed three bottles of strong port: the 'Three bottle Men' were well-known members of Cumberland society.

The practice of medicine was not a full time occupation for Heysham and his interests were diverse. Through inheritance, he was able to purchase or rent properties around the city: his farm to the north was one interest, whilst on the outskirts to the south, on John Wood's map of 1821, he is shown as owning four properties,[23] including being a partner in a cotton works (Cowan, Heysham & Co). In 1819, a large field belonging to Heysham was divided and sold for the building of the House of Recovery (Fever Hospital) and the Carlisle Gas Works: Heysham was appointed as Chairman of the Carlisle Gas and Coke Company in 1819; in the same year, the Carlisle Canal

Company was formed and Heysham was appointed Chairman. He had been a founder subscriber (1778) to the Subscriptions Library. He was appointed as a Commissioner for Assessed Taxes in the County and a Commissioner for Lighting and Improving Carlisle: he was a zealous supporter of the Police Establishment and at one time Chairman of the Commissioners. In 1808, he was appointed as a Justice of the Peace in the City and shortly afterwards as Deputy Lieutenant for Cumberland and Westmoreland.

As Magistrate, on market days he sat with Rev Dr Thomas Lowry at the Globe Inn, Scotch Street, Carlisle, on either side of the fireplace as the plaintiff made his case. On 30 April 1814,

> Richard Alder, who as the Guard of the Newcastle Mail Coach saith that on Monday evening 25th, John Carson of Caldewgate, did stop the Mail Coach with two horses and carts, he being asleep in one of them and did otherwise misbehave and used very gross and abusive language....

The magistrates fined him ten shillings for obstructing the turnpike road over the River Eden.[24]

On Saturday 22 March 1834, Heysham was unable to walk the short distance to hold court at the Globe Inn; instead Rev Lowry and he conducted the magisterial business at his own house in St Cuthbert's Lane. Next morning he was found moribund in his bed, and died before midday, in his eighty-first year.

In the *Carlisle Journal* his obituary took notice of his long medical career, though

> as a physician he had ceased to act for some years except in exceptional cases amongst his immediate friends....... he was indefatigable in the discharge of his magisterial duties..... In politics, we had frequent occasion to differ from him and his acts as Magistrate have been censored in this paper: but his strict integrity, his talents and his earnest endeavours to promote the best interests of the town, no man ever doubted.[25]

References

1. Lonsdale H. *Life of John Heysham MD*. London: Longmans, 1870.
2. Heysham J. Dissertatio Medica de Rabie Canina. *Medical and Philosophical Commentaries* 1777; *5*:43-52.
3. Fothergill J. The Case of a Hydrophobia. *Medical Observations and Inquiries* 1779; *5*:195.
4. Hutchinson W. *History of Cumberland.* Carlisle: Jollie, 1794; *II*:663-667.
5. Heysham J. *Observations on the Bills of Mortality in Carlisle.* Carlisle: Milliken, 1779-1787.
6. Heysham J. Remarkable Cure of Epilepsy and Dysphagia Spasmodica. *Medical and Philosophical Commentaries* 1780; *7*:349.
7. Heysham J. *An Account of the Jail Fever, or Typhus Carcerum: as it appeared at Carlisle in the year 1781.* Carlisle: Milliken, 1782.
8. *Plan of the Carlisle Dispensary.* Carlisle: Milliken, 1782.

9. Fothergill J. On a painful affection of the face. *Medical Observations and Inquiries* 1776; 5:129-42.
10. Hodgson J. *A State of Facts or Observations on Dr Heysham's Bills of Mortality for the year 1782.* Carlisle: Jollie, 1783.
11. Heysham J. *More facts or a Reply to a pamphlet entitled a State of Facts.* Carlisle: Milliken, 1783.
12. Pott P. *Remarks on that kind of palsy of the lower limbs, which is frequently found to accompany a curvature of the spine.* London: Johnson, 1779.
13. Monro A. *Observations on the Nervous System*. Edinburgh: 1783: 26,116.
14. Thornton RJ. *Facts Decisive in Favour of the Cow-Pock.* London: Symonds, 1802: 190-232.
15. Thornton RJ. *Vaccinae Vindiciae.* London: Symonds, 1806:81.
16. Hutchinson W. *op cit* addend 1-38.
17. Macpherson HA. *A Vertebrate Fauna of Lakeland.* Edinburgh: Douglas, 1892: xviii-xxii, 179.
18. Village Population. *Cumbria Library, Carlisle.* M839.
19. Hutchinson W. *op cit I*:522.
20. Milne J. *A treatise on the valuation of Annuities and Assurances on lives and survivorships.* London: Longman, 1815.
21. *First Annual Report of the Registrar General of Births, Deaths and Marriages in England (1838).* London: HMSO, 1839: 16-17.
22. Barnes H. Presidential Address, 64th Annual Meeting BMA, Carlisle. *BMJ* Aug 1896:250.
23. Wood J. Map of City of Carlisle from actual survey. Edinburgh 1821.
24. *Plaintiffs appearing before Rev T Lowry and Dr J Heysham 1814-15.* Cumbria Records Office, Carlisle. D/MH/1/15.
25. Obituary for Dr J Heysham. *Carlisle Journal*, 29 March 1834.

Chapter 10

THOMAS TROTTER 1760 – 1832

Physician to the Fleet

Joan Carmichael

My interest in Thomas Trotter was kindled some years ago by finding among the papers of Dennis Embleton[1] some brief notes about Trotter, taken from the account given by Mackenzie:[2]

> Dr. Trotter discharged the difficult and important duties of this office with unexampled diligence and ability. He reformed the arrangements in royal [Naval] hospitals; abolished the fine for cure of lues venera [*sic*] in ships; and, in 1801, induced the government to shut up 2000 gin-shops in Plymouth-dock, on account of the prejudicial effects these nuisances produced on the health of seamen.
>
> It is also told in the naval circles, that, when the late Earl St. Vincent was boasting of the many good things he had done for the navy, Admiral Sir Edward Thornborough replied, 'True, my lord, you did much; but there is one man still living who did more for the navy of the country than you or any person that ever existed, and that man is Dr. Trotter, who has been shamefully neglected'.

More recently, I was fortunate in being able to peruse a collection of letters to Dr Trotter, given to the National Maritime Museum by his great-granddaughter. These spanned the years 1795 to 1835 and included one to his widow from Earl Spencer a month after Trotter's death, saying it would be useless for her to apply to the Admiralty for a pension.[3]

These letters throw light not only on his naval activities, but on his life in Newcastle after leaving the navy in 1802.[4]

Trotter was an energetic, courageous and compassionate man, untiring in his efforts to reform the evils and injustices in the navy of his time and passionately dedicated to his life's work. The romantic side of his nature found expression in his poems[5] and a five act tragedy in verse.[6] His zeal to reform may have made him officious in manner at times with consequent alienation of those in authority, but the religious belief underlying his actions, which probably arose from his Scottish background and upbringing, was evident when he wrote in middle life 'it is inculcated by divine revelation and impressed on our very nature, to exert every faculty of mind and power of body to prevent or mitigate the ills which flesh is heir to'.[7]

He was baptized at Melrose in Roxburghshire on 3 August 1760,[8] the second son of a baker, John Trotter and his wife, Alison, and the third of five children. His younger brother, Andrew, became a surgeon and practised at North Shields. When he was seventeen, after schooling at Melrose and Kelso Academy, Thomas went to the University of Edinburgh and attended the class of Anatomy and Surgery of Alexander Monro *secundus*. Although only

17 years old, he was already contributing poems to the *Edinburgh Magazine*. It is probable that he was also a pupil of Dr Buckham of Wooler at this time.[9]

In 1779, he joined the Navy as a Surgeon's Mate, and was appointed to the *Berwick* of the Channel Fleet, sailing for the West Indies in the spring of 1780 when the War of American Independence was at its height. The squadron was hit by a hurricane off Bermuda; Thomas lost most of the contents of his medicine chest, all the ships were dismasted and some were lost. On the homeward voyage scurvy and dysentery broke out among the crew of the *Berwick*, 40 of whom died and 200 needed hospital treatment. Trotter himself suffered severe dysentery and he gives a vivid description of his own symptoms in the first volume of *Medicina Nautica*.[10]

A year later the *Berwick* was distinguished in the fight at the Battle of Dogger Bank and Trotter received public thanks from the commodore for his services to the wounded. He was promoted to the rank of surgeon the following year and appointed to the *William* but in February 1783 the *William* ran aground at the mouth of the Mersey and the crew were paid off.

There was a general disarmament at this time and Trotter was one of the 750 Naval Surgeons who were dismissed. He had to join the merchant service as surgeon on a slave ship, the *Brookes*.[11] This voyage lasted fourteen months, carrying slaves from Guinea to the West Indies. His experiences on this ship filled him with profound disgust at the slave trade and converted him into an ardent abolitionist. He later gave evidence before a House of Commons Committee on behalf of the petitioners for the Abolition of the Slave Trade.[12]

On his return to England in 1784 Trotter left the sea and practised for about three years at Wooler in Northumberland where he was Apothecary and Surgeon.[13] During this time he attended Dr Cullen's lectures in Medicine at Edinburgh and in 1787-8 studied clinical medicine, materia medica and botany there with James Gregory, Francis Home and Daniel Rutherford.[14] He received the degree of Doctor of Medicine from Edinburgh University, in 1788. His thesis was on drunkenness *De ebrietate, eiusque effectibus in corpus humanum*. At the graduation ceremony, Dr Cullen introduced the thesis with many compliments and concluded by saying of the author: 'Certe non ebrius erat, qui hanc dissertationem scribebat'.[15] Trotter was extremely proud of this qualification, as he was the only surgeon on the Navy list with an MD degree. Later he noted that only three Naval Physicians had obtained a regular degree, all others including Sir Gilbert Blane having obtained theirs by proxy.[16]

Surgeon and physician with Admiral Roddam

At Christmas 1789, he was appointed to the *Barfleur* – the flag ship of his friend and neighbour, Admiral Roddam, of Roddam Hall, about 6 miles from Wooler.

The Admiral's letter book for 1789-90 contains several references to Trotter and gives an idea of his duties at this period and of the Admiral's high opinion of him.[17] The first letter in the book (18 March 1789) from the Navy Board says,

> We have received your letter of the 16th inst., recommending Mr.Thomas Trotter to be appointed surgeon... of the Barfleur, and in return acquaint you that as soon as the three years for which Mr. Thompson was appointed surgeon are expired, (October 1790), or he can otherwise be provided.

In the event Trotter was appointed to the *Barfleur* at Christmas 1789.[18]

In March 1790 there was an outbreak of a contagious fever among troops on board the *Gorgon* lying at Portsmouth and the sick men were moved, on Trotter's orders, to a nearby hulk. From the numerous letters referring to this, Trotter must have been kept very busy – here is a typical example showing Trotter's concern for the diet of his patients:[19]

> 13.3.1790, from Sir Philip Stephens — Secretary to the Admiralty, to Admiral Roddam -
>
> Sir, I have communicated your letter submitting the expediency of ordering a supply of sago, currants and spices for the use of the sick men on board the hulk, as proposed by Dr. Trotter in his letter which you enclosed, and I am commanded by their Lordships....directing you to cause such quantities of these articles to be purchased....keeping a distinct account of the expense, that application may be made for repayment thereof.

It is clear from the records that Trotter sent reports to the Admiralty on the state of the sick troops every three or four days. It is good to note that two months later Sir Philip Stephens wrote to Admiral Roddam, 'that Dr. Trotter's vouchers for his expenses in attending the sick soldiers on board the *Gorgon* will be sent to the Secretary of State with a proposal for some extra allowance being made him for his attendance and trouble on that occasion'.[20]

In a letter to the Admirality on 4 Oct 1790, Admiral Roddam wrote:- 'Mr Trotter is a regular bred physician, and one, whom their Lordships may remember, to have given very successful proof of his professional skill on two or three similar occasions'.[21]

Second physician at Haslar Hospital

From 1789 until 1793, Trotter served on the *Barfleur*, the *Edgar*, the *Royal William*, the *Duke*, the *Centurian*, and the *Vengeance* on a cruise to the West Indies.[22] In 1793 he was appointed second Physician at Haslar Naval Hospital, and at once set about reforming every department with characteristic zeal.

Ten years earlier, at the age of twenty two, he had written to the Navy Board complaining of the cruelty, impolicy and disgrace of charging fifteen shillings to the seamen for the treatment of venereal disease.[23] He had again emphasized the evils of this charge in a pamphlet addressed to the First Lord of the Admiralty (1790), in which he suggested other reforms, such as the appointment of a Physician General for the Navy.[24] In his journal for 6 March 1795, Trotter noted that

> In my general visit to the ships, after our arrival at Spithead, many recent facts..... supported the former arguments I have employed against the charge.... for the cure of venereal disease..... In some of the ships were men who undertook to cure the disease in all its stages, and had more than one or two patients under their care.... A medicine, often fatal, even in the best hands, was a popular remedy with them — [Hydrarg Muriat].
>
> Some consulted itinerant quacks, who flock to the sea ports, and had paid largely for their advice; while simple local complaints were converted into a confirmed lues.... Several had with-held the knowledge of the disease from the surgeon, till the most excruciating and dangerous symptoms had supervened, and thus they became objects for a hospital.......

Trotter put the facts before Earl Howe and Sir Roger Curtis, Admiral and Captain of the Fleet respectively, and an immediate stop was put to the charge. The surgeons were remunerated appropriately.[25]

> .....Thus terminated a perquisite, illiberal from its institution, inhuman in its practice, and impolitic from its continuance....[26]
>
> It forms an epoch in Naval improvements, for hundreds of seamen have annually fallen victim to its effects.[27]

He was a Physician at Haslar for only four months – but he set out his plans for reforms in *Remarks on the Establishment of Naval Hospitals and Sick Quarters*, (1795). In this he made an eloquent plea for an establishment of Naval Officers at Haslar Hospital to maintain discipline; and also for a much larger and surgical staff – 'posterity will wonder that a hospital able to contain 2,000 seamen, should be without a single Naval Officer to preserve order and discipline among the men, who, on so many occasions, appear only as children of a larger growth'. He suggested a Captain as Governor, with Lieutenants to assist him (early lay administrators), saying:

> it appears to me that a Government in our hospitals, such as I have represented, would be one of the first and most certain checks to that system of defection, by invaliding improper 'objects', [by this he means sailors feigning illness], which has been the bane of the Navy....It must readily appear to every discerning person that so few physicians and surgeons, [two of each with some assistants] for such an immense business, must be utterly unequal to the task.
> No man.....can suppose that one Physician is capable of doing justice to four or five hundred patients in one day.... but it is not merely the time spent at the sick bed, where he is to do justice to his patients, there must be hours left for study and reflection. Diseases will now and then appear where every thoughtful mind would wish to turn over Authors on the

subject, and to canvas opinions, in order to give preference to a decided method or cure.[28]

The number of patients attended by one Physician — ought to be no more than he can visit with ease in a forenoon — that he may be enabled — at different times of the day to see those who require more frequent visits.

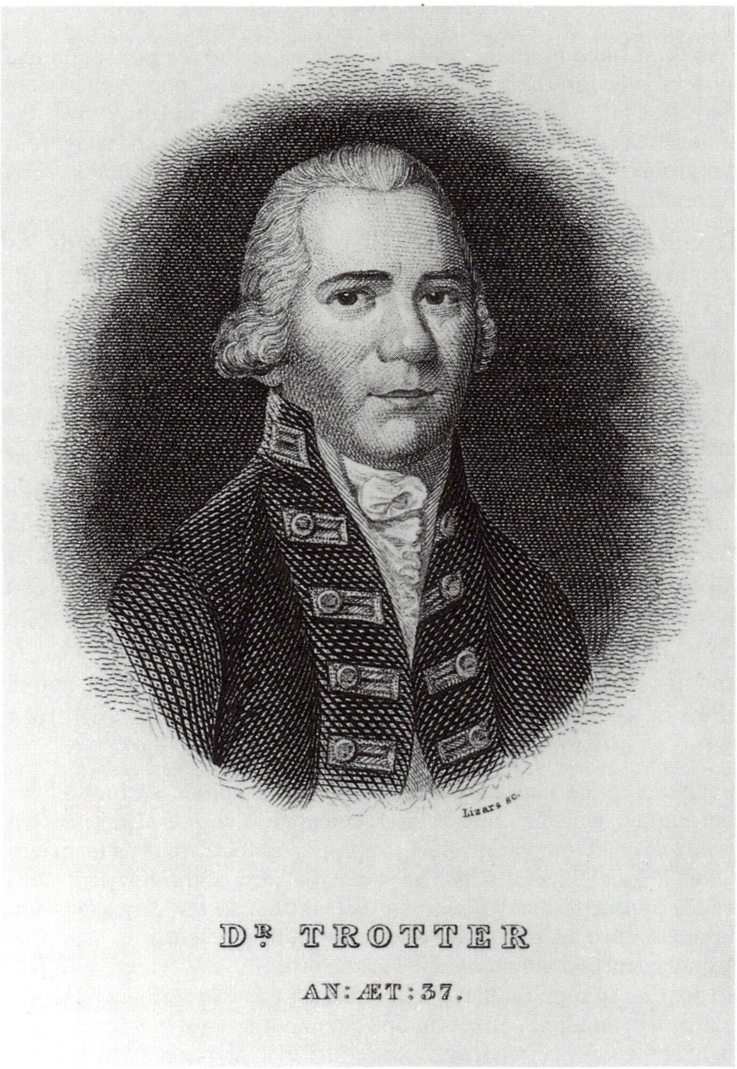

Figure 1. Trotter in about 1797, but in a uniform of a style adopted in about 1805.

After suggesting at least twice as many staff on increased salaries, he goes on to advise that in peacetime, two physicians and surgeons would be retained on full pay and the rest permitted to retire on half pay to be called on when necessary – 'that no narrow adherence to mistaken economy may ever be brought in competition with the sacred duties of sick bed attendance'.[29] He also recommended, with detailed plans, a medical library and clinical lectures.[30]

Physician to the Channel Fleet

In April 1794, Trotter was appointed Physician to the Channel Fleet by Admiral Howe, 'in compliments to his professional studies devoted to the health of seamen'.[31] It was a post he held for eight years. He attended the Fleet in the inappropriately named hospital ship the *Charon* and took great pride in the way she was fitted out.[32] Lloyd says that 'Admiral Howe's tactics at the beginning of the war' [1793 – the 20 years war with France] 'allowed for frequent returns to port for replenishment, but if the cruise was a long one, Trotter accompanied the Fleet in the *Charon* in order to supervise victualling'.[33] His appointment occurred two months before the famous Battle of the Glorious 1st June, when Admiral Howe defeated the French Fleet off Brest and took seven prizes.[34]

A year later, during the Quiberon expedition, when there was a tremendous swell of the sea, Trotter injured himself while climbing up the side of the *Irresistible* to attend to the Captain, who was severely wounded. He developed a hernia, a common condition among seamen. Lloyd says that 'of all the occupational hazards – and there were many – to which seamen were exposed in the days of sail, the commonest was that of hernia, and from the number of trusses issued, something like 1 in 7 of those serving must have been in some degree ruptured'.[35] This hernia prevented Trotter from doing active duty on boats and he had to lie down for some hours daily to relieve the pain. For the next seven years he served mainly ashore, still as a physician to the fleet, continuing to direct and advise the surgeons, and receiving their reports. It was during this time that he compiled his principal work *Medicina Nautica* which will be referred to in greater detail later.[36] He refers to his 'painful affliction' in later writings near the end of his life, saying that he 'found by the time he quitted the Navy in 1802, that he was incapable of ascending ships as he had hitherto done, without pain and hazard'.[37]

Medicina Nautica

In his book, *The Health of Seamen*,[38] containing extracts from the writings of Dr James Lind, Sir Gilbert Blane and Dr Thomas Trotter, Professor C C Lloyd says that although Trotter was not as eminent as the other authors,

> he was even more deeply imbued with a sense of sympathy and consideration for those under his charge. His enthusiastic personality, his reformist activities on behalf of his colleagues, and his genuine

> concern for the common seaman, illuminate with the warmest colours every page of his principal work, *Medicina Nautica*.

Lloyd points out that many of the works of Lind, Blane and Trotter from which he quotes are almost as rare as manuscript materials – and that despite Nelson's dictum that 'the great thing in all military service is health' – the subject has been largely neglected by naval historians.[39]

Trotter was widely read and made a point of keeping abreast with the medical literature of his day. Writing at the end of *Medicina Nautica* (vol 3) he says,

> Few persons can measure the degree of fatigue in body and mind, and the expense which attend pursuits of this kind, amidst the bustle of naval life. My official postage has often exceeded seven shillings per day and a new medical publication frequently taken my last guinea.[40]

Lind had published his *Treatise of the Scurvy* in 1753, and his *Essay on the most Effectual means of preserving the Health of Seamen* four years later. He had proved, by the first dietetic experiment on record, that lemons or oranges were the best available cure for scurvy. His specific for the disease was not adopted by the Admiralty until 1795 at the instigation of his disciples, Gilbert Blane and Thomas Trotter. Lloyd says,

> Lind's influence is to be discerned not so much in his own day, as in that of the next generation, which revived his teaching, and learned the experimental method from his books. Of those who made it their business to get his precepts adopted, Thomas Trotter is pre-eminent. He not only fought more energetically than anyone else for improving the conditions of his fellow surgeons, but in the warmth of his humanity he seems to stand nearest his master.[41]

Sir Gilbert Blane was the most distinguished and influential naval physician of his time. Unlike Trotter's, his was an Honorary MD degree. As personal physician to Admiral Lord Rodney, he had accompanied him to the West Indies Station in 1780, and he was responsible for the remarkable improvement in the health of the West Indies fleet during the last three years of the American War. Blane wrote of his experience in *Observations on the Diseases of Seamen* (1785). Because of his influence in high places he was able to instigate reforms more easily than his humbler colleague. As Commissioner of the Admiralty Board in 1795 he was responsible for the issue of antiscorbutics to the naval ships on a more generous scale than ever before[42] and he achieved the official issue of soap to the Admiralty the following year, although surgeons were still complaining of shortages ten years later.[43] He emphasized the importance of prevention of disease, and with his contemporary, Dr R Robertson, pioneered the presentation of statistics in naval medical records.[44]

Trotter followed his example and encouraged his ships' medical officers to do the same. He said,

> I have endeavoured to imitate Dr Blane in calling upon the surgeons for occasional remarks; and much valuable information has been received from that quarter; which I have thrown into the form of notes.....the extension of navigation and commerce has given rise to a new train of distempers; some of which had been little known if at all, in the ancient world.....We must on that account come nearer our own times to reap much information, and Dr Lind may be justly styled the father of Nautical Medicine.....his works have succeeded those of Robertson and Blane; it may also be proper to mention with them, Dr Clarke, who was a surgeon of an Indiaman, and wrote on the diseases of seamen.[45]

Later in writing on *The Health of Seamen*, he refers his readers to 'the very valuable observations to be found in Dr Blane's publication on *The Diseases of Seamen*, and to a most valuable work from the humane and learned, Dr Lind' – written with 'a view to preserve the health of our seamen'.[46]

Trotter offers the authors the 'tribute of his unfeigned gratitude', and recommends that

> the works of Lind and Blane should occupy the first place in the library of every Captain of a Man of War....for a careful perusal of them will teach him the way to render healthy, comfortable and happy the men over whom he is appointed to command.[47]

The first volume of *Medicina Nautica – An Essay on the Diseases of Seamen*, from which the above quotations are taken, was published in 1797, when he was still active as Physician to the Fleet. It is dedicated to 'Richard, Earl Howe, Admiral: The Flag Officers, Captains, and other officers of the Fleet'. No doubt he hoped that it would find a place in the Captain's Library beside the works of Lind and Blane. In his introduction he aims straight at his readership:

> the operations of a large fleet in Channel service offer a field for observation of the first importance to the Medical inquirer..... Ships newly commissioned, by receiving raw landsmen, and drafts of seamen from crowded guard ships, tenders and hospitals, are the most liable to suffer from infection; and are generally employed, at first, on home stations. Hence this subject has engaged much of our attention.....My accounts of different diseases... will be found useful to Medical readers in general. They abound with facts that could be met with nowhere else; and being compiled from a number of cases, they bring into one view an endless variety of symptoms.

He goes on to condemn the use of the 'gasses' (in vogue to fumigate ships) as 'hurtful' in the extreme.

> To a hyperoxygenated atmosphere, or one possessing its due proportion of oxygen, we look for security against infection; not as acting by chemical combination or contagious miasma; but as supplying the human body with a quality that enables it to resist the offending power — We do not rest this preference on an appeal to first principles only

> as we have witnessed its success on a larger scale of experience than has usually fallen to the share of one observer.[48]

His writings 'were compiled from notes taken as opportunity offered....the studies of a Naval Physician are something like the soldier's prayers; they must be said when and where he can'.

The book begins with two 'discourses'. In the first he describes recent reforms in the Medical Department of the Navy. These include many suggestions already made in *Remarks on the Establishment of Naval Hospitals* relating to the pay of medical officers, comparing it unfavourably with that of physicians in private practice and making a plea for parity with the army medical officers. He also emphasises that the supply of medicine to HM Ships should be at government expense, and 'not interwoven with the pay of medical officers' and 'the source of multifarious abuse'.[49]

In addition to a medical library he suggests a suite of baths, a pigeon house, a poultry farm and gardens and orchards around the hospitals for the use of the sick. 'How delicious an apple, a plumb or a pear after a long sickness on board?' Trotter's 'directions for the conduct of officers in the wards under his charge were a model of their kind'.[50] He concludes this section with the regulations he had drawn up for the visiting Apothecary and Assistant Dispensers in the wards of Haslar Hospital.[51]

The second discourse includes an account of the characteristics of the British sailor, his follies and vices (including methods of feigning sickness) and his virtues of courage, loyalty and sincere friendship. Trotter condemns the evils of impressment, about which he was to publish a book much later in life.[52] As Lloyd observes, 'once Trotter began to take the slightest interest in a problem, he invariably followed it through to the bitter end'.[53]

He gives a detailed description of a suitable uniform for sailors.

> A general uniform for seamen has been mentioned in the valuable works of Lind and Blane, and supported by arguments so conclusive that nothing can be offered against them. Amidst so many improvements in the Navy, we are surprised that ...... this has never been brought into universal practice.[54]

In fact nothing was done about this until 1857. He and his predecessors said that, in addition to the sanitary advantages of a uniform, it would be considered an honourable distinction, engender *esprit de corps*, and render desertion less easy.[55]

Excerpts from Trotter's Journal follow in a 'General Abstract of the Health of the Fleet from January 1794 to December 1796, and of the weather during that period'.[56] This section gives vivid pictures of the conditions under which seamen lived (and died) at that time. It also shows the untiring zeal with which Thomas Trotter tried to improve the conditions of the seamen under his care and his concern for the welfare of his fellow medical officers. When he was appointed Physician to the Channel Fleet on 9 April 1794 it consisted of thirty-two sail of the line, eight frigates, a sloop and a fire-ship......

Only two weeks later he had visited all the ships and reported their state to the Commander in Chief.[57] On 1 May he was able to say

> The whole of the Fleet may now be said to be in perfect health.
> May 13th — This day one man in small pox and another in measles. Both in a state of eruption, were sent on board the *Charon* from the *Gibralter*. These diseases did not extend to any other person. Six seamen and a gunner's child, were inoculated in consequence, on board the hospital ships..... all of whom had the disease in the mildest degree.[58]

Trotter's journal entries give a vivid picture of events at the time of the famous battle of the Glorious 1st June.

> May 19 (1794) This day Earl Howe received intelligence that the French Fleet was at sea; when the signal was made for the ships to prepare for action. Our course was therefore shaped for the enemy's fleet which was cruizing to protect their homeward bound American convoy, a long way to the Westward.During this pursuit, a number of vessels belonging to our Lisbon and Newfoundland trade were re-taken with two corvettes and a cutter, all of whom were immediately set on fire, and the people taken out.
>
> May 27th Two French prisoners in fever, were sent to the *Charon* from the *Thunderer*. One of them died next day. They came from a corvette....bearing dispatches to the French Admiral.
>
> May 28th The enemy's fleet were seen to windward.
>
> June 1st The details of this glorious battle, so honourable to the British Navy, will fall to the share of some more able historian. We were left in possession of seven sail of the enemy's line. One of them, the *Vengeur*, sank the same evening.

This is followed by tables showing the numbers of killed and wounded on both sides (including the names of the British Officers), a list of the surgeons present and their respective ships.[59]

> June 8th The Admiral having been informed that the French prizes were sickly, ordered me to visit them as soon as the situation of the Fleet would permit. The number of killed and wounded in these ships was very great — they were also sickly, and from being dirty to an extreme degree, a contagious fever had carried off many.[60]

Trotter reports later that the French ships

> were well supplied with medicines, surgeons and assistants. The necessaries carried at sea for the use of the sick consisted of many articles of comfort unknown in our Navy; they had even livestock on board for this purpose — (sheep, goats and poultry), which, when bestowed on our sick, must come from the tables of their officers.[61]
>
> June 13th This day we arrived at Spithead with our Prizes.....The wounded men were landed immediately...... It deserves to be recorded to the immortal honour of the officers of this Fleet, that the stock of their messes, consisting of sheep, poultry, with all the delicacies which

> their tables afforded, was cheerfully resigned for the support and comfort of the wounded. But their goodness did not stop here; they learned that the diet of the hospital was deficient in some articles which a wounded sailor could wish for; and sums of money were sent to procure them. My heart warms with indescribable emotions, while I relate a fact that deserves to be recorded with the pen of an angel.[62]

Trotter lost no time in dealing with the threatened spread of infection from the French prisoners.

> Being fully sensible of the danger to which the greatest part of our ship's had been exposed from a general contagion, I did not wait for reports from the surgeons.....but made it my business to see the whole.[63]

The following is an example of a Surgeon's report quoted by Trotter and shows the successful treatment of an outbreak of fever among the crew.

> From Robert Dunn, Surgeon of the *Circe*, June 1794.
>
> During the early part of the cruize there were few complaints of a serious nature. Several prisoners from a French Corvette and other prizes were sent on board the *Circe* and two were soon attacked with symptoms indicating an alarming fever. Some of our best men became daily affected in a similar manner: want of appetite, nausea, a foul tongue, some degree of tension of the skin, with costiveness, were the most observable appearances. Emetics were administered daily in these cases, and blood letting avoided where there were no violent symptoms of inflammation. Purgatives were necessary to clear the intestines, and relaxation of the surface was kept up by antimonials, sometimes combined with opiates. Three or four days illness was sure to induce great debility. A free use of wine was highly relished by them all and they soon gained their usual strength.[64]

The measures Trotter ordered to stop the infection included keeping the decks clean by dry methods, white-washing the inside of the ship, cleanliness of clothes, bedding and personal cleanliness of the men.

> Fires were kindled in pots in the hold, well, and bread-room; care was taken that the circulation of air through the wings should not be interrupted;....so that every corner below was pure and completely perflated by air......
>
> The immediate separation of the infected was what I most depended upon; and not even the slightest cases were allowed to remain on the ship.
>
> The Surgeons were directed to order their mates to walk frequently round the deck; and to watch those men who, while sitting in their berths, appeared dejected or solitary. This was always my practice in an infected ship, because seamen will sometimes withhold their complaints for a day or two, under the idea that an incipient fever is only a common cold.[65]

The fact that the whole Royal Family was able to visit the Admiral's Flag Ship, the *Queen Charlotte*, with impunity, twelve days after her arrival at Spithead, was due to these measures.[66] Trotter had sent all prisoners with the least symptoms of indisposition to the *Charon* at sea — one of them died next morning.

> How far every ship might have availed themselves of this salutary precaution, I cannot pretend to say, but it ought to be attended to in future, and an hospital ship provided sufficiently large to accommodate the sick of a large fleet, in similar emergencies.[67]

After this victory, Trotter drew the attention of Admiral Earl Howe to the important part played by the Surgeons and their Assistants. He was instrumental in getting the surgeons to present a petition to Howe containing the numerous defects in conditions of pay in the Medical Department of the Navy. The immediate result of this was that 200 surgeons were added to the half pay-list.[68]

There is no space to consider his accounts of diseases common to seamen — including typhus, yellow fever, catarrh, smallpox, scurvy and intoxication. He planned to 'extend' his writing on this last condition, which had been the subject of his MD thesis, but the outbreak of war prevented this until 1804.[69] The sections on dysentery and rheumatism contain vivid accounts of Trotter's personal experience of these diseases.[70] He says of dysentery:

> a medical man....sometimes acquires professional knowledge from personal sufferings. The danger which I had escaped, and the distress that I underwent, made me resolve to pay particular attention to this disease in future.[71]

Scurvy

It is worth considering scurvy in more detail as Trotter made a notable contribution to the conquest of this disease, 'the most malignant of sea-diseases in the 18th century, and killed more men and paralysed more fleets than any series of naval actions'.[72]

Trotter's journal and several contemporary letters give a vivid picture of the problems he and his colleagues faced, and of his untiring efforts to prevent and treat the disease.

Lind's 'sovereign cure', lemon juice, had actually been rejected by the Sick and Hurt Board in 1754. Although Sir Gilbert Blane had asked the Admiralty in 1781 for a supply of fruits, especially lemons, to be available to seamen, it was not until he was on the Naval Board 14 years later that he was able to persuade the Admiralty to sanction the official issue of lemon juice and fruit on a more generous scale than ever before.[73]

Trotter had published his *Observations on the Scurvy* in 1786, concluding as Lind had done that 'fresh vegetables of all kinds will cure it, but those fruits abounding with acids such as citrus class, are more effective than others'.[74]

During the severe winter of 1794-5, when beef was expensive because so many cattle had died, Trotter reports that

> the Victualling Board....thought proper to dispense with the usual allowance to the ships and reduced it to one day's fresh meat in the week. Whether there was more economy, ...in giving salt provisions rather than fresh, is a matter of doubt with me; but this I well know, that such a change in the victualling of a large Fleet ought never to have taken place without consulting the officers on the spot.[75]

He thought the long period of extreme cold predisposed the body to scurvy, and apart from this, the frost had destroyed all vegetation in the neighbourhood of Portsmouth.

> In this State of the Fleet, my fears were very early alarmed. I recommended the immediate stop to be put to the use of salt provisions, and laid before the Admiral what changes of diet I thought would be useful under the present circumstances — in lieu of butter and cheese — let cocoa and sugar be allowed for breakfast — or let sugar and molasses be mixed with oatmeal gruel, that the use of them may become general by being made palatable. Query — why is oatmeal supplied if seamen refuse to eat it?[76]

The Victualling Board did not approve his recommendations – except the molasses – and in any case the supplies did not arrive in time.[77] Towards the beginning of April 1795 scurvy 'had made very considerable progress' in the Channel Fleet – despite Trotter's endeavours. Trotter had demanded 'a supply of lemon juice or the fruit in its entire state, to be ready on board the hospital ship to serve the squadrons as they went to sea'. This supply did not come in time, so Trotter purchased at Portsmouth seventy pounds worth of lemons and oranges. 'The consequence of these precautions were that many cases of scurvy were cured at sea without a single death'.[78]

There were advantages of curing cases at sea; the ships remained ready for service, desertion was prevented, and 'indolent habits' soon learnt in hospitals were not so apt to appear under the eyes of their own officers. Indeed 3000 cases of scurvy were cured on board ship between March and June 1795.

> In my official letters, I took care to inform their Lordships that I had attended the vegetable stalls on market days as well as the gardens in the neighbourhood and had there found abundance for our consumption. We were (from 31st May), supplied with 5000 cwt of salad every day, which was distributed under my own eye, to the.....ships at Spithead. The good effects of these refreshments were astonishing; we had only to regret that they were not sent sooner.[79]
>
> The reader may smile at the idea of a Physician of the Fleet attending the stalls at a vegetable market, or perambulating the country to acquire the produce; but it never appeared to me below the dignity of the profession; nor did I consider it a mean task to serve the salad with my own hands from the *Charon*'s quarter deck.[80]

His determination to obtain supplies brought him into conflict with the local people, as he explained:

> A lady of rank, who was in the custom of giving large dinners to small parties, complained that she could no longer procure oranges and lemons for her company. She said, 'it is a shame that the nation's money should be expended in this way, Captain P. tells me that these things are not good for sailors, and what is worse, this Physician can persuade Lord Howe to do anything'.[81]

The truth is that ships would have been paralysed if such action had not been taken, and the blockade strategy as practised by St Vincent and Nelson, would have been impracticable.[82] Trotter concluded that:

> The late occurrences in the Channel Fleet have sufficiently established the fact that scurvy can always be prevented by fresh vegetables, and cured effectually by the lemon or the preserved juice of the fruit.......We contend that recent vegetable matter imparts a 'something' to the body, which fortifies it against the disease.[83]

It was over a century later that this 'something' was discovered to be Vitamin C.

By the end of the Twenty Years War, scurvy had almost disappeared from the navy. On 1 Feb 1796, Trotter was able to record in his Journal, 'No sickness of any kind in the ships of the Fleet'.[84]

Trotter was always ready to explore new ideas, such as the use of lemon juice in crystalline form (as advertised by Mr Coxwell of Temple Bar).[85] The preservation of the fresh juice had long presented great practical problems. He made trials of the crystals, which he found effective, and received many encouraging reports on their use from other surgeons in the fleet. When he recommended the adoption of the crystals to the Admiralty, they first directed that trials should be made on two ships, but finally concluded that their use would be too expensive.[86] 'I can already see that the Naval Service is not likely to be soon benefitted by this ingenious discovery', wrote Trotter, 'there is a worm that cankers the bud of all improvements here'.[87]

Approbation and conflict

In June 1797, after the publication of the first volume of *Medicina Nautica*, the surgeons of the Good Hope Squadron presented Thomas Trotter with a gold snuff box, 'in testimony of professional abilities successfully directed to the Welfare of the British Navy, and in gratitude for long and unwearied exertions on behalf of the surgeons'.

George McCallum, a Senior Surgeon and longstanding friend of Trotter, was commissioned to present the gift.[88] In the long complimentary letter accompanying it he says that the surgeons

> have already observed with the most heartfelt satisfaction, a considerable improvement in the Medical Department of the Navy, and in their hitherto neglected situation, they do not despair of seeing the plan of improvement which he has pointed out,[89] ultimately covered with compleat success.

Trotter must have been cheered by this gift and by the support of his colleagues. The same year his friend and patron, Admiral Howe, retired because of his age (71) and gout. He wrote to Trotter,

> It will always be a matter of grateful reflection to me that I was the means of nominating you to your present station. And I may justly congratulate yourself and the country on the important changes which have taken place in the ships and hospitals by your advice and exertions; and the zeal and activity which have been spread throughout the service by your example.

He thanks Trotter for the copy of *Medicina Nautica* he has sent him and concludes, 'I do not think the retirement of a weak invalid like myself can effect [*sic*] your appointment, from which on all occasions I received such effectual co-operation'.[90] In fact Trotter did miss the support and influence of his old chief and unfortunately incurred the displeasure of Howe's successors. Several letters in the National Maritime Museum show the cordial relationship between the two men.[91] Trotter wrote of Howe:

> With this good and great man, the health and comfort of his people were his first objects. In the exercise of my official duty, I was commanded to makes use of his name on every occasion, and in all my interviews with him, I never came away disappointed.

Trotter refers briefly to the mutinies which took place this year (1797), but in a later work, *A Practical Plan for Manning the Royal Navy* (1819), he expresses his conviction that if Howe had not been ill and absent, the earlier petitions would have been enquired into and the mutiny would not have occurred.[92]

He writes with understanding and sympathy about the causes of the mutinies and in his journal records the psychological aftermath when he visited the Fleet in August 1797:

> there appeared an unusual despondency and dejection of spirits among the patients in the different sick beds. The outrageous fury of late proceedings had subsided; and the horror induced by some awful examples of punishment was now operating [50 were sentenced to death of whom 29 were executed. Trotter observed] frequent fits of hysteria, accompanied by convulsions, immoderate risibility, weeping and delirium.[93]

In 1797 Trotter received a peremptory command from Admiral Bridport to 'repair on board *H M Atlas*, as his hospital ship, the *Medusa* was to be taken over for a troop ship'.[94]

On the *Medusa* he had been able to provide the sick with the same 'improved diet' as was customary on the *Charon*, with the addition of a milch cow, 'which may be considered the best article of comfort that we can suggest as practicable to be carried to sea'.[95] He records his feelings at the dismissal of the *Medusa* in *Medicina Nautica*:

> The dismissal of the hospital ship cut off much of my communication with the fleet; and in some parts I appear rather the historian of the afflictions of the sick than their physician — Lord Bridport ordered all the stores of that ship, which had been the pride of our service to complete, to be landed without ever consulting me, whether anything ought to be reserved lest the fleet came to action, or for other eventual malady......The consequence has been that the number of deaths at sea has been very great beyond the preceding seasons, and the sick deprived of all the comforts which the Admiralty under Earl Spencer had so bountifully granted.[96]

This unfortunate feud and clash of personalities between Trotter and Admiral Bridport had other consequences; eight ships were disabled by typhus, there were overcrowded hospitals, Trotter was unable to remedy the lack of an operating theatre at Plymouth Hospital,[97] even scurvy reappeared. He had retired to Plymouth saying 'some persons were glad to get quit of me on any terms'. Bridport even ordered the Governor of Plymouth Hospital to refuse to allow Trotter to enter; however this was rescinded on Trotter's application to the Admiralty.[98]

He had written to his friend, Sir Roger Curtis, telling him of his unhappy situation and asking that the surgeon of the *Medusa* should be removed to another ship, and had received a sympathetic reply:[99]

> Immediately upon receipt of your letter I wrote to the Sick and Hurt Board to solicit that the Surgeon of the *Medusa* might be removed to another ship..... By the appropriation of the *Medusa* for a troop ship, I think it is.... not intended to have another hospital ship attached to the Channel Fleet. Your situation is not certainly as pleasant as it used to be.

Trotter's concern for his medical officers is shown in a letter from him to the Lord Commissioners of the Admiralty, appealing on behalf of three surgeons who had served on the *Medusa* and, in his opinion, had been unjustly treated following the dismissal of the ship. He had kept a copy, which is the only letter in his own hand in the collection in the National Maritime Museum.[100]

Bridport was replaced as commander of the Channel Fleet by Admiral St Vincent in 1799, 'largely because the state of the Fleet had deteriorated to the point when another mutiny seemed possible'.[101] St Vincent was a formidable disciplinarian who had just left the Mediterranean Fleet in a state of greatly improved health due to his stringent measures.

Trotter lost no time in writing to his new Admiral. He suggested, and St Vincent agreed to, the replacement of the old hog-sties in the bows of the ship by the new Markham Sick Berth.[102] He also reported disturbing conditions he had found at Plymouth Hospital, where there were number of sailors 'feigning illness' and patients he had seen on board ship with typhus and contagion, directly traced to a man sent from the same hospital who 'brought with him to the boat his clothes in as dirty a condition as he had carried them ashore'.[103] St Vincent replied by assuring Trotter of his support 'in the discharge of the important office you fill', and stating that

> an order shall be issued to the surgeons of the squadron to report to you monthly, the state of their sick, from the date of my taking command. I conclude that you have reported to the....Admiralty the observations you have made on the conduct of Plymouth Hospital — (over which I have no jurisdiction) lest you should not have done so, I have sent an extract of that part of your letter......[104]

Unfortunately the zealous Trotter and his Commander in Chief soon came into conflict.[105] St Vincent thought that Trotter had exceeded his powers in retaining convalescents on shore and detaining ships until they were fully recovered. He wrote to Trotter on 9 July 1800, highly commending his exertions towards procuring vegetables....etc., 'at the same time, I must advise you will discourage....the propensity to remain in Port on account of sickness.... Ships companies will be far more healthy at sea, particularly now that lemon juice and sugar is directed to be supplied.....[106].

Four days later he sent off what Trotter called 'the following laconic epistle':[107]

> Sir, I very much disapprove of your officious interference to prevent H.M. ships under my control from putting to sea the moment their below water provisions are completed, this is ordered to be done with the utmost possible despatch, and I desire you will discontinue this practice.

'One of the broadsides St Vincent was in the habit of firing at anyone who interfered with his plans',[108] Trotter wrote in his journal: 'on.... first perusing this letter, I was....at a loss to conjecture what it alluded to. I suspected it concerned reports I'd given *re* scurvy on the *Temeraire* and *Superb*'. He decided it would be useless to reply, although in his view the letter was incorrect, as a medical officer had no power to detain a ship; he had acted in compliance with the second officer on the spot and had not intended that the ships be 'detained a single hour in port'.[109]

St Vincent refers to the quarrel in 1803, 'in terms which reflect the rectitude of the man'. Writing to his successor, Cornwallis in 1803, he says the post of Physician of the Fleet is unnecessary, but if a superintendent is required, he may have Dr Trotter, 'and it is fair to confess that he is thought very highly of by many of our brother officers, although he took offence at my presuming to differ with him in opinion touching the length of time it was necessary to detain the ships in port'....[110]. However, by this time, Trotter had retired to private practice in Newcastle upon Tyne.

Nelson

In January 1801, Trotter wrote in his journal,

> Vice Admiral Lord Nelson complained of a violent ophthalmia in his only eye, with a membraneous substance.....spreading fast over the

pupil. ...All persons round felt for his Lordship's indisposition and many quack collyria were recommended and sent to him. I prescribed a dark room — and bathing the eye every hour with cold spring water, which in 24 hours had a surprising effect, and in two days the inflammation was entirely gone. Cold spring water, I have long thought the best eye water'.[111]

Writing two years later, Nelson thanks Trotter for telling him where to get his latest book (*Medicina Nautica* Vol III) and adds: 'From what I have heard the Naval Service is under very great obligations to you....and I am sure I am, for your attention to me at Plymouth'.[112]

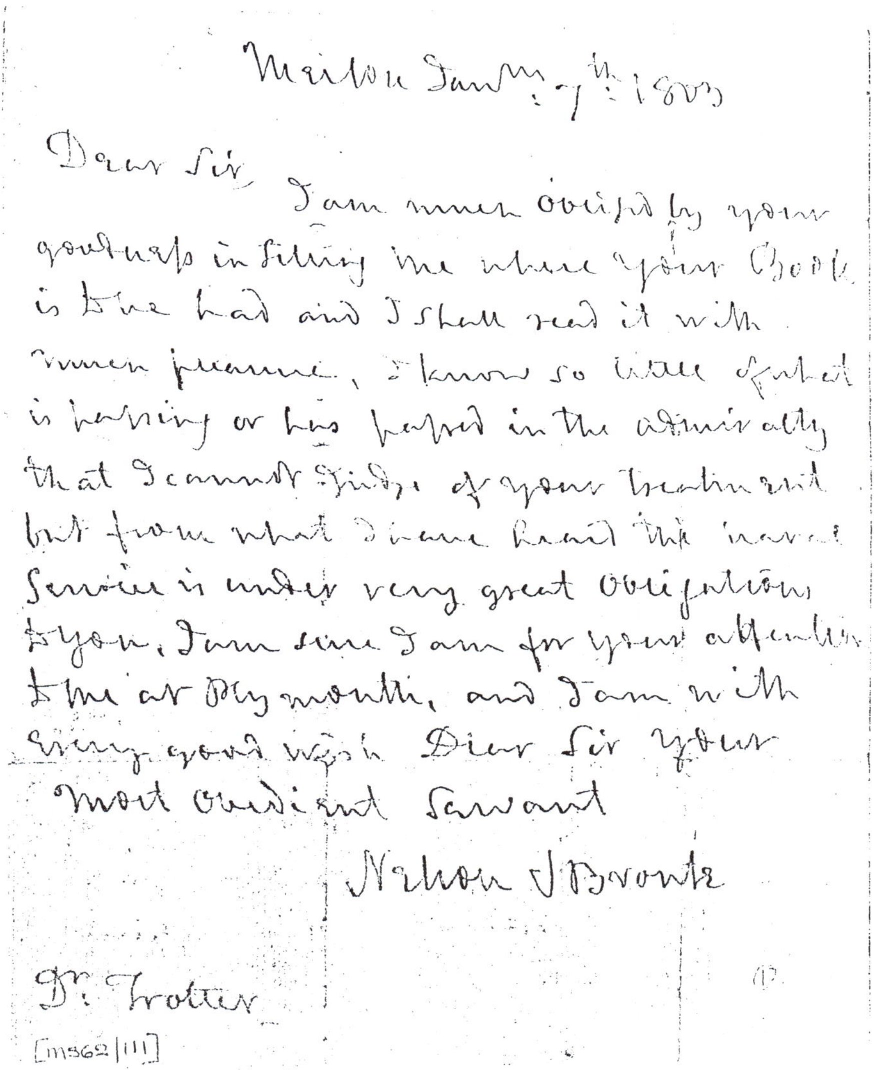

Merton Jany: 7th: 1803

Dear Sir,
I am much obliged by your goodness in telling me where your Book is to be had and I shall read it with much pleasure, I know so little of what is passing or has passed in the admiralty that I cannot judge of your treatment but from what I have heard the naval Service is under very great obligations to you, I am sure I am for your attention to me at Plymouth, and I am with every good wish Dear Sir your most obedient Servant

Nelson & Bronte

Dr. Trotter

[MS62/111]

Figure 2. Letter from Nelson to Trotter, 7 January 1803.

Jenner

Trotter, for whom the 'rules of Prevention of Disease' formed the great outlines of his code of health,[113] was an enthusiastic supporter of Jenner, whose *An Inquiry into the causes and effects of the Variolae Vaccinae* had been published in 1798. In 1801 he organised a subscription among the surgeons of the fleet to present Jenner with a gold medal from 'The Medical Officers of the Navy'.[114] This was the first 'public compliment' received by the discoverer of vaccination and was accompanied by a long complimentary letter written by Trotter.

> It comes from ....officers.....connected with the most brilliant period of our Naval Annals.... They thus offer their warmest support to the cause. The progress of truth is sometimes slow but always certain.

Jenner in his letter of acknowledgement said

> if anything could enhance the estimation in which I shall ever hold such a mark of distinction....it is that it has been presented to me by a man who has cultivated the most useful science with so much success and introduced so many valuable improvements in to the Navy of Great Britain.....[115]

He was grateful for Trotter's encouragement and thus began a most friendly correspondence which continued for over 20 years until Jenner's death.[116]

Practice in Newcastle

On leaving the Navy in 1802, Trotter came to live at 103 Pilgrim Street, next door to Bell's Court, later the first home of the Newcastle upon Tyne School of Medicine. He was no stranger to Newcastle. The Revd William Turner, writing to him ten years earlier, refers to 'that pleasing intercourse from which I had promised myself so much pleasure, had you been permitted to fix your residence in Newcastle' and says that the scheme for a Literary Society, will soon be 'put upon a pretty respectable establishement'.[117] (The Literary and Philosophical Society was founded the following year, 1793.) He asks that Trotter will secure for them any little 'curiosities', and will transmit the observations he may make upon the productions, and the climates etc., of the countries he visits. He goes on to request 'any little essays or papers....particularly could you furnish us with your paper on preserving water fresh at sea by mens of charred barrels.' 'I know.....that you will readily comply, exclusive of the tendancy of such communication to keep up your interest here.'

Trotter became a full member of the Lit and Phil in 1803, a member of the Committee in 1804, and had been an Honorary Member from its inception, but there is no record of his having complied with Turner's requests.

In the same year as the letter from William Turner (1792), he had addressed the Governors of the Dispensary on the importance of a dietetic department.[118] His proposal was warmly supported. He said 'the town....abounds with affluence and is noted for its charity and Christian virtues.' 'If it ever should be my fortune to return, when I have discharged my duty to my Sovereign, my Country, and her Defenders, I shall not fail to revive the subject.'

When he did return, in 1802, he had received no public recognition from the Naval Authorities for his valuable work for the Naval Medical Service.[119] Lloyd says of his naval career: 'to the end, this true friend of sailors was rebuffed and his services ignored by all except his fellow surgeons and the men under his care'.[120] His fellow officers of the Naval Medical Service did show their appreciation of his efforts on their behalf, by presenting him with an elegant and valuable set of tea-plate suitably inscribed in Latin.[121]

In 1805 when there was a general increase in half-pay for Naval surgeons, he was excluded. Without Trotter's knowledge, his friend, Admiral Sir Roger Curtis, asked the Board of Admiralty 'if there was anything against Dr Trotter that he was excluded from the new emoluments', and was told there was 'nothing against him'. Trotter made several personal applications to the Admiralty for an increase in his pension (which was £200 per annum), without success. He pointed out (referring to his hernia) that he was suffering from 'hurts obtained in actual duty'.[122] One reply (in 1808) acknowledged that 'their Lordships are fully sensible of the merits of your services'.[123] This treatment rankled with him until the end of his life. He felt it was 'the reward for his tireless badgering of the Naval powers-that-be on behalf of crews and surgeons'.[124]

Despite this 'personal calamity', as he called it, he embarked upon the second half of his professional life with the same vigour and determination which had characterized his naval career. The third volume of *Medicina Nautica* was published in 1803 – similar in format to the second volume which had appeared in 1799, and likened to a 'precursor of the modern *Journal of the Royal Naval Medical Service*' by Lloyd.[125] It included many reports from ships' surgeons, and extracts from Trotter's Journal from January 1799 to 13 April 1802, when the Medical Staff of the Fleet were discharged by order of the Admiralty at the Peace of Amiens.[126]

Marriage and domestic tragedy

The *Dictionary of National Biography* is incorrect in saying: 'he does not appear to have married'.[127] In fact he married twice. His first marriage must have been in 1802 shortly after leaving the Navy, as Rear Admiral Sir Edward Thornborough sent his 'regards to Mrs Trotter' in a letter to Thomas written on 3 Jan 1803.[128] He married Elizabeth Juliana, daughter of Captain Michael Everitt of Botley in Hampshire. Their son was born on 20 April 1804. He was called John Everitt Howe Roddam Trotter after his maternal grandfather and the two Admirals who had done most to promote his father's naval career.[129]

Elizabeth Juliana died 11 days after his birth, at the age of 29 years, presumably from puerperal fever.[130] Her death must have been a grievous loss for Thomas. He wrote a long epitaph in verse for her gravestone in St. Andrew's Churchyard. There is no sign of it today.[131]

Left with an eleven day old son, Thomas would have needed a housekeeper, possibly a member of his family, to help him to rear the child, especially as he was actively engaged in private practice at the time. No doubt he cherished high hopes for his first born son. The only reference to John in his writings occurs in 1807, when the boy was three years old. On the feeding of infants, Trotter recommends breast-feeding to the age of nine months, when cow's milk may be substituted.

> A child that is brought up by the 'pan and spoon', as it is called, ought to have the milk in the best perfection. This is a practice which is too lightly given into in families. I have weighed its merits fully in rearing my only child in this way, to fulfill the last wishes of an affectionate mother. But though my darling boy has surmounted his loss with the best possible health, I would not recommend this mode of nursing, on any terms, if it can be avoided.[132]

Records show that John Trotter was admitted to the Morningside Lunatic Asylum, Edinburgh in 1841, nine years after his father's death, and died there in 1879 at the age of seventy-four. The note on admission (10 Feb 1841) says 'Mr Trotter had been insane for several years before his admission into the Asylum. Few particulars are known of his history. His profession was that of an Accountant – requiring considerable mental application..... His mental condition approaches to fatuity. He is very gentle – almost childish in his manners'.[133]

Six years after Julia's death, in 1810, Thomas married Isabella Dixon in St John's Church, Newcastle upon Tyne.[134] They had two sons, William Curtis (born 1812) and Thomas Dixon Marr (born 1815), and a daughter, Alicia Alison (born 1816).[135]

His years in Newcastle were full of activity. In addition to his medical practice, he wrote books, pamphlets and numerous letters. He was a member of the Royal Medical Society and the Royal Physical Society of Edinburgh and from 1792 a member of the Philosophical and Medical Society of Newcastle upon Tyne. In addition to poetry including a *Monody on the death of Earl Howe* he wrote a verse tragedy in five acts, *The Noble Foundling* or *The Hermit of the Tweed*, which was performed at the Theatre Royal.[136]

> When a vacancy occurred in the Infirmary, he tendered his services, but finding he was expected to go round and ask for votes, he withdrew his offer. He opened his own home to give gratuitous advice to the poor on Tuesday and Saturday mornings, and immense numbers availed themselves of this privilege.[137]

In 1804 he produced *An Essay, Medical, Philosophical and Chemical on Drunkenness and its effects on the Human Body*; Trotter called this 'a comment' on his MD Thesis [of 1788], corrected and enlarged, and also the 'second edition'. In this work, he developed his belief that 'the habit of drunkenness is a disease of the mind'.[138] It has been recently published in the

Tavistock Classics in the History of Psychiatry series, with an introduction and commentary by Dr Roy Porter. Porter considers that the *Essay on Drunkenness* is 'a land-mark in the history of thinking about drunkenness, alcoholism and addiction', but that 'Trotter's perceptive grasp of the psychological under-pinnings of habitual drunkenness .... was hardly so original as he thought', and quotes from the writings of Lettsom, Cheyne and others to illustrate his point.[139]

There is evidence that before Julia's death Trotter was unsettled in Newcastle and had ambitions to practise in London. He must have asked his friend Jenner if he could find an appointment for him. Writing from London in March 1803, Jenner says,

> I have often been on the look-out for you, but cannot see a situation which would provide you that comfort to which you are so justly entitled. Heaven forbid I should make a thorny pillow for that head which ought to repose on one of down. Success in this great metropolis is not insured, you know, by medical talents; almost the whole hinges upon interest,.... an indescribable something which so highly varnished talents of mediocrity....as to give them a dazzling kind of lustre, and render their charms and attractions (especially among the great who are not always the most discerning) irresistible.

He concedes that there are many physicians 'who are in every respect entitled to the stations they fill'.... 'I should be happy to see you and converse with you on a subject of so much moment to your future happiness'.[140] In fact the year after receiving this letter, Trotter's 'future happiness' was shattered by his wife's death, and understandably he abandoned his ambition to practise in London.

In 1804 he published a pamphlet, A proposal for destroying the *Fire and Choak damp of Mines*, which involved him in a bitter row with two other pamphleteers who disagreed with his suggested methods for preventing gas explosions in pits.[141] He recommended an effective ventilation system, applying the same principles as those he had described in the chapter on 'Ventilation in Ships', in *Medicina Nautica, Volume III*.[142] He produced a second pamphlet on the subject in 1806, '...In confutation of two pamphlets lately circulated in the neighbourhood of Newcastle'.[143] In the same year there was published a book of much greater importance; this was *A view of the Nervous Temperament, being a practical enquiry into the increasing Prevalence, Prevention and Treatment of those Diseases commonly called Nervous, Bilious, Stomach and Liver Complaints, Indigestion, Lower Spirits, Gout etc*. Roy Porter calls it 'in many respects his most wide ranging and intellectually ambitious medical work.'[144] In this Trotter enlarges on many of the observations he had made in the article on Spasmodic Affections in *Medicina Nautica* vol III.[145] For example he recommended that seamen should be able to have music and dancing when off duty on board ship:

To a set of human beings confined for months together...the exhilarating powers of music could not fail to produce the most salutary effects.[146]

In *A View of the Nervous Temperament* he affirms that 'at the beginning of the nineteenth century....nervous disorders may be justly reckoned two-thirds of the whole with which civilized society is afflicted'. He attributed many nervous diseases to the degenerate habits of contemporary society, emphasizing the physical effects of emotional disturbance, and analyzing various complaints which would be now called psychosomatic.[147]

In 1808, he bought a house and small farm at Easter Housebyres near Melrose and apparently engaged in planting trees in addition to his many other activities. Roger Curtis (by then Commander in Chief, Portsmouth), wrote to him:

I am pleased you have a taste for planting trees, but remember one thing, planting will come to nothing unless the trees are well secured from intrusions of cattle after they are planted. My present office is a most laborious one. I have not time to write long letters'.[148]

Writing later (10 Dec 1812), after the birth of William Curtis Trotter, named after him, he says:

I rejoice at your prosperity. You show yourself a planter of eminence — two boys and more than one hundred and twenty thousand trees. God prosper thou His handy works — you have named one of your sons after a great man who was old when he died, [Howe] and the other after a man of much less worth — who though he yet lives is become old.....much less active than when you saw me leap and run at Gatcombe many years ago; and yet I have been eminently blessed in my journey through life.[149]

Sir Roger Curtis died in 1816.

Trotter wrote many letters to local and literary journals. Writing to the *Courant* in July 1816 on the subject of the re-appearance of small-pox in Newcastle and addressing the Mayor, he urges the need for some legal enforcement of vaccination.[150] In a second letter on 14 Sept he reserves any further remarks for another work, 'the publication of which is suspended from the importance which the subject has acquired in its progress, the daily acquisition of new matter'. This book was to be called *Medical Reflections on the Diseases of the Labouring class, including the Diseases of Women and Children etc.*, but there is no record of its ever having been published.[151]

There is evidence that, as late as 1818, he still aspired to return to the Naval Medical Service. Sir Graham Moore, First Naval Lord, writing in November that year says 'I have not a word to say to the kind of appointment on which you apply to me. Lord Melville keeps them entirely in his own hands, and whosoever may succeed Dr Robertson at Greenwich Hospital will owe me no thanks'.[152]

Trotter's last serious work *A Practicable Plan for Manning the Navy without Impressment* was published in 1819.[153] He distributed copies among his friends or told them where it could be obtained. Lord Exmouth, Commander in Chief, Portsmouth, to whom it was dedicated, wrote in his letter of acknowledgement: 'There can be but one opinion on the propriety and justice of putting an end to a system so truly revolting to every feeling of humanity....'[154]

William Wilberforce said that he was 'glad to find an old acquaintance and fellow labourer is employed in a manner so congenial with our former object, as you now are'.[155]

His last publication, *Sea Weeds, poems written on various occasions chiefly during a Naval Life*, appeared in 1829, two years after he had retired from medical practice in Newcastle to his farm at Easter Housebyres. Although 'the Doctor's poetry was not of a high order',[156] this book is of particular interest because of the autobiographical preface outlining his achievements, and in some detail describing his unfair treatment by the Naval Authorities. It also contains an engraving of Trotter at the age of 37 by Lizars, in a uniform which was not worn officially by Naval Medical Officers until 1805 (Figure 1).[157]

In 1830 he left Easter Housebyres and after living in Edinburgh for a short time, returned to Newcastle where he died on 5 Sept 1832 at 15 Leazes Terrace.

Writing of Trotter five years before his death, Mackenzie says:[158]

> a navy surgeon once expressed to the writer his belief, that more lives had been saved in the navy, during the late war, by the regulations and practices introduced by Dr. Trotter, than had been lost in battle.

Certainly his achievements were considerable. He played a major part in the great advance of naval medicine at the end of the 18th century, and was a pioneer, with his colleagues, in laying the foundations of preventive medicine.

Acknowledgements

I am grateful to the Trustees of the National Maritime Museum and to Miss Chrissie MacLeod of the Manuscripts Department, to Professor KA Fowler of the University of Edinburgh, Dr M Barfoot, Archivist to University of Edinburgh and Lothian Health Board, Dr L Gordon and Mr R Firth of the Robinson Library, University of Newcastle upon Tyne, all of whom have provided me with valuable material.

Notes and references

1. The MS notes for: Embleton D. Biographical notices of members of the Philosophical and Medical Society of Newcastle one hundred years ago. *Proc Northumb Dur Med Soc* 1890-1; 195-6.
2. Mackenzie E. *A descriptive and historical account of the Town and County of Newcastle upon Tyne......* Newcastle upon Tyne: Mackenzie and Dent; 1827, Vol 2 p 507. Mackenzie wrongly gives Trotter's first name as James in this account. He was also wrong about the gin shops, there were 200 not 2000 at Plymouth Docks!

3. National Maritime Museum. MS 62/111 (113) Letter from Earl Spencer to Mrs Trotter. 2 Nov 1832.
4. National Maritime Museum. MS 62/111 and MS 74/073.
5. Trotter T. *Sea Weeds. Poems written on Various Occasions, Chiefly During a Naval Life.* London: Longman; 1829.
6. Trotter T. *The Noble Foundling or The Hermit of the Tweed. A Tragedy in five acts in verse.* London; 1812.
7. Trotter T. Reappearance of the natural small pox in Newcastle. *Newcastle Courant.* Letter to the Right Worshipful the Mayor of Newcastle. 6 July 1816.
8. Porter IA. Thomas Trotter M.D. Naval Physician. *Med Hist* 1963, *7*: 155-64.
9. Trotter T. COW-POCK Inoculation in Newcastle upon Tyne. To the Editor of the *Newcastle Courant* — 18 Nov 1822..... "about 45 years ago when I was pupil to the late Dr Buckham of Wooler".....
10. *Medicina Nautica; an Essay on the Diseases of Seamen.....* Vol I. London: T Cadell and W Davies; 1797, 380-2.
11. Trotter T. *Observations on the Scurvy with a review of the opinions lately advanced on that Disease and a New Theory defended on the approved method of cure and the induction of pneumatic chemistry....* London: T Longman, J Watts; 2nd edit 1792: xxix,48,50,55.
12. *An abstract of the evidence delivered before a Select Committee of the House of Commons in the years 1790 and 1791 on the part of the Petitioners for the Abolition of the Slave Trade.* Newcastle upon Tyne: The Society in Newcastle for the Abolition of the Slave Trade; 1791:11, 21, 44.
13. *Book of rates. For the poor in the Parish of Wooler, January 1783.* Northumberland Record Office. "Mr Trotter's House £14..." ET 33/27/1786 "Dr Trotter's House £14..." ET 33/27/1787.
14. Porter IA. Thomas Trotter M.D., Naval Physician. *Med Hist* 1963; 7: 155-64. (from Class lists — University of Edinburgh).
15. *ibid.*
16. Trotter T. *Medicina Nautica...* Vol III. London: Longman and Rees, 1803: 45 footnote.
17. National Maritime Museum. Roddam letters ROD 6/1 p 1-2; ROD 6/3 p 2.
18. National Maritime Museum. Roddam Letters Bk 1 ROD 6/1, p 216-219, 222
19. *ibid* ROD 6/1 p 223.
20. *ibid* p 246
21. *ibid.* Letter from Vice-Admiral Roddam to Philip Stephens 4 Oct 1790.
22. Trotter T. *Medicina Nautica* III *op cit* note 16:217; I:186.
23. Trotter T. *Sea Weeds....op cit* note 5. Preface, xiii.
24. Trotter T. *A Review of the Medical Establishment in the British Navy with a Method of Reform Proposed.* London: J Bew, 1790.
25. Trotter T. *Medicina Nautica* I *op cit* note 10:111-112.
26. *ibid* p 113.
27. *ibid* pp 113-114 and footnotes.
28. Trotter T. *Remarks on the Establishment of the Naval Hospitals and Sick Quarters with HINTS for their Improvement.* Mowbray; 1795, 15.
29. *ibid* p 21.
30. Trotter T. *Medicina Nautica* Vol II. London: Longman and Rees, 1799: 3-6.
31. Trotter T. *Sea Weeds...op cit* note 5, Preface, xiv.

32. Lloyd CC. *The Health of Seamen. Selections from the Works of Dr. James Lind, Sir Gilbert Bland and Dr. Thomas Trotter.* London: Navy Records Society; 1965, 214.
33. Lloyd C, Coulter JLS. *Medicine and the Navy.* Edinburgh: Livingstone, 1961: *3*:159.
34. Trotter T. *Medicina Nautica* I *op cit* note 10:71.
35. Lloyd and Coulter, *op cit* note 33, 3:352.
36. Lloyd CC. *The Health of Seamen*. *op cit* note 32, 214.
37. Trotter T. *Sea Weeds... op cit* note 5, Preface, xix.
38. Lloyd CC. *op cit* note 32, 214.
39. *ibid*, Preface, vii.
40. Trotter T. *Medicina Nautica* III *op cit* note 16:505.
41. Lloyd and Coulter. *op cit* note 33, 3:43.
42. Lloyd CC. *op cit* note 32:132-3.
43. Lloyd and Coulter. *op cit* note 33, 3:79.
44. *ibid* p 46.
45. Trotter T. *Medicina Nautica* I *op cit* note 10:10-11.
46. *ibid* pp 455-456.
47. *ibid* p 457.
48. *ibid* p 3.
49. *ibid* p 19.
50. *ibid* p 26.
51. *ibid* pp 28-34. Many of these regulations were adopted at a later date.
52. Trotter T. *A Practical Plan for Manning the Royal Navy and Preserving our Maritime Ascendancy without Impressment*. Newcastle: Longman, 1819.
53. Lloyd and Coulter. *op cit* note 33, 3:288.
54. Trotter T. *Medicina Nautica* I *op cit* note 10:48.
55. Porter IA. Thomas Trotter, Naval Physician. *op cit* note 14, 162.
56. Trotter T. *Medicina Nautica* I *op cit* note 10:56.
57. *ibid* p 64.
58. *ibid* p 69.
59. *ibid* pp 71-73.
60. *ibid* p 76.
61. *ibid* p 77.
62. *ibid* p 78.
63. *ibid* p 79.
64. *ibid* p 80.
65. *ibid* p 81.
66. Trotter T. *Sea Weeds... op cit* note 5, Preface, xv.
67. Trotter T. *Medicina Nautica* I *op cit* note 10:83.
68. *ibid* p 17.
69. *ibid* pp 400-401.
70. *ibid* pp 380-381, 393.
71. *ibid* p 383.
72. Lloyd and Coulter. *op cit* note 33, 3:293.
73. *ibid* p 321.
74. Trotter T. *Observations on the Scurvy*. *op cit* note 11, 215.
75. Trotter T. *Medicina Nautica* I *op cit* note 10:407.

76. *ibid* pp 114-115.
77. *ibid* p 408.
78. *ibid* p 410.
79. *ibid* pp 128, 414.
80. *ibid* p 129 footnote.
81. Trotter T. *Medicina Nautica* III *op cit* note 16:5 footnote.
82. Lloyd and Coulter. *Medicine and the Navy. op cit* note 33, 3:324.
83. Trotter T. *Medicina Nautica* I *op cit* note 10:423, 424.
84. *ibid* p 152.
85. Trotter T. *Medicina Nautica* III *op cit* note 16:391.
86. *ibid* p 399.
87. *ibid* p 76.
88. National Maritime Museum. MS 62/111 (17).
89. Trotter T. *Medicina Nautica* II *op cit* note 30:7-10.
90. Trotter T. *A Second Address to the Owners and Agents of Coal Mines; on Destroying the Fire and Choke Damp*. Newcastle upon Tyne: Edward Walker, 1806: 27.
91. National Maritime Museum. MS62/111.
Trotter T. *Medicina Nautica* II *op cit* note 30:19.
92. Trotter T. *A Practical Plan for Manning the Royal Navy.....op cit* note 52: 28.
93. Trotter T. *Medicina Nautica* II *op cit* note 30:28-29.
94. National Maritime Museum. MS 62/111 (93) Letter from Admiral Bridport to Dr Trotter. 16 March 1798.
95. National Maritime Museum. MS 62/111 (94) Letter from the Lords Commissioners of the Admiralty to Dr Trotter at Portsmouth. 23 Dec 1796.
96. Trotter T. *Medicina Nautica* III *op cit* note 16:13.
97. Lloyd and Coulter. *op cit* note 33, 3:165, 238.
98. *ibid* pp 288-289.
99. National Maritime Museum. MS 62/111 (126).
100. National Maritime Museum. MS 62/111, Copy by Thomas Trotter of a letter sent by him to Sir Evan Nepean, Secretary to the Admiralty, 1 Dec 1798.
101. Lloyd and Coulter. *op cit* note 33, 3:165.
102. *ibid* p 165.
103. Trotter T. *Medicina Nautica* III *op cit* note 16:223.
104. National Maritime Museum. MS 62/111 (98), Letter from Lord St. Vincent on the Ville de Paris of Ushant, 14 May 1800.
105. Lloyd and Coulter. *op cit* note 33, 3:166.
106. National Maritime Museum. MS 62/111 (117).
107. Trotter T. *Medicina Nautica* III *op cit* note 16:73-74.
108. Lloyd and Coulter. *op cit* note 33, 3:166.
109. Trotter T. *Medicina Nautica* III *op cit* note 16:74-75.
110. Lloyd and Coulter. *op cit* note 33, 3:166.
111. Trotter T. *Medicina Nautica* III *op cit* note 16:107.
112. National Maritime Museum. MS 62/111. Letter written on 7 Jan 1803 in Nelson's own (left) hand.
113. Trotter T. *Sea Weeds...op cit* note 5, Preface, xviii.
114. Trotter T. *Medicina Nautica* III *op cit* note 16:115-121.

115. National Maritime Museum. MS 62/111. 18 April 1801. Letter from Edward Jenner thanking Trotter for the Gold Medal.

116. Brown WG. Letters of Dr Jenner. *Edinb Med J* 1859; *5*:92- 3.
National Maritime Museum MS 62/111. Letter from Jenner to Trotter 26 Nov 1822.

117. National Maritime Museum. MS 62/111. Letter from Revd William Turner (Jr), 19 Jan 1792.

118. Trotter T. *Medicina Nautica* I *op cit* note 10:279.

119. *Local Biography*. Vol 1: p 75 (anonymous newspaper cuttings), Newcastle City Library.

120. Lloyd and Coulter. *Medicine and the Navy*. *op cit* note 33, 3:44, 28- 29.
Gardner JA. *Recollections of James Anthony Gardner*. London: Navy Records Society; 1906: p 91. He described Trotter as 'a most excellent fellow with first rate abilities, an able writer and poet'.

121. Trotter T. *Medicina Nautica* III *op cit* note 16:31-33.

122. *ibid* p xxii.

123. *ibid* p xxiv.

124. Porter R. Introduction to *An Essay Medical, Philosophical, and Chemical on Drunkenness and its Effects on the Human Body*. London: Routledge, Tavistock Classics in the History of Psychiatry, 1988: p xx.

125. Lloyd and Coulter. *op cit* note 33, 3:44.

126. Trotter T. *Medicina Nautica* III *op cit* note 16:143.

127. *Dictionary of National Biography*. XIX:1181.

128. National Maritime Museum. MS 62/111 (125).

129. Parish Register. St Andrew's Church, Newcastle upon Tyne.

130. *ibid*.

131. *Local biography*. *op cit* note 119, I:75-77. The whole verse is quoted.

132. Trotter T. *A View of the Nervous Temperament being a Practical Enquiry into The Increasing Prevalence, Prevention, and Treatment of those Diseases commonly called Nervous, Bilious, Stomach and Liver Complaints, Indigestion, Low Spirits, gout., etc*. Newcastle: Edw. Walker, 1807: 239.

133. Records of Royal Edinburgh Asylum. Case books – Feb 1841 – Nov 1855, Aug 1870 – June 1879. Medical Archive Centre, Edinburgh University Library; HB/42/1. Note on 6 July 1846 'Mr Trotter's state is that of dementia in the form of fatuity'. Regular monthly records that 'bodily health is good'. Note on 31 Jan 1847 'He is a moody, taciturn old man'. 13 June 1879. Died – Death certified as due to 'Cerebral Ramollissement and Atrophy'. Post-mortem carried out; no report available.

134. Parish Register. St. John the Baptist Church, Newcastle upon Tyne.

135. Parish Register. St. Andrews Church, Newcastle upon Tyne.

136. Hughes E. *The Diaries of James Losh*, Vol I. Durham: Surtees Society 1962 *174*:19. 8 Jan 1813 – 'Went to see what was called a Tragedy written by Dr. Trotter, the most wonderful Farrago of nonsense ever exhibited upon any stage...'

137. *Newcastle Journal*. Obituary 8 Sept 1832.
Local Biography. *op cit* note 119, I:75-77.

138. Trotter T. *An Essay......on Drunkenness... op cit* note 124: 172.

139. Porter R. Introduction to *An Essay....on Drunkenness.... op cit* note 124, xvii, xv.

140. *Edin Med J* 1859; *5*:92-93.

141. Trotter T. *A Proposal for destroying the Fire and Choak-Damps of Coal Mines....addressed to the Owners and Agents of Coal Works* 1805.

Dewar Henry MD. *A letter to Thomas Trotter MD... containing chemical and general strictures on that work*. Manchester: J Murray; 1806.

142. Trotter T. *Medicina Nautica* III *op cit* note 16:269-291.
143. Trotter T. *A Second Address to the Owners and Agents of Coal-Mines; on Destroying the Fire and Choke Damp. In Confutation of two pamphlets, lately circulated in the Neighbourhood of Newcastle*. Newcastle: Edward Walker; 1806.
144. Porter R. *op cit* note 124, xxi.
145. Trotter T. *Medicina Nautica* III *op cit* note 16:360, 381.
146. *ibid* I:226-7 and footnotes.
147. Porter IA. *op cit* note 14, 161.
148. National Maritime Museum. MS 62/111 (9).
149. National Maritime Museum. MS 62/111 (36).
150. Trotter T. *op cit* note 7. Letter of July 1816.
151. Trotter T. Letter to the Editor of the *Newcastle Courant* re Smallpox in Newcastle. 14 Sept 1816.
152. National Maritime Museum. MS 62/111.
153. Trotter T. *A Practical Plan for Manning the Royal Navy...op cit* note 52.
154. National Maritime Museum. MS 62/111 (170). Lord Exmouth writing on 20 May 1879.
155. *ibid* MS 62/111 (110). William Wilberforce.
156. Local Biography. *op cit* note 119, I:77.
157. Porter IA. Thomas Trotter — Naval Physician. *op cit* note 14, 162.
158. Mackenzie E. *op cit* note 2, Vol 2: 507.

Chapter 11

THOMAS MASTERMAN WINTERBOTTOM MD
1766 – 1859

S W Stuart Menzies

Introduction

Most medical textbooks when discussing African Trypanosomiasis (Sleeping Sickness) mention 'Winterbottom's Sign' – enlargement of the posterior cervical glands. Whilst in Sierra Leone at the end of the 18th century, Winterbottom had recorded that:[1]

> Small glandular tumours are sometimes observed in the neck before the commencement of this complaint (severe lethargy) though probably depending rather upon accidental circumstances than upon the disease itself. Slave traders, however, appear to consider these tumours as a symptom indicating a disposition to lethargy, and they either never buy such slaves, or get quit of then as soon as they observe any such appearances.

Readily accessible information relating to Winterbottom is sparse,[2] and sometimes misleading.[3] For a period of four years 1792–1796, he was Physician to the Colony of Sierra Leone. Returning to England in 1796 he took over his father's medical practice and settled in South Shields, Co Durham. He married in 1805, and retired from active practice in 1820. On retirement he removed to the nearby village of Westoe, and spent the next 39 years actively involved in most of the educational and philanthropic ventures in the town. In his will he left a sum of money sufficient to erect and endow a School for Mariners. The South Shields Marine and Technical College remains to this day.

Family background and education

Thomas Masterman Winterbottom was born on 26 March 1766 in a house situated about 150 yards north of the Parish Church of St Hild, South Shields, in the County of Durham.[4] The land before the house belonged to the church, but in 1768 was sold to the Town Council, which erected a Town Hall in the centre, and laid out the surrounding land as a Market Place, and so it remains to this day, although the property in which were Winterbottom's birthplace, early home and professional premises, is no more.[5]

Thomas' father, James Winterbottom, was born in Whitby in 1744, and apprenticed to William Ingram, a Whitby surgeon, in 1758. He came to South Shields in 1760 and set up in practice as a surgeon-apothecary. On 16 May 1765 he married Lydia Masterman, the daughter of a prosperous shipowner of the town, who also originated in Whitby. Thomas (1766) was their first child, and others followed in quick succession, Anne Masterman (1768), Elizabeth Masterman (1769), Matthew (1771–1794), Lydia Masterman

(1773), Mary Masterman (1776) and John Hall (1779–1838).[6] Thomas however outlived them all, dying on 8 July 1859 in his 94th year.

James Winterbottom is the only South Shields medical man listed in the Medical Register until 1783, when his name is joined by those of Messrs Simpson and Cockerell. However, as Dr Simmons' Medical Register had no official status, it is quite possible that there were others practising medicine and surgery in this town at that time, although their names are not included in the Register.[7] By 1790 further changes had occurred, and the South Shields medical fraternity included Messrs Winterbottom, Colvin, Simpson, and Lee. All four were appointed as medical assistants in the Preservation Department of the Newcastle Dispensary (instituted 1777). This particular department had been set up to preserve '... the lives of persons apparently dead by drowning, noxious vapours in the coal mines, and suffocation from other causes.' Receiving houses for the reception of supposedly drowned persons were set up at several towns and villages on the banks of the Tyne. Physicians and surgeons were appointed as medical assistants at North and South Shields, Howdon Pans, Newcastle, Lemington, Swalwell and Winlaton and were requested to 'communicate the cases they may attend, and the means made use of to Mr Wilkie at the Dispensary' (Wilkie was the resident apothecary at that time).[8]

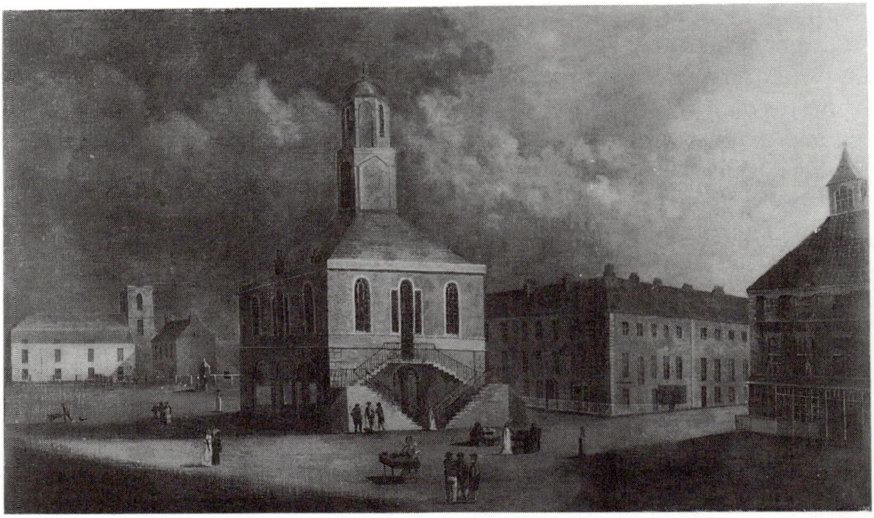

Figure 1. The Market Square and Town Hall, South Shields about 1800, artist unknown. Original in South Shields Museum & Art Gallery.

Education

Thomas Winterbottom's early education was in the hands of the Rev Hugh Brown, assistant curate at St Hild's Church,[9] only a stone's throw from the Winterbottom home. It is likely that he was then apprenticed to his father for a short time before undertaking a more formal study of medicine in Edinburgh.

Edinburgh in the 18th century was one of the great centres of medical learning and many students from several parts of the world enrolled there. The Edinburgh school had been founded by pupils of Boerhaave, so much of his philosophy and teaching methods were enshrined in the new school. The emphasis was on clinical teaching: cases were presented by the lecturer, symptoms and signs demonstrated, diagnosis, prognosis and method of cure were discussed. Teaching was carried out at the Infirmary, and students had much closer contact with patients than was usual at that time. There was no set curriculum, the students only enrolling for such classes as they felt would benefit them. Non-medical students were also able to enroll for classes, and thereby swell the numbers. The average anatomy class in the 1780s sold 340 tickets, which reflected the numbers attending.

The University of Edinburgh records show that Thomas Winterbottom enrolled there for the session 1787-8 in classes for Anatomy, Surgery, Chemistry, Practice of Physic and Clinical Lectures.[10] The Clinical Lectures at the Royal Infirmary at that time were conducted by Dr James Gregory, Professor of the Institutes of Medicine, and were clearly demonstrations of patients, for Thomas Winterbottom quotes examples from his student notes when writing later about urticaria.[11] At the time Alexander Munro *secundus* held the chair of Anatomy, Joseph Black the chair of Chemistry, and William Cullen was Professor of Physic. It is probable that Winterbottom was also a pupil of Alexander Wood, an eccentric surgeon who conducted his rounds accompanied by a tame raven and a sheep.[12]

The Glasgow University records show that Thomas Winterbottom also attended a session in London, probably after 1788, before presenting his MD thesis in Glasgow.[13] There is no evidence, however, that he ever studied in Glasgow. Circumstantial evidence suggests that his London studies were with Robert Willan at the Public Dispensary in Carey Street. Willan was a Northerner – his father practised in Sedbergh – and Robert, after graduating in Edinburgh in 1780, practised in Darlington until 1782, when he went to London. The following year he was appointed Physician to the Public Dispensary in Carey Street, London, where he remained for the next twenty years.[14] A bond of friendship developed between Robert Willan and Thomas Winterbottom, and the latter dedicated his MD thesis to his friend Willan 'on account of innumerable services conferred'.[15]

A number of Winterbottom's books were given to him by Willan and bear his hand written testimony of friendship; his copy of Willan's *On Vaccine Inoculation*, 1806, bears the inscription on the title page, 'In amicitio atq observantio testimonium. R.W.'

On 2 March 1792 Thomas Winterbottom presented his MD thesis *De Morbo Puerperali* to Glasgow University for their approval. The title page of the dissertation suggests that he had a Master of Arts degree (AM), but nothing seems to be known about this; certainly neither Glasgow nor Edinburgh conferred it upon him. The thesis was accepted, and he received his medical degree on 7 March 1792.

It is generally held that Thomas Winterbottom then worked with Willan in London, but that cannot have been for more than a week or two, for he applied for and obtained the post of Physician to the Sierra Leone Colony, arriving there around 1 Aug 1792.[16] As the journey took six to eight weeks, he must have left England sometime in May, only two months after graduating.

Sierra Leone

Sierra Leone was intended as a new homeland for freed American slaves. An earlier attempt at settlement at Granville Town in 1780 had not proved successful, but the second expedition was better organised, and the new site at Freetown was more suitable. In March 1792 John Clarkson arrived from Nova Scotia with some 1200-1400 freed American slaves, and a hundred or so employees and members of the Sierra Leone Company, who were to administer the new colony. The Company members in London were largely members of the Clapham Sect, a group of Evangelical Anglicans with a strong social conscience, and some less pious, hard-headed businessmen. Men involved in pressing for the abolition of slave trading, such as Wilberforce, Granville Sharpe and the Clarkson brothers, were also associated with the Sierra Leone colony.

At the time of Thomas Winterbottom's appointment, John Clarkson was Governor. There were a number of conflicts within the Company, possibly because the Court of Directors comprised philanthropists, and businessmen. The terms laid down by the Court of Directors for governing the Colony were impractical and led to differences of opinion with their executive officers at Sierra Leone, and failed to settle properly differences between the executive officers themselves. A new governing body was set up to replace the original Council of eight men and a Superintendent or Governor.[17] This was to comprise a Governor and two Councillors. When Winterbottom arrived, Clarkson was expecting also the arrival of one of the two new Councillors, William Dawes, a former lieutenant of the marines. Clarkson transcribed part of a letter from Henry Thornton, one of the Directors in London, into his diary for 29 August 1792:[18]

> ...We have sent a sealed letter respecting the succession to the Government in case of total failure of our new Governor and Council. I will tell you confidentially that Dr Winterbottom will stand at the head, and two others the least objectionable in our eyes will be joined with him in case of such an event.....

Shortly afterwards Clarkson returned to London, and Dawes succeeded him as Governor. Dawes was later ably assisted by his deputy, Zachary Macaulay, who arrived in January 1793.[19] In March 1794 when Dawes' health broke down, Macaulay became Governor.

Winterbottom's predecessor, Dr Bell, had come over with Clarkson, and had never been sober since his appointment.[20] His death on 13 March 1792 was unlamented, although for appearances' sake he was given a ceremonial funeral, much to the disgust of John Clarkson.[21] During the first year of the colony, out of 119 original members 57 died and others left, so that only 40 remained, and many of them were constantly indisposed due to sickness.

With Winterbottom, in August 1792, came supplies for the Colony and a large prefabricated building, some 300 feet long, which was intended for use as an hospital, although there was an opinion expressed by some that it would be of more use as a storehouse. Almost as soon as he came ashore, he was asked to attend the widow of one of the Company's European traders. In her journal Anne-Marie Falconbridge describes her illness and recovery:[22]

25th August 1792

> ......I was confined three weeks with a violent fever, stoneblind four days and expecting every moment to be my last. Indeed, I most miraculously escaped the jaws of death, fortunately, just as I was taken ill, a Physician arrived, to whose attention and skill I consider myself principally indebted for my recovery.

In Freetown Thomas Winterbottom had the care of some 1400 persons – or 400 families, but he was also consulted by local tribesmen, some of whom, when his fame had later spread, would walk a hundred miles or more to see him. He also engaged in medical tours through surrounding neighbourhoods. In all this he had the assistance of an apothecary and two or three surgeons.

He seems to have been a diligent and caring doctor, for he was everywhere highly spoken of, by the company officials, the settlers and the native Africans. Fifty four years later, when in retirement in South Shields, he had a visitor from Sierra Leone, with an affectionate address from 34 of the original settlers, expressing their good wishes and thanks for his earlier services. In return Winterbottom, clearly moved by their action, sent each one a Bible.[23]

Other friendships developed, such as those with Macaulay, and with Afzelius. Between Macaulay and Winterbottom a very close friendship grew, and the latter was later to become Macaulay's confidant, taking his good wishes back to England to Macaulay's fiancée, Miss Selina Mills. From the letters he wrote to Miss Mills we are able to judge Macaulay's feelings for Winterbottom.[24]

> ...from Winterbottom I was not used to conceal a thought of my heart. I have therefore told him, under strong injunctions of secrecy of our relation to each other, and I have also requested him, should he visit Bath, to call upon you. Winterbottom has seen me in every different situation in which it is almost possible for a man to be placed and he certainly knows my interior as well as any one, myself excepted....

> Dawes and Winterbottom will come to see you as soon as they arrive in England, and our secret will be safe with them. Dawes is one of the salt of the earth... I believe I love Winterbottom still more. He is certainly far from having attained the distinguished eminence of Dawes, but there is so much warmth of affection in him, and the expression of it so often bursts from him involuntarily, that one is constrained to love him. Besides, I was accustomed to look up to Dawes for advice and assistance while Winterbottom, on the contrary, has been in the use of looking to me for counsel, and as you know how naturally a dependence of that sort begets, in a degree, all the feelings of parents to children. He is a man of general science and great professional skill. He is also a sincere enquirer after truth; and though his religious principles are by no means so fixed as Dawes, he may be fairly reckoned a disciple of Christ. He has four sisters to whom he is so warmly attached, that, he would scarce think it too much to drudge all his days in a coal mine for them.

Winterbottom's other friend, Adam Afzelius (1750-1837), was a Swedish botanist, a pupil of Linnaeus and a protegé of Sir Joseph Banks, who had recommended him to the Sierra Leone Company. It was Afzelius' task to develop and maintain botanical and herb gardens for the colony. He was also engaged in preparations for an atlas of the flora of Sierra Leone, but although he did much preparatory work, the atlas never materialised.[25]

Disaffection amongst the settlers, who complained that the promised plots of land had not been staked out, nor had the promised houses been built for them, resulted in numerous irritations in relations between the settlers and the Company employees. These and other infringements of common law were dealt with by Dawes and Macaulay, but from time to time Winterbottom also had to act in a judicial capacity in the Court of Sessions which was held every three months. The cases were generally trivial, but the jurors took so long to reach a verdict that much time was taken up by the proceedings.

Despite his medical and judicial activities, Thomas Winterbottom found time to carry out research and to write. He continued his custom of recording cases, as in Edinburgh days, and was able to contribute a short note on pemphigus to *Medical Facts and Observations* in 1792. This was followed a year later by *Notes on Urticaria or Nettlerash*. Although he described only four cases, he noted that urticaria may be precipitated by eating crab, shellfish, strawberries and sweet almonds. He himself developed urticaria after eating almonds, although not if they were blanched. Porter also could precipitate urticaria, as could wallflowers and insect stings.

Throughout 1793, Thomas Winterbottom made observations of the weather and climate, and later (1800) published his findings and methodology in *Medical Facts and Observations*. Prior to sailing for Sierra Leone he had purchased a number of meteorological instruments: barometer, Fahrenheit thermometer, rain gauge and two hygrometers. The latter were whalebone slip hygrometers.[26] In this instrument a thin sliver of whalebone, cut across the bone fibres, is fixed to the base of the instrument and at its other end, indirectly, to a pointer. As the whalebone absorbs moisture it lengthens, and as it dries out it contracts, and accordingly the pointer moves back.

Winterbottom set out his meteorological station thus:[27,28]

> Barometers and hygrometers were kept in a room some 60 feet above sea level, the doors and the windows were always open, but the instruments were not in any draught. The hygrometers were each enclosed in boxes pierced with holes, and the lids of the boxes were removed two minutes before readings were taken. The rain gauge was set out in the open, well away from house and trees on a stand four feet from the ground. The thermometer was suspended six feet from the ground in a shaded open passageway. Observations were made at set times, four times every day throughout 1793, and the results recorded in his meteorological journal. Each line of entry recorded Hour; Date; Air pressure; Temperature; Humidity; Moon's age; Prevailing wind; Appearance of the sun; Rainfall; Relative air temperature with respect to feelings.

The next year, 1794, was a momentous year both for the settlers and for Winterbottom. In March, Dawes returned to London ill, and Zachary Macaulay was appointed Governor. In May, one of Thomas Winterbottom's brothers, Matthew, and Mr Watt, another Company employee, returned from a 450-mile expedition to Teembo, the capital of the Fulah tribe. This expedition had been taken with a view to establishing trading links, especially at Labe and Timbo, but a number of climatic observations were made en route.[29] Two months later Matthew Winterbottom was drowned when his boat capsized as he was going ashore at Fort Dix, on the Gold Coast.[30]

The greatest crisis, however, was the visit of a French squadron towards the end of September. The French Revolution was in full swing, and coup had followed coup since 1789. On 21 Jan 1793 Louis XVI had been executed, and in that year also, the British were blockading French ports with serious consequences for their trade.

Early on the morning of Sunday 28 September 1794, seven large and well-armed vessels appeared off Freetown. By their rig and by their colours, they were British, but illusions were soon dispelled when they opened fire upon the town. As the town was unarmed, Maucaulay had little choice but to run up a flag of truce. This was ignored however, and the bombardment continued until evening, when the French came ashore. The inhabitants of Freetown meanwhile had fled into the bush, and some took refuge at Granville Town. The raiders looted and smashed all before them; livestock was slaughtered, Company buildings, including the Governor's house, were fired and destroyed. Nor were the homes of black settlers immune. Afzelius' carefully cultivated botanical gardens were uprooted and plants destroyed, as were his botanical collections and most of his drawings. The church in particular was the object of their revolutionary zeal; pulpit, clock, hymn-books and Bibles were all destroyed. In the town library, books were scattered on the floor, and many removed to the French ships. Bibles and books looking like Bibles were torn up. The apothecary's shop was destroyed with all its contents and stores.[31] Thomas Winterbottom's instruments, and many of his written case notes were destroyed, as he sadly noted in one of his communications to *Medical Facts and Observations*.[32]

Earlier in September, and further up the coast, the French had captured a number of English vessels, including some belonging to the Sierra Leone company. It was under the guidance of a disgruntled American slave trader named Mariner, that the French were able to enter Freetown and wreak so much damage. On 9 October the Company's relief vessel the *Harpy* appeared off Freetown. Before she was able to put about and make her escape, she too was captured by the French, and her cargo, worth some £10 000 destroyed. The passengers were robbed, and despatches and letters were flung into the sea, along with a large botanical collection from Kew. Macaulay had tried to reason with the French Commodore, and his officers who had treated him civilly enough. He pointed out their common desire for liberty, freedom and equality and that Freetown was a settlement for freed slaves. It was obvious however that normal naval discipline had broken down, and that the French officers were unable to control their men.[33]

Throughout this period, Winterbottom worked hard and long amongst the survivors of the raid, but he was hampered by lack of medicines and stores, and by the difficult circumstances in which they were all situated.

The colony was able to rebuild slowly, aided greatly by the friendly relations which had been established with most of the neighbouring natives. The earlier establishment of farms around Freetown also helped to provide food for the devastated colony. Macaulay, in his journal, records his opinion that some £400 000 worth of damage had been done. In some ways however, the French raid served to unite the settlers at Freetown, and this was reinforced by subsequent rumours of further impending attacks.

After the French invasion, Winterbottom, encouraged by Macaulay, engaged in further writing, and on Christmas Eve 1794 submitted a paper entitled 'Some observations relative to Angustura Bark' to Dr Simmons, the editor of *Medical Facts and Observations*. The paper was not immediately published but appeared in Vol VII in 1797. In this paper Winterbottom recorded his experience with Angustura (or Venezuelan) bark in the treatment of remittent and intermittent fevers. He endeavoured to show that it was as effective as Peruvian bark, and was considerably cheaper. Unfortunately it proved to be more prone to produce nausea and vomiting. The opening remarks relating to assessment of new drugs are worth quoting:

> A long time is, in general, required before the merits of a new treatment can be duly ascertained: for while some extol it to the skies as a cure for every disease others are equally fond of depreciating the powers that it actually possesses. Experiments frequently repeated are therefore necessary, before we can form a just estimate of the effects of any remedy.

It is likely that his paper 'Observations on the Use of Arsenic in the Intermittent fevers of a Tropical Climate, etc' was written about this time also.[34] He describes some 19 cases, many of which had splenomegaly. He found arsenic of some value, but not as good as bark, in effecting a cure for intermittent fevers. Nevertheless as arsenic was cheaper than bark, he concluded it would be 'especially valuable in ships whose surgeons have to supply the necessary medicines at their own expense.'

At the request of the Sierra Leone Company, Winterbottom as their appointed Physician, was asked to prepare medical advice 'for the use of such trading vessels in the service of the Company as were unprovided with surgeons'. This he did, writing purposely, he tells us 'in a plain manner of order to render them more intelligible and more easily applicable to practice.' Technical terms were carefully avoided. This must have been a successful project, for he later expanded these notes, adding illustrative case histories and one or two other items. It was then published in 1796 under the title *Medical Directions for Navigators* etc. A second edition was called for and published in 1803.[35] With the approval of the Director of the Board of Trade for the Colonies, it was translated into Dutch, and used on Dutch vessels also.[36]

The period after the French invasion was also used by Winterbottom to collect details of the habits, customs, beliefs and languages of the local native Africans. Of special interest to him were their medical notions and practices. This culminated in his magnum opus *An Account of the Native Africans in the Neighbourhood of Sierra Leone, to which is added an Account of the Present State of Medicine among them*. Although advertised between the 1803 and 1804 Reports of the Court of Directors of the Sierra Leone Company, as a single volume of about 600 pages, it was ultimately published in two volumes costing 15 shillings in 1803.[37]

Macaulay returned to England on leave in May 1795, and Dawes was reappointed Governor. Macaulay returned in April 1796; Winterbottom and Dawes, who had become ill, then left Sierra Leone and returned to England. A letter from Mr Dawes to the Court of Directors, dated 23 April 1796 noted:[38]

> .... Dr Winterbottom having requested leave (as you will see by his letter No.9) is also coming home on the *Mohawk*, along with Governor Dawes — It is much our and we believe the united wish of every person in the colony that Dr W. might be prevailed upon to return to Sierra Leone, at the same time from what he has intimated to us we almost despair of again seeing him here.

Macaulay charged them with the pleasant task of visiting his fiancée, Miss Selina Mills, who was at that time staying with the Misses More, assisting them in their village schools project at Cowslip Green, near Bristol. This they did and on 23 June Winterbottom wrote to tell Macaulay of their visit.[39] Selina also wrote to tell Macaulay of the visits paid to her by his former colleagues.

South Shields

Shortly after this, Winterbottom returned home to South Shields and joined his father in medical practice in the Market Square, but only for a year or so as James Winterbottom died on 16 Sept 1797.

Thomas succeeded his father in the practice, and lived with his mother in the Market Square house. Like many other doctors of his day, Winterbottom took apprentices or pupils; the names of two are known, Dr John Aitken who settled in practice in Edinburgh, and Dr Davidson, who later practised in Woolsingham. Years later Dr Davidson attended his mentor's funeral as the oldest living medical pupil of Dr Winterbottom.

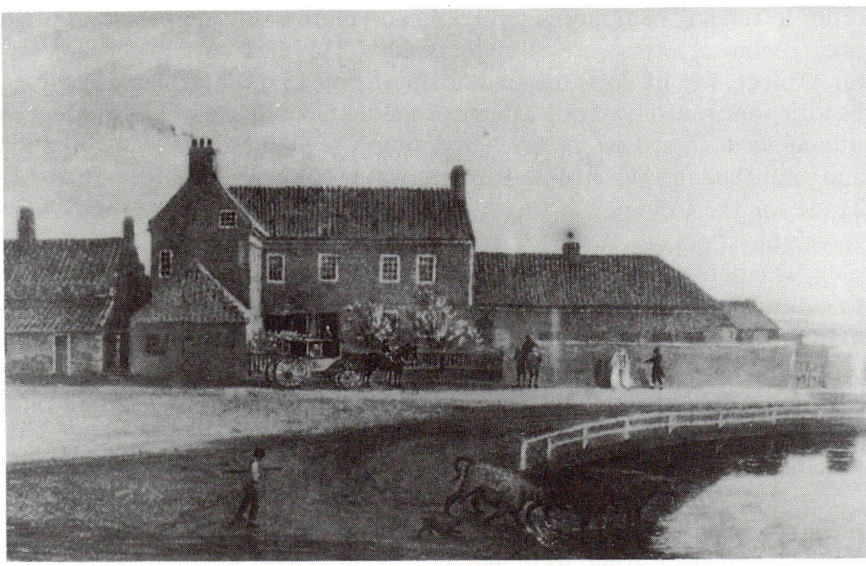

Figure 2. Watercolour painting of Winterbottom's Westoe home, by Newby Lawson (South Shields Museum & Art Gallery).

On 5 Oct 1805 just sixteen days before the battle of Trafalgar, and when England expected an invasion at any time, Winterbottom married Barbara Wardle, the 45-year-old widow of James Wardle, shipowner. His bride was one of the two daughters of Joseph Hunter of North Shields. Barbara had married James Wardle in 1794, her sister married James' brother Matthew in 1794. The girls had a cousin named John Hunter, who was a barber-surgeon, known to, and possibly an assistant of, James Winterbottom. It is probable that this is how Thomas Winterbottom and Barbara met.

It is more than likely that Winterbottom's considerable affluence derived from his wife, since she was both the daughter and the widow of shipowners. She was also the owner of the house in Westoe village, South Shields, to which Thomas presently moved. There is in the South Shields Museum and Art Gallery, a delightful watercolour painting depicting a scene outside the Westoe house. According to a paper label attached to the back it was:

> painted by Newby Lawson Esq. a pupil and friend of Turner R.A. Dr Winterbottom on horseback, Mrs Marshall in the carriage: her daughter Mrs Wallis sitting opposite to her (Walter driving) Mr Archer talking to Miss Isabella and Miss Fanny Green, Mrs G. Ridley (in a calash) going to dine with the doctor and Mrs Winterbottom, and her servant with her.

Winterbottom threw himself diligently into medical practice and also the social and cultural life of South Shields. When he retired from full time practice around 1822, he retained a considerable interest in medicine and his patients, attending for instance, the children of Mr and Mrs Fox who lived opposite.[40]

For thirty-five years or so after his retirement, he enjoyed an annual continental tour,[41] during which time he frequently purchased books to enlarge his library, and souvenirs, many of which he presented to the Literary, Mechanic and Scientific Institution in South Shields. It was during the return voyage and subsequent time spent in quarantine in Stangate Creek in 1822 that Winterbottom began to question the necessity of keeping in quarantine a vessel which had been at sea for some weeks without any of the occupants having shown any evidence of illness. He wrote a long article about this which was published in two parts in the *Edinburgh Medical & Surgical Journal* in 1828 and 1829.[42] In this article he points out the absurdity of prolonged quarantine in vessels that have been at sea for several weeks, and the inconsistent application of quarantine rules in many places. He also presents a history of quarantine regulations and demonstrates their wide divergence from country to country.

It was after his retirement that Winterbottom's influence in South Shields affairs was chiefly felt. He was interested in the fields of education and welfare in particular. The first project in which he was involved was the South Shields Literary, Mechanic and Scientific Institution, which was founded on 23 November 1825, with 'the object of diffusing useful knowledge generally, but especially the arts'. From the Institution's foundation until his death in 1859, Winterbottom was an Honorary Vice-President, and occasional lecturer. He promoted the interests of the Institution in conversation, by many financial gifts, and the presentation of several books to its library.

In 1828 he read an interesting paper on 'The Ocean, its depth, its boundaries, the formation of rocks and islands, marine plants and animals'. Eleven years later he gave a lecture entitled 'Navigation of the Ancients, in parts of the Mediterranean with especial reference to the trading enterprises of the Syrians, Phoenecians and Israelites'.

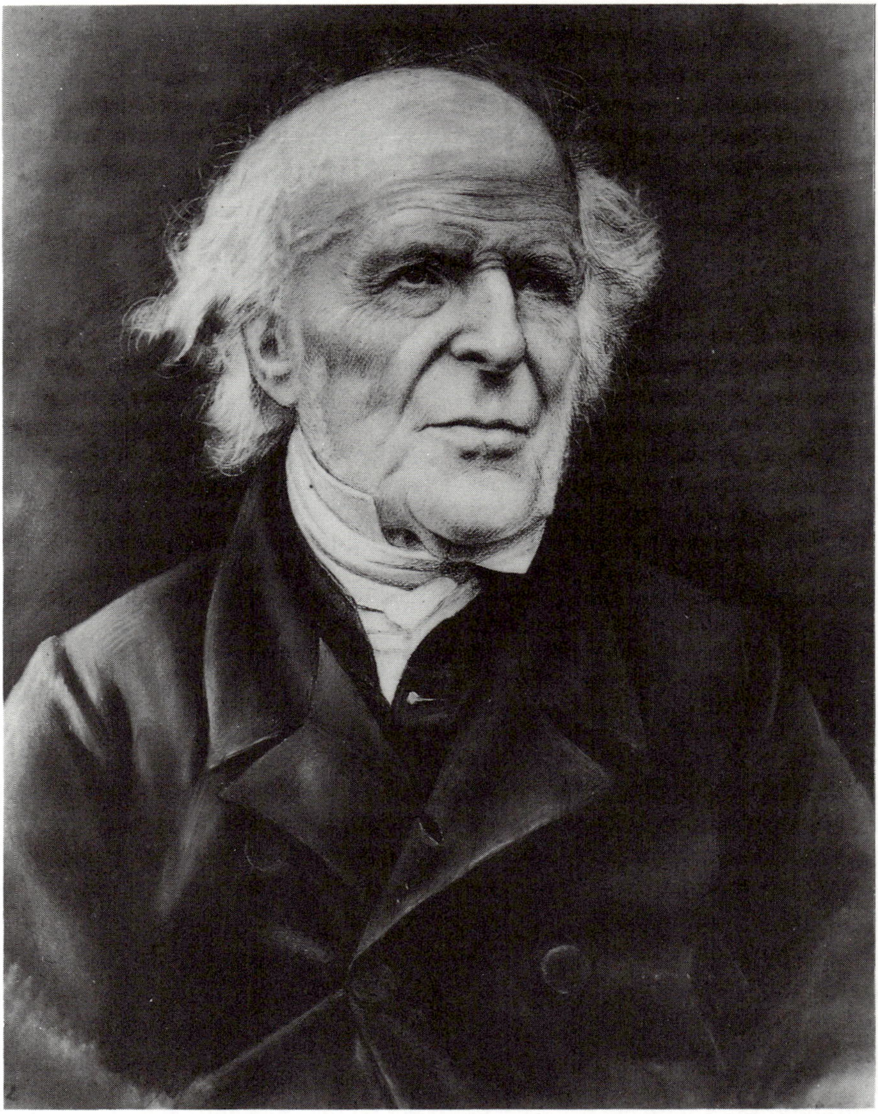

Figure 3. Thomas Masterman Winterbottom (South Tyneside MBC).

At the request of the committee, in 1843 he gave an account of his recent continental tour, with many interesting anecdotes illustrative of the habits of the peoples he had visited. He also offered practical advice to would-be travellers as to their behaviour towards local inhabitants. At this meeting he presented facsimiles of writing in the languages in which the Scriptures were originally written....and a Greek newspaper.

The 1851 annual report of the Institution records that their 'ancient and venerable friend' had presented to the Institution a medal which had been given to him as their representative at a meeting of an Italian Literary Society.

In addition to his interests in promoting the education of adults in South Shields by the L M & S I, Winterbottom was interested in the education of children. In 1834 he was elected Vice-President of the South Shields Committee of Union Schools. This committee included both Anglicans and Dissenters, and administered the Union Schools. Here children over 5 years old paid 1d per week tuition fees and had to undertake to attend the place of worship which their parents or guardians themselves attended or selected.

In the 1830s many shipowners wished for some test of competency of Master Mariners and in 1838 the Marine Board instituted examinations. Anticipating this Winterbottom had the previous year unveiled his carefully thought out plans for a Marine School at South Shields. It was the first school of its kind in Britain. Winterbottom intended that youths over 17 years of age, who had spent at least one year at sea, and who could read and write and do simple arithmetic, should have free tuition. A great many subjects were to be offered.

For a suitable fee and if the headmaster permitted, others could be admitted to classes. Although ladies could attend, mixed classes were thought to be inadvisable. Winterbottom drew up detailed rules for the running of the school. The constitution of the board of trustees was outlined and shares to the value of £21 000 were set aside for the project, although Winterbottom himself and his three surviving sisters Ann, Elizabeth and Mary, were to have the first claim on the money. A site was earmarked for the school buildings. Fortunately for the school, Winterbottom's sisters predeceased him, and on his death work was quickly put in hand. The site, being found unfavourable, was sold and another and better plot in Ocean Road was secured. As it was not clear how the school would develop, rooms were hired in the the new L M & S I building immediately opposite the site in Ocean Road, and the school opened on 26 March 1861, almost two years after Winterbottom's death.

Still pursuing his interest in the welfare of mariners, in January 1839 Winterbottom founded the Master Mariner's Asylum and Annuity Society for aged, infirm and poor mariners. Later that year the Master Mariners' Cottages were opened. At a total cost of £200, 21 cottages were built, forming the north side of a square. They are still standing, occupied and in good repair – a fitting memorial to the philanthropy of Dr Winterbottom. In 1849, a further 17 similar cottages were built, under the auspices of Robert Ingham MP, to form the south side of the square.

Later in 1839, on Friday 28 June, there was a great explosion in the St Hilda mine, two miles from the pit bottom. Fifty one men and boys were killed, including one man who, having escaped, returned to seek his son who was also a victim. Three days later, on the Monday, a public meeting was called and at Winterbottom's suggestion a subscription was raised to help the widows and families of the dead miners. Within a month over £1000 had been raised.

A major result of this accident was the setting up of the South Shields Committee to consider safety in the mines. Winterbottom and the successor to his practice, the surgeon WK Eddowes, Robert Ingham and other prominent men were members of this committee. Three years later, after having visited several pits and talked with many witnesses, a most valuable report was produced. It subsequently became a textbook of pit safety, was translated into several languages and was widely distributed. On the recommendation of the South Shields Report, Inspectors of Mines were appointed, and a more scientific approach to the problem was adopted. Perusal of this report however, fails to identify any contribution at all by Winterbottom.

Mrs Winterbottom died on 12 February 1841 at the ripe old age of 81. There were no children of the marriage. Thomas lived on another 17 years in Westoe Village. His philanthropy continued unabated, further charities were endowed and contributions given to many others than those listed here.

1. Master Mariners (enrolled) Asylum and Annuity Society. This society provided cottages and annuities; a secondary endowment was added later to pay for maintenance of the gardens and paint work.
2. Winterbottom's South Shields Fund for the Relief of Deserving Widows of Mariners. This charity provided annuities for the relief of the widows of mariners.
3. The Unmarried Female Servants' Reward Fund made two awards annually.
4. East Chester Ward Agricultural Society Ploughboys' Award.
5. Christmas Coals to the Poor in Westoe Village.
6. Old Scullermen's Annuity Society, which provided annuities for the Watermen of the Tyne.
7. Loyal Standard Association of South Shields Seamen, which provided members with annuities, and investment opportunities.
8. The South Shields Marine School.

The annuities and awards were not great by today's standards, producing on average perhaps £2–£6 for rewards and £5–£10 for annuities. Consider, however, that the Mariners' cottages cost just under £10 each to build!

Apart from the occasional attack of ague in the 1790s Winterbottom enjoyed good health. There is a story told that once when listening to a lecture on Sierra Leone, he heard the speaker expatiate on the deadly climate of the colony and declare that no European had ever come back alive, Winterbottom sprang out of his seat and shouted 'I am proof to the contrary'.

By 1855 however, the old man, now in his ninetieth year, began to fail. He developed cataracts, a great trial to such a bibliophile. 'Ah those are all sealed books to me now' he would say to friends who came to read to him, 'but I must not murmur, Providence has been very kind and I feel humbly thankful'. In the early part of that year (1855) he suffered from a prolonged bout of bronchitis, and for the first time since 1822 he was unable to make his annual continental tour, and had to content himself with a visit to Folkestone, and his sister in London.

In 1857 a visitor from Sierra Leone stayed with him for a while. At Christmas time the local newspaper recorded that 'The benevolent Dr Winterbottom has distributed 28 cartloads of the best coals, carriage free, among the poor of Westoe, in addition to his presents of warm clothing'. His last outing appears to have been on 30 April 1859, when he took a cab to South Shields to cast his vote for his friend Robert Ingham. On 12 June he developed abdominal pains suggestive of intestinal obstruction, and later peritonitis. He lingered on for some four weeks, sometimes rallying, sometimes worsening. He was exasperated with his inability to get the prognosis right; for several times he had announced that he was 'nearly arrived' or 'on the very point', only to improve again. Characteristically he remarked that he had 'never been so out in his prognosis before'. Thus his first and last confinement to bed since his return from Sierra Leone 65 years earlier ended on 8 July 1859, and South Shields mourned the passing of her greatest philanthropist.

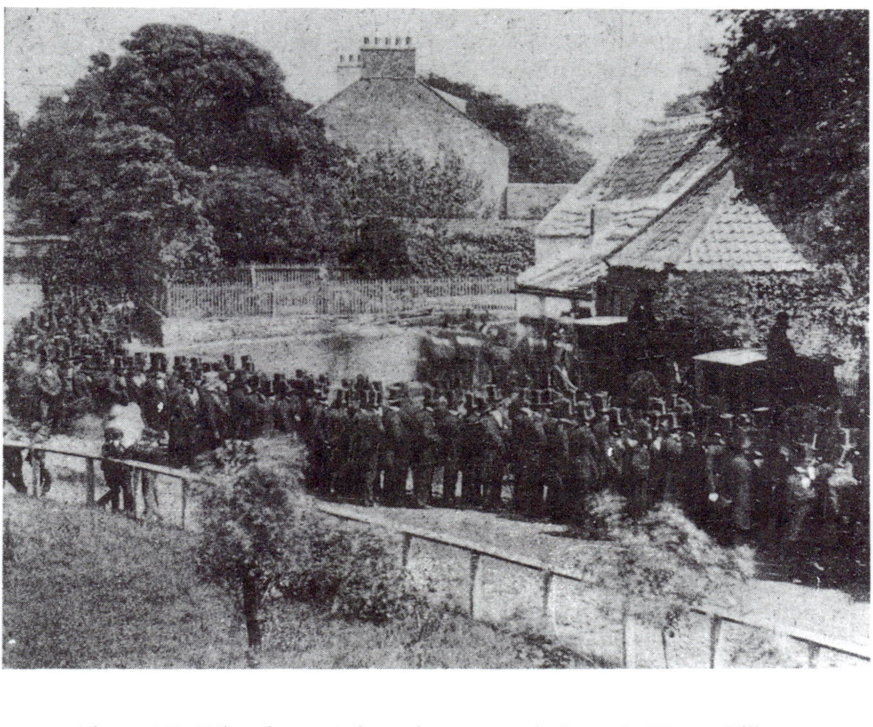

Figure 4. Dr Winterbottom's funeral cortege at the house in Westoe Village (South Tyneside MBC).

He was the first notable local man to be buried in the new Westoe Cemetery, and his grave is at the very centre. The attendance at his funeral was estimated to be about 10 000, and those following the cortège stretched over half a mile. Admission to the cemetery grounds, a mile from his house, was by ticket only, although when all ticket holders had been admitted, the gates were opened to all. As a mark of respect, all the shops in the town closed for 3-4 hours, and ships in the lower reaches of the Tyne flew their flags at half mast. All the doctors in South Shields attended the funeral, with others from neighbouring North Shields, Earsdon and Newcastle. Dr Davidson, his oldest surviving pupil, came over from Woolsingham.[43,44]

After his death Winterbottom's house in Westoe village fell into disrepair and in 1936 passed into the hands of the Convent of the Helpers of Holy Souls. Subsequently it was joined by a covered passage to the neighbouring house, and came into the ownership of the Mission of Medical Sisters. More recently it has become a Careers office.[45]

Acknowledgements

I am grateful to South Tyneside Metropolitan Borough Council and to the Tyne and Wear Museums Service for permission to reproduce the illustrations.

Notes and references

1. Winterbottom TM. *Account of the Native Africans in the Neighbourhood of Sierra Leone to which is added An Account of the Present State of Medicine among them*. (2 vols). London 1803; *2*:30 (Reprinted: Frank Cass & Co Ltd. London 1969).

2. Emmerson JS, Thomas Masterman Winterbottom, MD. *Univ Durh Med Gaz* Dec 1955; Bett WR, Historical Notes. The Medical Press 1959; *242*:32; Elliott JH, On Observation & Interpretation, with special reference to Thomas Winterbottom. *Bull Hist Med* 1942; *12*:137-144. Of these by far the best as far as information relating to the life of Winterbottom is concerned, is that by Miss Joan Emmerson, then Medical Librarian at King's College Library, Newcastle upon Tyne.

3. *DNB* gives date of birth as 1765 instead of 1766, as does Garrison & Morton; *Dict Mod Eng Biog* gives date of birth as 1764 or 1765; Duggan A, Tropical Medicine. In Gibson W C, ed. *British Contributions to Medical Science*. London: Wellcome Institute, 1971:73, overlooks Winterbottom's appointment as Physician to the Colony of Sierra Leone, and possibly confusing him with his seafaring brothers, refers to him as a mariner.

4. Salmon T, *Memoir of T.M.Winterbottom, Esq.,M.D.*, printed at the local newspaper office *North & South Shields Gazette*. Not dated but probably published just after Winterbottom's death. Salmon was the Town Clerk of South Shields and a relative of Winterbottom.

5. An oil painting executed about 1800, depicting the Town Hall, Market Place, St Hild's Church and incidentally Winterbottom's birthplace now hangs in the South Shields Museum & Art Gallery (formerly the home of the Literary, Mechanic & Scientific Institution). A coloured picture post card reproduction is available from the Museum. Winterbottom's early home and other buildings on the North side of the square, were demolished in the early 1960s. The area is now covered by a block of offices and shops.

6. St Hild's Parish Registers. (Central Library, Newcastle upon Tyne) Baptisms Vol 1 1683-1774; Vol 2 1775-1812; Burials Vol 5 1785-1812; Matthew Winterbottom became mate on one of the Sierra Leone Company vessels. He drowned at Fort Dix Cove, Gold Coast, when the boat bringing him ashore, capsized 7th July 1794. (Winterbottom *op cit* note 1:33). John Hill Winterbottom was an officer on HMS Champion when he died of gunshot wounds in the West Indies in 1838. The exact circumstances are not known. His only son had died when young. Masterman & Everritt. *Masterman & Heath Family Pedigrees*. nd 19.
7. Simmons SF. *Medical Register*. London: 1779, 110; 1780,130; 1783,96.
8. Anon. *The History & Statutes of the Newcastle Dispensary*. Newcastle: 1790, 28-31.
9. Salmon T. *op cit* note 4:1.
10. Hall JTD, Sub-Librarian, Special Collections, Edinburgh. University Library, 1984: personal communication. Hargreaves JD & Backett JD eds. for reprint of Winterbottom TM, *Account of the Native Africans &c. op cit. 1*:xiii.
11. *Medical Facts & Observations* 1794; *5*:61f.
12. Kay J. *Edinburgh Portraits*. Edinburgh: 1877 quoted by Guthrie D. *A History of Medicine*. London: Nelson, 1945; 229.
13. Dow DA, Archivist, Greater Glasgow Health Board, 1984; personal communication.
14. Munk W. *The Roll of the Royal College of Physicians of London*, Vol 2. London: Roy Coll Phys, 1878: 350. MacCormac H. Robert Willan (1757-1812). In: D'Arcy Power, ed. *British Masters of Medicine*. London: Medical Press & Circular, 1936: 71-78.
15. Roberto Willan, M.D. propter innumera in se collata beneficia, animi haud ingrati testimonium, hanc dissertationem medicam sacram esse voluit auctor. Winterbottom TM. *Dissertatio Medica De Morbo Puerperali*, Glasgow, 1792: 2. (Thesis G55156).
16. Falconbridge Anne-Marie. *Narrative of Two Voyages to the River Sierra Leone 1791-3*. London: 1802:154. (2nd edit, 1802 reprinted London: Frank Cass, 1967.)
17. Report of the Directors of the Sierra Leone Company. London: 1794:9.
18. *Sierra Leone Studies* 1927, *Old Series 8*:1-114, Extracts from John Clarkson's Diary.
19. (1768-1838). Father of Lord Macaulay, the historian.
20. Haliburton G. The Nova Scotia Settlers of 1792, *Sierra Leone Studies* 1957, *New Series* : 24. Wilson EG. *John Clarkson and the African Adventure*. London: Macmillan, 1980:85.
21. Wilson EG. *op cit* note 20:85-6.
22. Falconbridge A-M. *op cit* note 16:154.
23. *Shields Gazette and Telegraph*, South Shields. 11 Oct 1930.
24. Holland M, Viscountess Knutsford. *Life & Letters of Zachary Macaulay*. London: Arnold, 1900:135-6.
25. Widstrand CG. A Note on Adam Afzelius. In Kup AP, ed. *Adam Afzelius' Sierra Leone Journal 1795-1796*. Studia Ethnographica Upsaliensia *XXVII*, London: 1967.
26. Winterbottom TM. *op cit* note 1: I:290; De Luc. *Phil Trans Roy Soc Lond* 1792; *81*:20-42, diagram p 42.
27. Winterbottom TM. *op cit* note 1: I:280-291; *ibid*. Some Observations relative to the Climate and Diseases of Sierra Leone. *Medical Facts & Observations*, 1800; *8*:56-110.
28. It is not clear what Winterbottom means by this last entry line 'Relative air temperature with respect to feelings' unless he refers to his own comfort or discomfort. Thus 'close and sultry', 'the temperature of the air, though little different in absolute heat from that of the preceding month, was rendered more agreeable to the feelings, by the fresh breezes which prevailed...' *op cit* note 27.
29. Watts' Journal, 1794. MS copy in Rhodes House, Oxford, MS Afr.s.22.

30. Winterbottom TM. *op cit* note 1. *1*:33;
Afzelius' Journal, *op cit* note 25. Footnote 73r (1) p 161.

31. Afzelius' Letter to Chevalier von Engstrom, Swedish Ambassador in London. Reproduced in Hoare P. *History of Sierra Leone and Memoirs of Granville Sharpe*. London: 1820: app X, xxii.

32. Winterbottom TM. Angostura Bark. *Medical Facts & Observations* 1797; *8*:61,62.

33. Report of the Court of Directors, London 1795;1-31.

34. Observations on the Use of Arsenic in the Intermittent Fevers of a Tropical Climate, to which is added an Account of the Weather at Sierra Leone, during the Season in which such Fevers are most Prevalent. *Medical Facts and Observations* 1795; *6*:1.

35. Winterbottom TM. *Medical Directions for Navigators and Settlers in Hot Climates*. London:1796.

36. *London & Provincial Medical Directory*. London: 1859, 764.

37. Republished in 1969 by Frank Cass at £50.

38. PRO 268/5/137.

39. Knutsford. *op cit* note 24: 141.

40. One of these children, William (1812-1893), became Prime Minister of New Zealand and received a knighthood.

41. His passport visa, dated 29th July 1854, is in the possession of the South Shields Marine & Technical College. A marginal annotation records that at age 88 his height was 5 feet 4 inches.

42. Winterbottom TM. Thoughts on Quarantine and Contagion. *Edinb Med Surg J* 1828; 61-102, 1829; 92-107.

43. Obituary. *Lancet* 1859; *2*:76-7.

44. Accounts of funeral in *Lancet* 1859; *2*:101;
Salmon T. *op cit* note 4.

45. Flagg AC. *A History of Westoe Village*. Vol 2: Village Houses and Some of their occupants. Typescript MS 1965; 108-114. Original in South Shields Public Library.

Chapter 12

NEWCASTLE'S MEDICAL SCHOOLS

Gordon Dale

It is not generally realised that Newcastle is one of the oldest university towns in England and is the only one where university teaching began in the faculty of Medicine.[1] Indeed it might have beaten Durham into fourth place if the paper 'The Expediency of Establishing in Newcastle an Academical Institution of the Nature of a College or University for the Promotion of Literature and Science' given to the members of the Literary and Philosophical Society on 5 April 1831 by local surgeon, Mr TM Greenhow, had met with success.[2] In common with several of England's provincial universities, established just after the 1832 Anatomy Act, Newcastle Medical School has recently celebrated its 150th anniversary. The celebrations, in 1984, coincided with the opening by Her Majesty Queen Elizabeth the Queen Mother of the School's latest building – its ninth, counting the occupation in the 1930s of the old Dame Allan's School as an annexe. Substantial parts of all but one of these buildings still survive.

Bell's Court

The first formal course of medical lectures was given in a converted auction room overlooking Pilgrim Street. In 1832 Mr (later Sir) John Fife, surgeon and local politician, together with five of his colleagues, rented accommodation adjacent to his consulting rooms in the narrow lane called Bell's Court. They arranged a series of medical lectures which were attended by eight students, including John Snow – noted later for his work on cholera and his practice in anaesthesia. Although these lectures were rather haphazard, and meant to supplement rather than replace the apprenticeship system of medical training, they proved to be successful and were repeated in the following year. The front door that once opened onto the lane, and through which passed Fife's patients and students, was removed in 1939 and is preserved in the North Corridor of the Framlington Place Medical School. Now divided into offices, and without its original decoration, the Bell's Court lecture room still exists.

The Barber Surgeons' Hall

With the increasing recognition of the absurdity of the apprenticeship system, 'confining a young man for several years to the work of a shopman',[3] the continuing popularity of these lectures led to a search for suitable larger premises. The unused Barber Surgeons' Hall nearby was an obvious target. The Barber Surgeons' Company, which was already in existence on 10 October 1442,[4] had been housed in several parts of Newcastle before settling in the King's Manor Hall in 1652. It was visited in 1698 by Celia Fiennes, who described it in her journal:[5]

> I went to see the Barber Surgeons Hall which was within a pretty garden walled in, full of flowers and greenes in potts and in the borders; its a good neat building of brick, there I saw the roome with a round table in it, railed round with seates or benches for the conveniency in their disecting and anatomiseing a body and reading lectures on all parts; there was two bodyes that had been anatomised, one the bones were fastned with wires the other had had the flesh boyled off and some of the ligeaments remained and dryed with it, and so the parts were held together by its own muscles and sinews that were dryed with it; over this was another roome in which was the skin of a man that was taken off after he was dead and dressed and so was stuff'd the body and limbs, it look'd and felt like a sort of parchment; in this roome I could take a view of the whole town, it standing on high ground and a pretty lofty building.

The Hall was rebuilt in 1730 and is described in Bourne's contemporary *History of Newcastle*[6] as 'very beautiful and not a little sumptuous, it stands on tall piazzas under which is a spacious walk'. Its architectural style recalled that of the adjacent Holy Jesus Hospital, built in 1681. The ground floor was occupied by a lecture room 19 feet 10 inches by 16 feet 2 inches, fitted with six tiers of seats, together with a laboratory and dissecting room of similar dimensions. Probably the most important feature was the Anatomical and Pathological Museum which occupied the first floor; it looked down into a square garden containing four large stone statues representing Aesculapius, Hippocrates, Galen and Paracelsus, two of which were erected in 1710 and two in 1712. At the foot of this formal garden, and a little to the east, was the physic garden of medicinal herbs and a gardener's house (which was later used for making anatomical preparations).

In 1833 the Hall had been empty for some time. The Barber Surgeons' minute books, now in the Tyne and Wear County Archives Department, reveal that while the Company had rejected a bid for the hall to be rented as a Pestalozzian school, John Fife persuaded his fellow brethren of the Incorporated Company of Barber Surgeons and Wax and Tallow Chandlers of Newcastle on Tyne to support his plans for reformed medical education. The hall was permitted to be used 'for the purpose of giving lectures in the various practices of medical education', at an annual rent set at £12. On 26 May 1834, Fife submitted proposals for the glazing in of the open arches of the 'piazza', converting the space into a lecture room.

There was outside support for the venture; the corporation gave £100, the Duke of Northumberland £50 and Sir Matthew White Ridley £20 towards the formation of the anatomy museum.[3] The Newcastle upon Tyne School of Medicine and Surgery, the forerunner of the present medical school, was thus established in 1834; it was recognised both by the Apothecaries' Hall and the Royal College of Surgeons and the fee for the six months course was 40 guineas ('members of the medical profession and clergymen of every denomination, have free admission to all lectures'). By the late 1840s, student numbers had increased to 21 in the winter, when dissections could be carried out, and 14 in the summer.

There is now no trace of the Surgeons' Hall on the Manors. In 1847, George Hudson MP began negotiations with the Barber Surgeons' Company for the site as part of his plan to drive the North Shields and Berwick railway through Newcastle and link to the Central Station by a series of bridges and viaducts.

In a letter dated 11 May 1847 the Wardens of the Barber Surgeons Company wrote to Hudson at the House of Commons:

> The Railway which passes through the Town require the Hall and premises of the Fellowship of Barber Surgeons now occupied by the Newcastle upon Tyne School of Medicine and Surgery. The hall contains lecture dissecting and other rooms where an extensive museum of Anatomical and chemical preparations and other articles are deposited, open free of charge to the inspection of the public.
>
> There is a house also where the anatomical specimens are prepared with rooms for the Janitor and other erections used in connection with the School and about 2000 square yards of ground.
>
> So soon as the Fellowship of Barber Surgeons were informed that the Railway Co. required the premises they appointed a Committee to meet with the representatives of the Railway to negociate terms.
>
> At the request of Mr Dobson the Committee immediately entered into negociation with him for the disposal of the property when the Committee stated that the hall and other premises were everyway suitable for the School of Medicine and Surgery and there were capabilities of extending the accommodation by Buildings etc and under these circumstances it was agreed that the Railway Co. should erect a Building everyway convenient for the School containing suitable accommodation. The New Building to be of greater extent and an equivalent in value for the Building ground now belonging to the Barber Surgeons Company.
>
> The premises are held by lease for 61 years from the Corporation of Newcastle at an annual ground rent of 6/8 which has been twice received on payment of a fine of one pound for the house called the Gardeners House but no fine for the Hall or Ground.
>
> Under these circumstances and as there are still thirty six years of the lease unexpired it was agreed that the property to be given by the Railway Company was to be of freehold tenure.
>
> The Barber Surgeons Company consider the lease is renewable for ever but cannot guarantee this but as the proposed will be a public Building it should be of freehold tenure and in accordance with the Buildings of the present time.
>
> As Mr Dobson is now in London we considered it a good opportunity to write you that you might communicate with him on the subject and shall be glad to have your reply to lay before the Company as early as possible.
>
> *HB Lipton and William Turner.*

In exchange for the loss of the Hall, the Railway Company undertook to provide the Barber Surgeons, and therefore the Medical School, with a fine new one. It was to be sited on Rye Hill at the top of what was to become Victoria Street. As for many of Newcastle's important buildings at the time, the architect was John Dobson.

Once the decision had been taken to demolish the Hall, no further maintenance was carried out on it and the Secretary of the School was forced to complain to the Barber Surgeons' Company:

> *28 August 1850*
>
> I am obliged reluctantly again to draw your attention to the condition of the Medical School. The beginning of another session is close at hand and I assure you that I am quite at a loss to know what excuse to make to the students for again meeting in such an unwholesome place as our present accommodation is. For three winters I have assured them that the new building would be speedily in progress and yet we appear to be as unlikely to obtain it as ever, in consequence of which many are making up there minds to leave us, our loss already has been immense, our museum is going to wreck, our apparatus is being damaged and what is still worse we are losing credit with the profession. In fact the character and very existence of the school is in greatest jeopardy.
>
> I shall be much obliged if you will urge upon Mr Dobson the necessity of immediately proceeding with the building as the only chance of saving us, indeed if we should not be in a position to advertise that it is commenced with before October, I fear we will have few students coming to us.
>
> *W. Dawson.*

The New Barber Surgeons' Hall, Victoria Street

The New Surgeons' Hall was a splendid building, one of the finest of the new class of provincial medical schools. *The London Illustrated News* described it as

> ...admirably adapted for an institution of this description. On entering the building it is at once apparent that the architect has duly considered the facilities afforded by the favourable aspect on the south, on which side of the edifice is placed a private dissecting room, 21 feet by 13 feet; next, the library, 30 feet by 21 feet, and students' waiting adjoining, 21 feet by 14 feet; and above these rooms is a magnificent museum, 60 feet by 28 feet. This spacious apartment is lighted, not only by five windows on the south, but also from the roof... [There] is an excellent lecture-room, arranged as an amphitheatre. This room is 30 feet long and 25 feet wide, and is capable of seating 130 students. Adjoining it is the laboratory, 25 feet by 11. There are also in this part of the building, dissecting and other rooms.

> The elevation of the building is of the Italian style of architecture, and is divided into three bays, which rise from a noble basement. The windows in the upper stage are ornamental, having an arcade with imposts and archibolts. The arms of the Barber Surgeons' Company fill the spandrils, and the key-stones are decorated with Aesculapian Serpents.

The foundation stone of the new hall was laid on 6 February 1851 by Dr Charles Thorp, Warden of the University of Durham, accompanied by his senior colleagues together with the Mayor, Sheriff and civic dignitaries. After the ceremony the members of the Barber Surgeons' Company, the lecturers and representatives of the University all dined together, with Sir John Fife in the chair.

Unfortunately, before the transfer to the new building could be completed, a furious row broke out amongst the lecturers which led to the dissolution of the School. Dr Dennis Embleton, who had joined the School in 1839, was a guardian of the Poor Law Union and as a consequence was concerned with the appointment of medical officers to the districts. When a vacancy arose, his fellow lecturers expected him to support a colleague, Mr WR Sheill. Instead, he voted in favour of an old friend. In the angry meeting that followed, neither Sheill nor Embleton would agree to resign and the students and lecturers pledged support to one side or the other, splitting the school. Fife, together with the minority of students supporting Sheill, moved into the newly built hall as 'The Newcastle upon Tyne College of Medicine and Practical Science' – known colloquially as the Rye Hill College. A vitriolic exchange of correspondence is recorded in the *Lancet*.[7] Despite its admirable building, the Rye Hill College did not prosper and was to last only five years before the bitter animosity subsided and the rival schools became reunited.

The fate of the four statues from the Manors remains a mystery. A handwritten note of 24 October 1876 from the papers of Dennis Embleton in the Newcastle University Library suggests that they were 'taken down and buried in the ground of the New Barber Surgeons Hall, Victoria Street, Westmorland Terr. when the Hall was finished.' Whatever the reason for this burial, the statues, Newcastle's oldest, have not been discovered during the extensive building works that have since proceeded in the grounds of what is now St Paul's Church of England School.

The Gardener's House

The demolition of the Old Barber Surgeons' Hall began late in 1850 and was completed by the spring of the following year. In the meantime the 'majority' faction, headed by Dr Embleton, was homeless. In August 1851 the school obtained permission from the Finance Committee of the Corporation to occupy, at a nominal rent, the Gardener's House – the only building left standing on the Manors site. This was the janitor's house mentioned in wardens' letter to George Hudson. A temporary single-storey brick building was hastily erected to provide a dissecting room for the following winter.

Meanwhile the Barber Surgeons themselves had obtained temporary accommodation at 11 Nun Street for the storage of the specimens from the old anatomy museum. This was an important collection. Without it, neither of the rival schools, now locked in bitter conflict, would be recognised by either the College of Surgeons or the Apothecaries' Society in London. During the night of 28 August 1851, members of the minority school broke into the Nun Street store rooms and carried off the most valuable specimens, hiding them in a stable in Eldon Lane. Having discovered the loss, the angry majority attempted to salvage the remainder, only to have the minority group take away some of the residue in a second raid. The whole episode was recorded in a long mock-heroic ballad by John Cargill, 'The knights of St John and the Cross; or, the raid o' the Auld Musee':[8]

> But O what a show roun', aboon, an' below,
> O'livers a'steep'd in the briny bree!
> Lichts, stammacks, an' hearts, an' a' the parts
> That gie signs o' ilk human infirmitie!

Although the accommodation in the Gardener's House was, by any standard, miserable for the 16 lecturers and 24 students, it housed what was, at the time, Newcastle's largest medical school. The inaugural lecture on 1 October 1851 – the same night as that of the minority school – was given by Dr TE Headlam, who later became President. In view of the unsuitability of the building, the address was delivered in the lecture hall of the Literary and Philosophical Society.

After the formation of the College of Medicine and Surgery, earlier negotiations were resumed for a link with Durham University. In 1851 a *Lancet* editorial described Durham, England's fourth university, as 'comparatively unknown, and its influence is unfelt beyond the castle walls wherein it finds a peaceful yet dignified habitation'.[9] On 28 October of that year a deputation from the college was received by the Warden and Senate. The rival Rye Hill College vigorously opposed this move and also sent a deputation to Durham, hoping to persuade the Dean and Chapter, as Governors, to forbid the proposals. However, after appropriate revision of the constitution, agreement was reached and in January 1852 the medical school of the majority became the 'Newcastle-upon-Tyne College of Medicine in connexion with the University of Durham'. Their courses were recognised by the College of Surgeons and the Society of Apothecaries.

Although the future development of the majority school was assured by these moves, there was an urgent need to find better accommodation.

Unlike the old Barber Surgeons' Hall, of which it once formed a minor part, the Gardener's House still exists – on the south side of the City Road, between the abutment of the railway bridge and the Corner Tower of the Town Wall. The temporary dissecting room so hurriedly built in 1851, was finally demolished in 1984, although the chimney of the furnace used to incinerate the residues of dissections still survives.

Orchard Street

On 30 October 1851 the School approached the Corporation Finance Committee for a building site to the west of the old Infirmary (where the clinical training was conducted). Although the Committee recommended the sale to them of 690 sq yds at 14s a yard, the Infirmary objected to the move on the grounds that it would be insalubrious to have a medical school so close. No doubt Fife, politically powerful both in the hospital and the city, quite rightly saw the proposal as a very real threat to his Rye Hill college, which would then be rather more remote from the hospital than its rival.

Following this rebuff the majority school purchased Westmorland House, adjoining the Literary and Philosophical Society. Although not appropriate for academic accommodation, the old mansion, later renamed Neville Hall in view of its reputed connection with the Earls of Westmorland, was thought to be suitable for collegiate and domestic purposes. But it proved not to be so, and the building was sold to the Mining Institute, the profit from the sale enabling the College of Medicine to pay off its debt from the initial purchase. Meanwhile the title 'Neville Hall' was transferred to No 1 Leazes Terrace which was used as a hall of residence for medical students.

In the spring of 1852 the College commissioned Dobson to design a new school building in the former orchard of the mansion on what was to become Orchard Street. In appearance, the new building was simple in style and not unlike that of Dobson's Lying-in Hospital in New Bridge Street. An important consequence of developments at the eastern end of the Central Station was that a collection of academic institutes was beginning to grow around the Literary and Philosophical Society. The Museum and School of Design, the Natural History Society and the Mining Society (later to become the Mining Institute) pooled their facilities with those of the Medical School so that their overcrowded space could be more efficiently used.

Relationships between the various groups on the site were usually amicable although it was understandable that the proposal to construct connecting corridors for the convenience of the Medical School was vetoed because of the fear of smells emanating from the dissecting rooms. There was, however, unity against the common enemy on Rye Hill – although Wood, President of the Mining Society, judiciously retreated in the face of Burdon Sanderson's protests that the proposed addition of 'and Practical Science' to the title of the Institute of Mining was a further direct attack on the title of his college – which was already struggling to handle the pressure from Orchard Street. Not only had it an association with the University of Durham, but it was bigger and better organised. It had the benefit of adjacent library facilities; the Rosemary Lane Lying-in Hospital was 200 yards away and the proximity of the station meant that students could live at the coast.

It was becoming clear to everyone that Rye Hill could offer no serious competition to Orchard Street. Reunion of the rival colleges was inevitable and in 1857, the year that followed the establishment of the University of Durham Licence in Medicine, the brief and inglorious existence of the Rye Hill School came to an end with the reunion. Durham University celebrated the event by conferring honorary MA degrees on representatives of the former rival schools, Sir John Fife and Dr Frost. Hence the couplet from the *Comet*, Newcastle's comic paper:

And the blistering mustard of Durham was done,
For the Frost had been thawed by a tune on the Fife

By 1862, the college had grown to around sixty medical students, more than the combined faculties at Durham.[10] The newly formed General Medical Council carried out its first inspection in Newcastle in 1867 and noted that, while the examinations were satisfactory and 'noted especially for the practical character', the standard set for the pre-medical examination was unsatisfactory and did not include all of the required subjects. Appropriate corrections were made to the course. The loose connection with Durham University was proving to have some disadvantages for the school since other medical schools were refusing to recognise tuition received at Newcastle. However, in 1870 the College formally became part of Durham University as the 'University of Durham College of Medicine' and its teachers became professors and lecturers with representation on the senate. During this period the School grew to be the largest provincial medical school in England with an intake in 1879 of sixty new students.

The college adopted the motto, Scire usum medendi, from Virgil's *Aeniad* (XII, 396):

scire potestates herbarum usumque medendi

and acquired a badge which subsequently developed into the crest, used for many years but never submitted to the College of Heralds for approval. Perhaps the badge is best regarded as a parody, since what was intended as Aesculapius' staff, with single serpent, was in reality the winged caduceus of Mercury, with its two serpents, while what looks like a Maltese Cross was meant to be Durham's Cuthbert cross. The history of the error is difficult to piece together but it appears that in October 1870, following the incorporation into Durham University, the College Council resolved 'That a St Cuthbert's Cross, side by side with the Newcastle Tower and the Esculapean Serpent between the two, be adopted as the Armorial badge of this College....Mr JM Carr was instructed to prepare a sketch for the approval of the Council.' This sketch was not attached to the minutes. What was actually approved was a badge featuring the caduceus of Hermes — the messenger of the Gods, one of whose duties was to escort the souls of the dead to the world below!

Arnison, coauthor of the book written to celebrate the School's centenary, recalled what Orchard Street was like in 1888, when he became a student.[11] The entrance to the Orchard Street School was most insignificant, just opposite the site end of the Central Station Hotel. An apparently blind passage with a door on the right opened into a small room where the head janitor had his quarters, while a door further on led to stairs down to the chemical lecture room. Another passage went into the lower dissecting room, which 'was also used as a gymnasium for single stick, boxing etc.' On the first floor were the chemical laboratories and a large lecture hall where most of the lectures and demonstrations were given. The second floor, which had been added in 1881, contained a large dissecting room lit from the roof but having also windows running along the upper part of the west wall. Behind this room was the Museum of the Natural History Society, 'which was open for students to read and work in, but only had a small coke stove and was very cold in winter'.

Northumberland Road College of Medicine

As a result of its increasing popularity, Orchard Street became very overcrowded. By 1883 this was intolerable, and there was, no doubt, a sense of relief when it was learned that the North Eastern Railway Company proposed an extension to the Central Station that would require demolition of the School[12] – especially as the indications were that the company's compensation terms were likely to be generous. For the second time in its history, railway expansion caused the medical school to take stock of itself and to explore opportunities for change. Negotiations were protracted but an agreement was finally reached and the Council found a suitable one-acre site on Bath Road (later renamed Northumberland Road), by Northumberland Street. Although the proposed site had the considerable disadvantage of being distant from the Infirmary on the Forth Banks, in view of the dramatic growth in the size of the city and consequent overcrowding in the hospital, it was thought likely that a replacement hospital would soon be built on a site not far from the new medical school.[13] At an extraordinary meeting held on 12th April 1887, the Newcastle architects Dunn, Hanson and Dunn were commissioned to submit designs for the new building. Of the two styles offered, Gothic and Queen Anne, the members unanimously favoured the first. On 4 October Dr Heath, presiding over the last opening ceremony to be held in the Wood Memorial Hall, announced that they 'were absolutely engaged in the erection of a new college, which they trusted would be an edifice not unworthy of the city'.[14] The foundation stone of the new college was laid by the Duke of Northumberland on 3 November 1887. It was planned to have the anatomy block ready for occupation in January 1888, and remaining portion in the following October. It is a credit to the skill and speed with which buildings were constructed in those days that this very tight schedule seems to have been satisfied – certainly the College of Medicine calendar for 1887-88 records that:

> two sides only [of the quadrangle] have been built, the Main (north) Front in Bath Road, and the East Wing which contains the Anatomical

> Department.....The Main Front in Bath Road is 150ft long, and has a bold archway, above which is an oriel window two stories in height, corbelled out. Externally the front has two other features, a large bay window at the western end opening from the Council Room and the Library above it, and an angled turret corbelled out at the NE corner containing a staircase from the floor of the Museum to the Gallery.

To the left of the main tower was the Anatomy Wing, practically cut off from the rest of the building. Immediately above this room was the traditional steeply-raked anatomy lecture theatre, with the dissecting rooms further along the wing. The tradesman's entrance in this wing was through a yard, in which can still be seen at ground level the small square window in the wall through which coffins were passed into the embalming room where the bodies for dissection were prepared. By the end of the century, women students were attending in increasing numbers and a 'women's dissecting room' was planned (but never built).

The oil painting by C Kay Robertson of the President (Professor, later Sir, George Hare Philipson) addressing the 14 professors and lecturers in 1893 shows not only the appearance of the Council Room with its specially-commissioned oak table and chairs, still in use in the present School, but also just how few teaching staff there were in those days.

I am greatly indebted to Dr Tom Kirk for his memories of the Durham University College of Medicine seventy years ago. He wrote:

> Red brick? Very much so. A good example of turn-of-the-century architecture solid, functional, but with enough flamboyance in tower and window design to allow it to dominate Northumberland Road.
>
> That is how I saw it when, in the summer of 1915 I passed through the Entrance Hall and up the fine staircase to sit, with about 100 others (one third women) either for Entrance or for one of the two scholarships, the Pears and the University, in the big and most impressive Library, which was later to become the venue for all examinations. It was also used for the few social functions possible in war time — dances, concerts and even amateur theatricals.
>
> The presiding genius of the place was Robert Howden, a father-figure always affectionately known as "Bobby". He interviewed all entrants, dividing us into groups of four and allotting us bodies in the large well-ventilated dissecting-room at the back of the building. Once a week we submitted our dissections for "signing up" and frequently we listened to lectures, illustrated by beautifully-executed blackboard drawings, by Howden or one of his demonstrators. These were delivered in the steeply raked lecture-theatre.
>
> Day-to-day administration was in the capable hands of Warwick and Patterson who inhabited a small office on the left of the Entrance Hall, Botany and Zoology were taught either at the Hancock Museum, or in the College. Of the teachers, I remember the Professor of Chemistry, a little man called Sam Philips Bedson who did not suffer fools (of which

I was one) gladly. Physiology was taught by Menzies, a quiet methodical Scotsman who was part-author of a book on the subject.

In due course, the building like most of its predecessors, was overtaken by the inevitable overcrowding. Student numbers rose from 245 in 1927 to 432 in 1936.[15] The congestion was only partly relieved by an overflow into the vacant former Dame Allan's School opposite. The need for a larger building, preferably nearer to the Royal Victoria Infirmary, became increasingly urgent: the guess that the Infirmary would move from its site near to the Central Station had proved to be correct in itself, but the Leazes site was scarcely more convenient to Northumberland Road than the Forth Banks had been.

King's College Medical School, Queen Victoria Road

An ideal site for the new medical school became available on Queen Victoria Road, next to Armstrong College (formerly the College of Physical Science, established in 1871) and opposite the Royal Victoria Infirmary. Although the land was purchased with help of a loan from Armstrong College, the problem of raising the funds for a building proved to be difficult. When Robert Howden retired in 1927, the management of the College of Medicine devolved on Sir Robert Bolam as Registrar (and later, in 1935, President). It proved to be a turbulent period. Bolam, a considerable medical politician, enlisted as Treasurer Sir Joseph Reed – described by Bettenson as 'a hard-bitten business man from the local newspaper world'.[15] Both set out to tighten up the organisation, pay off the debt to Armstrong College and to raise the money to build the new medical school. 'Eventually they did all these things which was a considerable achievement, but in doing so they acted with a zeal that left little room for sensitivity'.[15] A serious dispute arose between Bolam and Hutchens, Head of the Department of Bacteriology, which was every bit as intense as that of the 1840s, and like it, raged for several years, polarising the staff into supporting one or other of the protagonists. A detailed account of the whole unedifying affair has been assembled by Bettenson.[15] A consequence of eight years of skirmishing was the setting up in 1934 of a Royal Commission which was followed in 1935 by the University of Durham Act. This completely redesigned the statutes and resulted in the merging of Armstrong College and the Medical College into what King George VI later agreed might be called 'King's College'.

Throughout the troubles, Sir Robert had pressed on with his plans to build the new Medical School on the Queen Victoria Road site opposite the Infirmary, assisted by a gift of £100 000 from Sir Arthur Sutherland. He was able to see the completion of the building before he died.[16] It was opened by King George VI on 21 February 1939, the event having been delayed by the growing international crisis.

The design of new building was criticised in the *University of Durham Medical School Gazette* as being reminiscent of 'a modern jam factory, albeit a very superior sort of jam factory.'[17] No doubt the student body was unaware of the very tight financial constraints imposed on Bolam when he set out to replace the splendid, but overcrowded, Northumberland Road School.

In the postwar years, the Goodenough report highlighted the shortcomings of teaching in medical schools. Careful deliberation led to the introduction, in 1962, of a new integrated curriculum, a notable feature of the course which has since been subjected to continuous evolutionary modification. The school prospered and its student numbers increased. Inevitably the building, which 50 years ago seemed to the Northumberland Road planners to be able to accommodate foreseeable expansion, itself became overcrowded and inconvenient. The 'extremely fine Medicine Theatre' and the more modern, but scarcely more comfortable, wooden-seated physiology lecture theatre had become gloomy and outmoded. The dissecting room, proudly described in 1938 as being 'like a prosperous barber's shop, with its gleaming fittings, and tiled walls and air of detachment' was no longer suitable for its purpose.[17]

Framlington Place Medical School

Perhaps a decade after the need became desperately apparent, and no doubt stimulated by the amicable separation of Newcastle University from Durham in 1963, the school moved once again, this time onto the Framlington Place site.

The new medical school was included in a plan conceived in the 1950s in which it was to combine with the Dental School (which had moved into the Northumberland Road building following the departure of the Medical School) and a new ward block of the Royal Victoria Infirmary on an adjacent site to the northeast of the hospital. The Dental School and Hospital were opened by His Grace the Duke of Northumberland in 1978. The ambitious medical school project, although not without problems and set-backs, was successfully completed by the design team headed by architects Robert Matthew, Johnson-Marshall & Partners. The building is in the form of linked blocks around courtyards, and consists of a reinforced concrete frame with clay brick external walls enclosing 33 000 square metres of usable floor area. It was officially opened by Her Majesty Queen Elizabeth the Queen Mother on 6 November 1984, almost exactly 150 years after its original foundation.

References

1. Bettenson EM. *The University of Newcastle upon Tyne: a historical introduction, 1834-1971.* Univ Newcastle upon Tyne: 1971.
2. Embleton D. *The history of the Medical School, afterwards the Durham College of Medicine at Newcastle upon Tyne, for forty years, from 1832 to 1872.* Newcastle-upon-Tyne: Andrew Reid, 1890: 5. (Address at the opening of the Durham College of Medicine, 1 Oct 1890).
3. Richardson MA. *The local historian's table book....of Newcastle-upon-Tyne, Northumberland and Durham.* Newcastle-upon-Tyne: Richardson, 1841-4. Historical Vol 4: 216-217.

4. Pybus FC. The Company of Barber Surgeons and Tallow Chandlers of Newcastle-upon-Tyne. *Newc Med J* 1929; *9*:147-163

5. Morris C (ed). *The journeys of Celia Fiennes*. London: The Cresset Press, 1947:211-2.

6. Bourne H. *The History of Newcastle upon Tyne...* Newcastle: John White, 1736:137-8.

7. Editorial. *Lancet* 26 July 1851; *1*:89.

   Embleton D, Charlton E. The Newcastle-upon-Tyne School of Medicine. *Lancet* 30 July 1851; *1*:143.

   Dale G, Miller FJW (eds). *Newcastle School of Medicine 1834-1984. Sesquicentennial Scrapbook*. University of Newcastle-upon-Tyne, 1984:17.

8. Grey Turner G, Arnison WD. *The Newcastle upon Tyne School of Medicine 1834-1934.* Newcastle: Reid, 1934:93-4.

9. Editorial. *Lancet* 1851; *1*:64.

10. Rose JD. The History of the Newcastle Medical School. *Med Illustr* 1952; *6*:187-9.

11. Grey Turner G, Arnison WD. *op cit* ref 8; 93-4.

12. Editorial: The Newcastle College of Medicine. *Lancet* 1883, *1*:651.

13. *Lancet* 1887; *2*:890.

14. *Lancet* 1887; *2*:717.

15. Bettenson EM. History of the Medical School. *In* Dale G, Miller FJW, Bramley K (eds). *Newcastle School of Medicine 1834-1984 Sesquicentennial Celebrations: Proceedings*. Univ Newcastle, 1985:10-17.

16. Green RB. The Medical School 1900-1950. *Univ Durh Med Gaz* 1950; *45*:4-7.

17. Editorial. *Univ Dur Med School Gaz* 1938; *33*:3.

Chapter 13

JOHN HUTCHINSON: INVENTOR OF THE SPIROMETER – HIS NORTH COUNTRY BACKGROUND, LIFE IN LONDON, AND SCIENTIFIC ACHIEVEMENTS*

E A Spriggs

This paper and the two which follow, by Dr B Gandevia and Mr P J Bishop, are concerned with a remarkable man who was born in Newcastle upon Tyne on 14 January 1811. He studied and practised medicine in London, and then emigrated to Australia in 1852, dying in Fiji on 16 July 1861. He was by no means the first to measure human ventilation, and the story of other attempts must be told elsewhere; but his adaptation for this purpose of the gazometer or gasometer of Lavoisier,[1] Watt[2] and Davy,[3] and particularly its exploitation in more than 4,000 clinical measurements, justify his reputation as the inventor of spirometry.

Genealogy

Hutchinson's paternal ancestors can be traced back to the seventeenth century in the parish records of Ryton, still a pleasant village though now partly suburban, a few miles up the Tyne from Newcastle and on the south side. His great-grandfather and grandfather were Parish Clerks.[4,5] They were farmers on a considerable scale as proprietors and tenants, and some plans remain of the family fields.[6] There was no professional man among the paternal relations, but our subject's uncle (also called John, 1779-1808) attended medical classes at Edinburgh in the session 1799-1800; he did not graduate but he read a paper to the Natural History Society of Edinburgh on 30 May 1799 'On detonation', which may still be seen in the Edinburgh University MSS.

The maternal forebears of our subject were gentlefolk,[7] the Collinsons of Aydon Castle, north of the Tyne, and indeed there is a tradition in the family, hard to substantiate, of descent from the great Earl of Clarendon. He was, of course, father of Anne Hyde, who married James Duke of York and bore him Queen Mary II and Queen Anne, but died before James became king.

Life in the North East

The parents, James and Anna Hutchinson, were living in Percy Street, Newcastle, when they took John to be baptised on his first birthday.[8] James

* Published in *Med Hist* 1977; *21*:357-364 and reprinted by kind permission of the Editor. The two following papers were a description of Hutchinson's subsequent life in Australia and Fiji[60] and a full bibliography of his works.[23]

was a 'coal fitter' or coal merchant[9] as well as a lessee of collieries.[10,11] He appears to have had his coal office in the yard behind the Custom House on Quayside.[12] He also had a partnership in a brewery at Stella[13] and owned a public house, the Lambs Arms, at Crawcrook[14] – both of these villages were in Ryton parish.

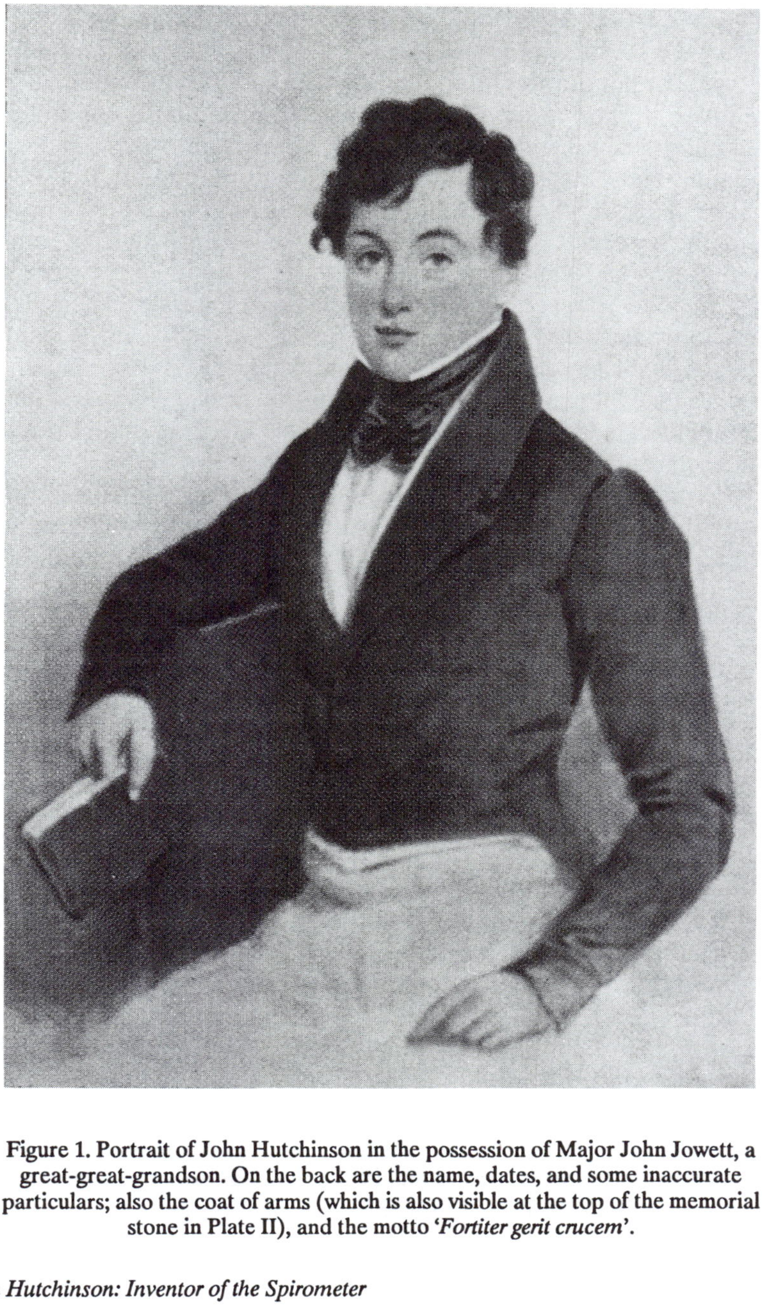

Figure 1. Portrait of John Hutchinson in the possession of Major John Jowett, a great-great-grandson. On the back are the name, dates, and some inaccurate particulars; also the coat of arms (which is also visible at the top of the memorial stone in Plate II), and the motto '*Fortiter gerit crucem*'.

From Percy Street, James and his family may have moved to Sheriff Hill,[15] south of Newcastle in a colliery area where he had an interest, and then not later than 1820 he bought from JH Wharton Esq MP, an estate at Hookergate[16] in the south-west part of Ryton parish, and built a house there[17] some time before his death in 1832 (the tombstone is shown in plate II). A valuation of this estate, comprising 142 acres, about the time of his death is still available[18] and the plan which probably goes with it. The Mansion House is valued at £216, and the lands at £3,092; John Hutchinson, being the only child, may be presumed to have inherited. The estate was then sold, however,[19] and the house was replaced by another building, called Beda Lodge, in the 1850s.[20] There were, when the Hutchinsons lived at Hookergate, a farm, granary, stables and 'fold yard'. The farming stock was also advertised when James Hutchinson died.[21]

It is not known where John Hutchinson went to school. There is no record of him at the Newcastle Royal Grammar School, Durham School, or Sedbergh. A recent Rector of Ryton suggests the Bruce Academy in Percy Street, where George Stephenson sent his son Robert, who was to become, like his father, a distinguished railway and mining engineer. Robert was eight years senior to John Hutchinson, and later said about his teacher John Bruce, 'it was from him that I derived my taste for mathematical pursuits and the facility I possess of applying this kind of knowledge to practical purposes.'[22] No list of pupils for the relevant time has been found.

The only fragments of knowledge we have about Hutchinson's early years are that his boyhood's favourite was (James) Cook; that his mind was early directed to mechanical engineering, of which he made ingenious constructions at an early age, and that he was in the habit of descending the coalmines on the Tyne.[23] He himself said that he had been not less than 200 or 300 times in the mines.[24]

That he returned regularly to the North East is suggested by his evidence to the House of Lords[25] on mining disasters. One wonders whether, when he went to Jarrow Colliery on 23 December 1845, he was up visiting his old haunts for Christmas. He is also said to have lectured to the Literary and Philosophical Society of Newcastle,[26] but that society has now no record of this.

London

No connection has been found with the Newcastle College of Medicine, but Hutchinson attended University College, London,[27] where he was probably taught by Sir Charles Bell, the celebrated anatomist, and by Dr Dionysius Lardner, Professor in Natural Philosophy and Astronomy. Mr WR Merrington, FRCS, tells me that on 2 October 1834 Hutchinson paid £3 for a course of Medical Jurisprudence by Dr AT Thomson; in January 1834 £3 for Materia Medica by Dr AT Thomson; in January 1835 £3 for Practice of Medicine by Dr Elliotson; and in February 1835 £4 for Chemistry. He took the MRCS in 1836[28] and became one of the Physicians to the Britannia Life Assurance Company,[29] and Surgeon to the Southampton Dispensary, Leighstreet, Burton-crescent,[30] not far from University College. He had given up this latter appointment by 1845.

In 1842 Hutchinson became a Fellow of the Statistical Society,[31] newly founded by Farr, and in 1848 he obtained the degree of MD Giessen on thesis and in absentia.[32] Then the London directories begin to change Mr Hutchinson, surgeon, to Dr Hutchinson, physician. And in 1850, for a brief two years, he became Assistant Physician to the Hospital for Consumption, Brompton.[33]

Hutchinson was married from 30 Gower Place on 23 April 1840, in St Olave's Church, Hart Street, City of London, to Ann Sarah, daughter of Henry Buckle, described as a merchant.[34] From 1845 to the time of his emigration he occupied a house at 105 Milton Street, now Balcombe Street, near Marylebone Station.[35,36] The house was built in 1844, but it is not possible to be sure from the rating records whether Hutchinson owned it or rented it from the Portman Estate. It has been replaced by modern buildings, but much of the street still preserves an early nineteenth-century air of some distinction.

They had three children, and I have been fortunate to meet a great-grandson, Field Marshal Sir Geoffrey Baker, GCB, CMG, CBE, MC, recently Chief of the General Staff, and his daughter Alexandra, now Mrs Thomas Bremridge.

Contributions to Medical Science

Hutchinson's water spirometer was much the same as the instrument we use today. It did not make a graphic record, and had the disadvantage that the patient or the observer had to turn off the stopcock at the end of expiration, to confine the air until the position of the index was read on the graduated scale. Volumes were measured at manometrically adjusted atmospheric pressure, and corrected by calculation for any deviation of room temperature above or below 60°F. Hutchinson defines the vital capacity as 'the number of cubic inches given by a full expiration following the deepest inspiration'.[37] He divides the quantity of air in the thorax into:

Hutchinson's term	*Corresponding modern term*
complemental air	inspiratory reserve volume
breathing air	tidal air
reserve air	expiratory reserve volume
residual air	residual volume

It is appropriate that one of Hutchinson's first presentations was to the Statistical Society.[38] He shows that there is a linear relationship of vital capacity with height, and draws frequency distribution curves.[39] He finds no relationship to weight, if correction is made for height – except that above a certain weight, for any given height, the vital capacity diminishes. The relationship between chest circumference and vital capacity is found to be irregular, if anything inverse. The vital capacity diminishes with age. 'I have found a dinner diminish the vital capacity to the extent of 12 and even 20 cubic inches.'

Both the content and the presentation of Hutchinson's papers seem to have been admired. At the Royal Medical and Chirurgical Society:[40]

> A Fellow of the Society having complied with the request to come forward and submit himself to experiment, his height was found to be five feet five inches, and, accordingly, the quantity of air he could expel should, by the tables, be 206 cubic inches (3,380 ml). The gentleman then breathed into the spirometer, and actually produced 205 cubic inches, which, making allowance for temperature, make it 206 cubic inches. This was so satisfactory, as to leave no doubt on the mind that these tables must have been calculated with care, and upon an extensive number of cases.

When Hutchinson took the circumference of the chest he usually deducted $^1/_4$ in. for the shirt and another $^1/_4$ in. for the flannel. Though he made measurements with the spirometer on women, he wrote 'We do not know the vital capacity of women, nor is it easy to determine it, because of their tight dress,'[41] though further on he comments 'We never heard a woman acknowledge that she wore her clothes tight'.

Hutchinson considered the spirometer useful in the diagnosis of disease, but he had in mind not so much, as we should today, conditions with airways obstruction such as asthma, emphysema, and chronic bronchitis. There were no cigarettes then, but he did observe the inspiratory sinking and expiratory bulging of the intercostal spaces and base of the neck in emphysema, commenting 'there must be some impediment in the air tubes'.[42] Rather, in spirometric measurements, was he concerned with the great killer of his time, phthisis, which diminishes vital capacity by destroying the lung tissue. In 1842 Freeman, the American giant, under whose skeleton one may still stand at the Royal College of Surgeons, came to England, and Hutchinson examined him before a prize fight.[43] He was 6 ft 11 $^1/_4$ ins high, and weighed 19 st 5 lb. He had the very large vital capacity of 434 cu in, 88 per cent of what one would now predict from his height and weight. Freeman spent a rambling and dissolute life for the next two years and then, when he became ill, weighed two stone less, and had a vital capacity of 344. He was taken to two 'physicians well skilled in auscultation', who could not detect organic disease. He died the next year, and autopsy showed phthisis.

All but the youngest physicians today will remember temperature charts where the nurses had twice daily, at the bottom, recorded respiratory rates '20-20-20...'. I was always puzzled by this figure, evidently taught in the nursing schools as one from which it was hazardous to deviate; for it is far too high for a resting healthy person who is not anxious. Hutchinson may be responsible.[44] He counted the respirations in 1,714 cases, in the sitting posture, and found both the median and average rates to come out at twenty per minute, though the range was from six to forty. The pulse rates were also high, at eighty, and it is probable that most of the experimental subjects were in a state of apprehension. It is curious that John Dalton (1813)[45] had found that in a state of quiescence he himself took twenty inspirations a minute. Hutchinson does note[46] that a man after a narcotic breathed twice in a minute.

He measured positive and negative pressures which could be produced by activity in the chest.[47] He also obtained, in two corpses, measurements relating pressure with volume.[48]

It is hard to believe that one of the great physiological controversies of the eighteenth century had been that between von Haller and Hamberger, who differed as to the function of the interosseous portion of the internal intercostal muscles. They agreed that the external intercostals and the inter-cartilaginous internal intercostals were inspiratory, but von Haller thought the interosseous internal intercostals were inspiratory, whereas Hamberger thought them expiratory. Hamberger (1749)[49] had a volume published in which Haller's *De respiratione* was interspersed with Hamberger's critical comments. On this controversy, Hutchinson quotes Haller: 'Let it be allowed me to deplore, among the miseries of human life, that such anger and bitter quarrels should be forced upon us on account of matters wherein we are so little personally concerned'. Hutchinson, on anatomical and mechanical grounds, took Hamberger's view, and has lately[50] been proved correct by electromyographic studies.

Hutchinson published figures on the familial disposition to phthisis.[51] He distinguished, on rather doubtful grounds, between the 'crackles' of consumption and what he calls the 'crepitations' of bronchitis and pneumonia.[52] He comments: 'If Laennec had done no more in his short space of time, than discover this crepitating sound, and the pathology thereof, Laennec had erected for himself a monument, more durable than any now standing, on the plains of Egypt'.

It is likely that much of Hutchinson's earnings in London came from insurance work. His last known publication *The spirometer, the stethoscope and scale-balance* is directed particularly to this aspect.[53] He regarded a family history of consumption, apoplexy or insanity as prejudicial to long life, and he held particularly strong views on alcohol.

Evidence before Select Committee of House of Lords

The minutes of Hutchinson's evidence on accidents in coal mines[54] deserve comment, because they bring the man to life – also because they reveal the shocking conditions in which miners worked, and not infrequently died.

Hutchinson pointed out to their lordships that, among deaths following explosions, the major part of the mortality was from suffocation: '...Haswell exploded in April 1845; there were 14 burnt and 81 were suffocated.' 'I have seen men frequently brought out of a mine (it was so in the case of Springwell, which happened 9th May 1833), close from beside the bottom of the shaft, with a perfectly placid and calm expression, without the slightest mark upon their persons of fire or violence....'.

It may be explained that, even within the memory of people still living, ventilation in these coal mines was achieved by underground furnaces causing air to rise. Hutchinson described the complicated arrangements which had to be perfected to make a continuous current of air. Often a partition, or brattice, of wood was all that separated two air streams in contrary directions, and an explosion causing a hole in the brattice could condemn to suffocation numbers of men far beyond. This he illustrated to the Select Committee: 'The Witness exhibits an experiment with a candle, over which he places a glass tube 20 inches long, and the candle almost immediately goes out; but on again lighting it, and introducing a division, representing a brattice, down the centre of the tube, the candle continues to burn clearly.' Having, one feels sure, impressed the committee by this demonstration, Hutchinson pointed out the engineering methods by which flimsy brattices could be avoided.

According to Hutchinson's evidence, Jarrow colliery exploded seven times in twenty-nine years: 'When I was going to that mine, I asked a miner "Which is the way to Jarrow colliery?" and he said "Sir, I do not know of any colliery; but there (pointing me in the direction of the colliery) is a butcher's shop;" and that was a man who did not know I was making any inquiries into the state of the mine....'.

But the Select Committee was to enjoy a second dramatic demonstration, that of Hutchinson's method of lengthening the time a rescuer can go without breathing poisonous gas: 'If any of your Lordships will look at your watch, as soon as I am ready I will strike the table.... (The Witness makes several deep inspirations and expirations, then held his breath for the space of a minute and a half)'.

Migration to Australia

Hutchinson left England in September 1852.[55] Why did he go? There is the hint of an explanation in the *Lancet* annotation of 1920, which refers to Professor G Dreyer's "recent" dedication to Hutchinson of a book on the assessment of physical fitness.[56] This annotation says that 'soon after the discovery in 1851 of gold deposits in Australia he [Hutchinson] left England'. Certainly Hutchinson was interested in mining, but this is hardly likely to be the whole story.

Another possible explanation is that Hutchinson developed consumption, for the journey to Australia was a recognized way of 'taking the cure' in those days.[57] There is no evidence that he was sick. Alcoholism is possible, and would fit in with some of the Australian escapades and with the rumours from Fiji about his end (see B Gandevia, 'Dr John Hutchinson in Australia and Fiji', pp 365-383).[60] Is it in favour of this hypothesis or against it that, writing of insurance examinations, Hutchinson inveighs against the drunkard? 'Domestic distress and grief may drive him foolishly to seek rest of mind, by intoxication.... Sobriety is an ornament; if this ornament is not in the applicant we should *decline the case*'.[58]

Another speculative suggestion (and of course more than one of these reasons may have been operative) is that Hutchinson's marriage was not happy. Dr Gandevia will deal with the interesting point that Hutchinson's will did not mention his wife or children (see pp 377-379). Mrs Bremridge, a descendant, tells me that the children succeeded to trust funds bringing in £500 p.a. each, but it is not clear whether these came from their father or their mother.

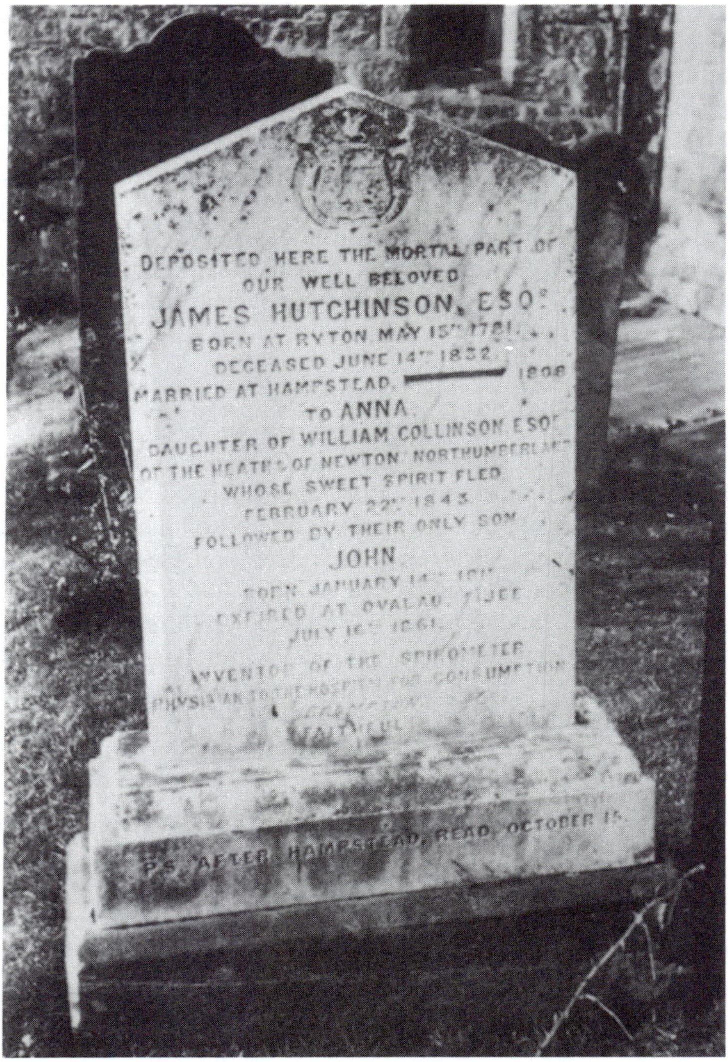
OUR WELL BELOVED
JAMES HUTCHINSON, ESQ
TO ANNA
DAUGHTER OF WILLIAM COLLINSON ESQ
WHOSE SWEET SPIRIT FLED
JOHN

Figure 2. There are two memorial stones in Ryton Church relating to John Hutchinson and his ancestors. That shown commemorates John Hutchinson himself, and his father and mother; 'the Heath' probably refers to Hampstead. Another stone nearby commemorates on the front and back several other relations.

The Man

From Hutchinson's achievements and writings, one pictures a precise, forceful and industrious personality. There is Australian evidence, (see Gandevia pp 371-373),[60] that he was aggressive in his later years. The *Medical Times* obituary[59] notes that he had an exquisite ear for music, his execution on the violin being masterly; that he had great ability as a draughtsman; that he sculptured admirably in basso relievo; and that he painted in oils. Some of his writings are illustrated by the most delightful silhouettes and one wonders whether he drew these himself. At the Royal Medical and Chirurgical Society he was asked whether he had examined any men of remarkably small stature. He replied that he had in the course of his observations, sought out the giant and the dwarf: 'He then handed a spirited sketch of a human being, whose height was under thirty inches – Don Francisco, aged 42'. One imagines that Hutchinson had made the sketch himself. The obituary also states that he conducted researches on vital statistics and meteorology and was noted for his dramatic and conversational powers.

It seems, in retrospect, a great loss to British medicine that Hutchinson should have emigrated, for reasons which are not clear, and ceased scientific work at the age of forty-one.

Summary

John Hutchinson (1811-1861) came from Newcastle upon Tyne and received his medical education at University College London. He practised especially in insurance work, and wrote about this, as well as about his celebrated spirometer, the functions of the intercostal muscles, ventilation in coal mines, and other subjects relating to respiration. He became Assistant Physician at the Brompton Hospital.

At the age of forty-one he left his wife and children, abandoned his professional position and scientific work, and migrated to Australia. We do not know why he did this, but his later career is taken up by Dr B Gandevia in the paper which follows.[60]

Acknowledgements

For much of the information about John Hutchinson I am indebted to the work of others, notably: Mr PJ Bishop and Dr Bryan Gandevia; Mrs Thomas Bremridge, Hutchinson's great-great-grand-daughter; Mr G Peaston, a patient who drew my attention to the memorial stone in Ryton churchyard; The Rev JLl Rowlands, lately Rector of Ryton; Mr P Bumstead and the History Sixth Form of Hookergate School; Mr G Nicholson of Ryton.

References

1. Lavoisier A-L, trans Kerr R. *Elements of chemistry*. Edinburgh: William Creech, 1790:308-19.
2. Beddoes T, Watt J. *Considerations on the medicinal use of factitious airs*. Bristol: Johnson & Murray, 1794, pt II: 1-10.

3. Davy H. *Researches*. London: Johnson, 1800:573-6.
4. Welford R. Local muniments. *Archaeol Aeliana* 1909; Ser 3, *5*:114.
5. *The general election roll for knights of the shire; to represent in parliament the County Palatine of Durham*. Newcastle upon Tyne: Akenhead, 1790:11.
6. Univ Durham, Dept Palaeography and Diplomatic. Gibson Deposit, plan No 146.
7. Hodgson JC. *A history of Northumberland*. Newcastle upon Tyne: Reid, 1902; *6*:135-7.
8. St Andrew's Church, Newgate Street, Newcastle upon Tyne. Baptismal register, 14 Jan 1812.
9. *A general directory for Newcastle upon Tyne, Gateshead, and places adjacent*. Newcastle, pr Francis Humble, Durham, for the publisher, 1824:70.
10. Gateshead Public Libraries. Cotesworth MSS, CA/2/158 & CA/2/160.
11. North of England Institute of Mining and Mechanical Engineers, Neville Hall, Newcastle upon Tyne. Letter from James Hutchinson to John Watson, Watson Collection, v 96.
12. Parson W, White W. *History directory and gazetteer of the counties of Durham and Northumberland*. Newcastle, 1827:46 & 106.
13. *Newcastle Courant*, 19 May 1821, p1.
14. *Newcastle Courant*, 1 Sept 1832, p 2.
15. Parson & White. *op cit* note 12.
16. Surtees R. *The history and antiquities of the County Palatine of Durham*. Sunderland: Hills, 1909:174.
17. Mackenzie E, Ross M. *An historical, topographical, and descritive view of the County Palatine of Durham*. Newcastle upon Tyne: Mackenzie & Dent, 1834; *1*:205.
18. Univ Durham, Dept Palaeography and Diplomatic. Gibson Deposit Paper No 122 & Plan No 68.
19. *Newcastle Journal*, 22 Sept 1832, p 1.
20. Personal communication from G Houlden Esq, who recently owned Beda Lodge.
21. *Newcastle Journal*, 1 Sept 1832.
22. Williamson JB. *Memorials of John Bruce and Mary Bruce*. Newcastle upon Tyne: Reid, 1903:241.
23. Bishop PJ. A bibliography of John Hutchinson. *Med Hist* 1977; *21*:384-96 (hereinafter cited as Bishop), No 33: (Obituary) The late Dr. Hutchinson. *Med Times Gaz* 1862; *1*:200-1.
24. Bishop No 19. Accidents in Coal Mines. *Rep Select Comm House of Lords on accidents in coal mines* Session 1 Feb-1Aug 1849; *VII*:140-164, 602-4.
25. *ibid*.
26. Bishop No 33. *op cit* note 23.
27. Bishop No 36. A pioneer in spirometry. *Lancet* 1920; *2*:563.
28. Records of the Royal College of Surgeons of England, 29 April 1836.
29. Bishop No 33. *op cit* note 23.
30. *The London Medical Directory*. London: Mitchell, 1845:84-5.
31. Bishop No 36. *op cit* note 27.
32. Personal communication from Leist W, Justus Liebig-Universitat, Giessen.
33. See description in Bishop No 36.
34. General Register Office, Somerset House, London. Certified copy of an entry of marriage, application no 8535D.
35. Bishop No 17 (j). Hutchinson J. Ventilation in general..., in relation to public health. *J Publ Hlth & Monthly Rec Sanit Improvement* 1849; *2*:113-7.

36. Archives Dept, Westminster City Libraries, London. Rating Records.
37. Bishop No 7. Hutchinson J. On the capacity of the lungs, and on the respiratory functions, with a view of establishing a precise and easy method of detecting disease by the spirometer. *Med Chir Trans* 1846; *29*:137-252.
38. Bishop No 3. *ibid*. Lecture in vital statistics. *Lancet* 1844; *1*:567-70.
39. Bishop No 7. *op cit* note 37.
40. Bishop No 9. Hutchinson J. On the capacity of the lungs ... *Lancet* 1846; *1*:630-2.
41. Bishop No 26. Hutchinson J. *The spirometer, the stethoscope, & scale balance*. London: Churchill, 1852.
42. Bishop No 25. *ibid.* Thorax. *In* Todd RB (ed.). *The cyclopaedia of anatomy and physiology*. London: Longmans, 1852; v4:1016-7.
43. Bishop No 7. *op cit* note 37.
44. *ibid*.
45. Dalton J. On respiration and animal heat. *Mem Proc Manchr Lit Phil Soc* Ser 2, *2*:26.
46. Bishop No 26. *op cit* note 41.
47. Bishop No 7. *op cit* note 37.
48. Bishop No 25. *op cit* note 42.
49. Hamberger GE. *De respirationis mechanismo et usu genuino.* Jena: Croeker, 1749.
50. Taylor A. The contribution of the intercostal muscles to the effort of respiration in man. *J Physiol (Lond)* 1960, *151*:390-402.
51. Bishop No 26. *op cit* note 41.
52. Bishop No 20 (c). Hutchinson J. Diagnosis and treatment of pulmonary consumption, No III. Abnormal breathing sounds. *Med Times* 1850; *ns 1*:250-53.
53. Bishop No 26. *op cit* note 41.
54. Bishop No 19. *op cit* note 24.
55. Bishop No 33. *op cit* note 23.
56. Dreyer G. *The assessment of physical fitness*. London: Cassell, 1920.
57. Thomas KB, Gandevia B. Dr. Francis Workman, emigrant, and the history of taking the cure for consumption in the Australian colonies. *Med J Aust* 1959: *2*:1-10.
58. Bishop No 26. *op cit* note 41.
59. Bishop No 33. *op cit* note 23.
60. Gandevia B. John Hutchinson in Australia and Fiji. *Med Hist* 1977; *21*:365-383.

Chapter 14

SCIENCE AND HEALTH: A SAFETY LAMP FOR MINERS

David Knight

Like plague, accidents in coal mines brought sudden death (particularly dreaded by our ancestors), and threw widows and orphans upon charity or poor rates. By 1800 coal mines could go deep because there were steam engines to pump out water from them, but this brought great danger from gas or 'damp': the explosive fire damp, and its residue, choke damp. In 1812 at Felling Colliery, 92 men were killed in an explosion in what was believed to be an up-to-date pit, an accident which was vividly reported,[1] and in 1813 a Society for 'preventing Accidents in Coal-Mines' was set up at Bishopwearmouth, now part of Sunderland, with the Rector, Dr. Robert Gray, as chairman. William Reid Clanny, an Irishman trained at Edinburgh, was the local doctor; appalled by the loss of over 200 lives in seven years, he had described a safe lamp of his invention to the Royal Society earlier in the year, communicating it through William Allen, the Quaker pharmacist and philanthropist.

Clanny's plan was to cut off the flame from the outside air: 'the idea of insulating the light, and also the plan which I have adopted for carrying this idea into effect, by the construction of the apparatus or lamp, are perfectly original'.[2] Air was pumped with bellows in and out of the lamp through water, the great antagonist of fire; an explosion inside would not therefore set off gas outside. The lamp was apparently a success at Harrington Mill, where there had been an explosion in October 1812, but it was a cumbersome device, even in Clanny's improved version which weighed 34 ounces. Even though Clanny received medals in 1816-17 from the Society of Arts, his invention (which required a boy to work the pump) never came into general use.

As was (and still is) usual in technical history,[3] Clanny's device was developed by evolution from familiar things, lamps and lanterns; it drew upon no recent science. Clanny identified the fire damp as 'inflammable air', the old name for hydrogen, and as 'carburetted hydrogen', which is marsh gas or methane – his chemistry was a bit vague. Because the invention was not perceived to have remedied the situation, Gray then wrote to Humphry Davy in the summer of 1815, the latter having just returned from the continent, after visiting Napoleonic France to collect a prize for his electrochemical researches.

Davy had come far since giving up his apprenticeship to an apothecary-surgeon in Penzance, exchanging the life of a country GP for a meteoric career in science (then a very risky business), and had been knighted in 1812. His great reputation depended both upon utilitarian studies of tanning and agriculture, and on his work on chemical affinity and on acidity. In bursts of activity, usually in the autumn after his holiday and before the lecture season at the Royal Institution began, he had proved the electrical nature of chemical combination, isolated sodium and potassium, and established that chlorine was an element. This demolished Lavoisier's view that oxygen was responsible for acidity, for there was none in the acid from sea salt. Davy was fighting the French wars in the laboratory.[4]

In his early studies on tanning and agriculture, Davy had followed the old pattern, using science to vindicate the best practice of the day. Now, with new confidence, he set out on a new programme. Two hundred years before, Bacon had written that 'experiments of fruit' (practical results) would follow from 'experiments of light' (the urge to understand), and Davy showed this to be true. Instead of beginning with lanterns, he started with analysis of the fire damp, and determined its properties. His crucial finding, in risky experiments carried out with few safety precautions, was that a high temperature was required to ignite it. His lamps were therefore devised to be cool: access to the flame was, in the earliest models, through metallic tubes which would disperse heat, and then in later models through wire gauze. This safety lamp was one of the first products of applied science, the use of new research in a practical device. Davy's lamp was also a scientific instrument (since the presence of fire damp was revealed by the character of the flame) which he used in studies involving catalysis.

Davy made fruitful contact with John Buddle, the manager or 'viewer' at Wallsend colliery, who tried out the lamps and became an enthusiast for their use. Though over his lifetime 800 men were said to have died in pits under his management, he was still a widely respected and trusted engineer, and a warmly sympathetic person in whom practice and science were joined.[5] The reputations of Davy and Buddle were such as to ensure that the Davy lamp became well known, and was introduced widely. Davy refused to patent it. He was awarded a baronetcy – Newton had only been a knight – but this was a useless honour for a childless man, and some pointed out that those generals and admirals who had been responsible for thousands of deaths were far better rewarded than the philanthropic Davy.

Sir Joseph Banks, President of the Royal Society, wrote him a magnificent letter:[6]

> To have come forward when called upon, because no one else could discover means of defending society from a tremendous scourge of humanity, and to have, by the application of enlightened philosophy, found the means of providing a certain precautionary measure effectual to guard mankind for the future against this alarming and increasing evil, cannot fail to recommend the discoverer to much public gratitude, and to place the Royal Society in a more popular point of view than all the abstruse discoveries beyond the understanding of unlearned people.

Davy's safety lamp made him the obvious candidate for President when Banks' 42-year reign ended with his death in 1820; the lamp was a shining instance of the benefits metropolitan science could confer.

Meanwhile, a more obscure mining engineer than Buddle, George Stephenson, had also been experimenting in the evolutionary, trial-and-error mode, and had come up with the Geordie lamp, in which access of air was restricted by admitting it through narrow tubes, later modified to a perforated metal plate. Both Davy and Stephenson were self-made men, but Stephenson was an unknown until his locomotives later made him famous; their reputations depended upon their discoveries, and both were sensitive about their intellectual property. In the story of this 'epidemic', if Davy is the London consultant, then Stephenson is the heroic local GP. Davy believed that Stephenson's lamp was unsafe, an exploding machine, until it was improved by copying that of Davy, but supporters of Stephenson attacked Davy for arrogance and declared his lamp ineffective. The scientific journal *Annals of Philosophy*, whose editor Thomas Thomson of the Glasgow Medical School was no friend of Davy, published polemic by supporters of Stephenson.[7] There seems no doubt that both had come up with very similar inventions, via different routes; Davy had understood the underlying physics and chemistry better, but Stephenson had, by systematic experiment, produced a very similar device. Such simultaneous discoveries are not uncommon.

Davy's critics declared that the lamp was not safe in the mine, whatever might happen in the laboratory, but Buddle tested it under quite extreme conditions, and was sure that, if properly maintained and used, it would not explode gas. Lamps came into use not only in Britain, but in Belgium and in the other coalfields of Europe. Unfortunately, deaths in explosions did not fall; in fact they rose, but not nearly as fast as did coal production. There seem to have been various reasons for this rise in deaths. One was that safety lamps were not used in pits believed safe – only after the horse had bolted was the stable door locked. Another was that they might be damaged: lamps might be poorly looked after, or opened to light a pipe; if the gauze was broken, gas could be ignited.

But the lamps could also fail. Improvements in ventilation, producing strong currents of air, might make a lamp unsafe by blowing the flame through the gauze. Davy's experiments had been carried out on methane collected by Buddle from a mine, but it transpired that this fire damp was not the only explosive material: coal dust mixed with air was also very dangerous, and could be set off at lower temperatures, for example by a lamp in which the gauze had become red hot. Safety was not absolute, but was a matter of degree. The original designs were therefore modified so that the flame was enclosed in glass, as in the lamps with which we are familiar, with gauze below and above; even when electric light came into the mines, such lamps were used as instruments to test the air. If mining death is regarded as a kind of epidemic, then it was brought under control by both applied science and by rational empiricism, but the disease did not disappear.

References

1. Hodgson J. An account of the dreadful accident which happened at Felling Colliery. *Ann Phil* 1813; *1*:355-65 & 438-47.
2. Clanny WR. On the means of procuring a steady light in coal mines without the danger of explosion. *Phil Trans R Soc Lond* 1813; *103*:200-5 & plate XV.
3. Basalla G. *The evolution of technology*. Cambridge: U Press, 1988.
4. Knight D. *Humphry Davy: science and power*. Oxford: Blackwell, 1992.
5. For Buddle, see *Dict Nat Biog*.
6. Davy J. *Fragmentary remains, literary and scientific, of Sir Humphry Davy, Bart*. London: Churchill, 1858:208.
7. Longmire JB. Remarks on the wire-gauze lamp lately constructed by Sir H. Davy. *Ann Phil* 1816; *8*:31-4;

   Children JG. Answer to Mr.Longmire's objections to Sir H. Davy's lamp. *op cit*: 265-8;

   Holmes JHH. On safety lamps for coal mines. *op cit*: 269-71;

   Knight W. Observations on Mr. Holmes's letter. *op cit*: 306-7;

   Murray J. Observations on the fire-damp of coal mines; with a plan for lighting mines so as to guard against its explosion. *op cit*: 406-20;

   Longmire JB. Answer to John George Children, Esq. on the wire-gauze lamp. *op cit*: 420-9;

   Holmes JHH. On safety lamps for coal-mines, in answer to the letters of Mr. Children and Mr. Knight. *op cit*: 429-33.

Chapter 15

DR GEORGE JOHNSTON, 1797–1855

GAC Binnie

George Johnston was a countryman by birth. His parents both came of Berwickshire farming stock; he himself was born at Simprim in the same county and shortly afterwards his father moved to another farm at Ilderton in north Northumberland. From there George went to Berwick Grammar School as a boarder. Many years later the school was endowed with the Johnston Prize, which is still awarded in the school which succeeded it. He was the tenth of 15 children but little is known of the rest of his family: a brother was an army colonel, a nephew farmed in Berwickshire, and Adam, his favourite brother, died aged 50 in 1847. Johnston commented in a letter to a friend in 1854 that he had not been to Ilderton since 1813, three years after the death of his widowed mother.[1]

It was as a child that he developed his interest in natural history which was to become a lifelong obsession and the source of his contemporary and lasting fame; he was a byword for being last home because he had been distracted by something botanical on the wayside. Perhaps because of his interest in natural history he became a medical student in Edinburgh, where he lodged with the Rev McCrie and was apprenticed to Dr Abercrombie, a leading Edinburgh physician, who was later to be Physician to the Queen in Scotland. He qualified LRCSE in 1817 and, after studying for a term with Dr Joshua Brooks the London anatomist, he went into practice briefly in Belford. There he met Catharine Charles, whose father had been an assistant surgeon in New York before the American Revolution; they were married in 1819. In the same year he took over the practice of Dr Robert Stevenson in Berwick and set up house and surgery in Bridge Street, moving to 35 Woolmarket in about 1827; after his death the Woolmarket house was named 'The Anchorage', supposedly because he had a share in a boat sailing out of Berwick. There he lived and practised for the rest of his life.

Also in 1819 he obtained his MD from Edinburgh University with a thesis entitled *De Hydrops* and in 1824 was made FRCSE with a dissertation on cancer. The latter was a very gentlemanly affair; the examiners seemed pleased to have a successful candidate. He was appointed a surgeon on the staff of Berwick Dispensary in 1819 (founded in 1814 and now Berwick Infirmary) and became physician to the Dispensary in 1831, apparently on his own proposition if the minutes of the meeting are a true record of the proceedings. He was senior physician by 1852 and often called out in consultation by his colleagues; his obituary commented that 'he never sought to earn his consulting fee by changing the treatment prescribed by the general practitioner who had referred the patient',[2] a tribute still applicable to present day consultant practice. In 1851 he wrote that he had 'had a very busy life, and would' ...have withdrawn... 'from all but consultation practice, had

I not, four years ago, lost the whole of my money; so I must go on working' – a reference to two failures of local banks in Berwick, which also involved Berwick Dispensary in financial loss. A year or two later he could write that his was the 'best practice in Berwick, or within twenty miles of it, and I look forward to discharge all claims on me in reasonable time;'...two years more would provide for his dependants.[3]

Achievements in natural history

Although interested in natural history as a schoolboy, he could remark that it was a study that he 'took up as a relief from the idleness of a young practitioner'. He had some 90 scientific publications which made him widely known throughout Britain. A fossil, *Sphenopteris johnstoniana*, was named after him 'as a mark of respect to a distinguished naturalist, whose writings and labours have added much to the history of our country', and PH Gosse named *Othonia johnstoni* after 'the father of our Marine Invertebrate Zoology'. Johnston himself made original findings, one of which, *Plumularia catharina*, was so named after his wife.[4,5]

Some of his early work was published in the *Transactions of the Plinian Society*, a student society which flourished in Edinburgh in the 1820s and which numbered Charles Darwin amongst its members. He was one of three founder editors of the *Magazine of Zoology and Botany* which was first published in 1835 and ran for about 10 years. He was largely responsible for the founding of the Ray Society in 1844 and was its first secretary: the society still exists to publish scholarly natural history works which might not attract a commercial publisher.

One of his most lasting achievements was the founding of the Berwickshire Naturalists' Club (in 1831) with nine founding members of whom seven were medically qualified. This was the first local naturalists' field club in the world and was followed by an explosive development of similar clubs elsewhere.

His first book was *A flora of Berwick-upon-Tweed*, published in two volumes in 1829-31, and was followed by works on *British zoophytes* (1838, 2nd edit 1847), *British sponges and lithophytes* (1842), *An introduction to conchology* (1850), *The natural history of the Eastern Borders* (1853), and as if these were not enough, his *A catalogue of the British non-parasitical worms* was published posthumously in 1865.

That his resultant fame was widespread in the British Isles shows in his correspondence, and he was very much a natural history consultant for others who were eminent in that field. This led to problems. He writes of receiving a parcel of worms, and also a bottle of worms that were the worse for wear, and frequently apologised for specimens left unexamined for months because of pressure of work – presumably these were less smelly botanical specimens. He collected specimens widely; he constructed a dredge to collect in Berwick Bay, met fishing boats on their return from the sea, exchanged specimens with other collectors and his botanical collection is still preserved in Edinburgh's Royal Botanic Garden. He was offered the chair of Natural History in Belfast in 1845 but declined for 'family reasons' – his wife had said 'No'. Later he applied for the equivalent chair in Edinburgh but, like Huxley and Hugh Miller, failed to be appointed. Despite having a supporting reference from Charles Darwin, he also failed in his attempt to get a British Museum fellowship, which he admitted would have lessened his financial anxiety about the future. It is almost an anticlimax to add that Aberdeen University awarded him an LLD (*Honoris Causa*).

Like many naturalists he found himself in some awkward predicaments. Once while he was botanising he was mistaken for a pedlar selling razors; he admitted to narrowly escaping being drowned in the Whitadder, and also to being almost submerged by the tide when returning from Holy Island with his family. His long-suffering wife Catharine regularly used a muff on their expeditions – it was very useful for concealing specimens; George kept some worms in her work-box for three years, presumably bottled. It was hardly surprising that she seems to have had a lot of psychosomatic illness, although she helped him by making drawings for future engravings. She had servants to help her look after her four children, but her husband was an inveterate entertainer of guests to stay overnight as well as for meals. And when he was not engaged in natural history in one way or another, he was busy with public works. Like so many in his profession it seemed surprising he had time to fit in any professional duties.

Civic duties

As if general practice and natural history were not enough, Johnston was heavily involved in civic duties. He was three times mayor of Berwick, and twice its sheriff; he was a JP, living only yards from the court house, and he became senior magistrate, with all the attendant entertaining. The Royal Highland Show was held in Berwick in 1841, and his work on its behalf was rewarded by its gold medal. His fellow citizens gave him an epergne, a branched ornamental plate centrepiece for the table.[5]

Family

The Johnstons had four children. Jane, the eldest, married an army officer, the son of a doctor, but he died after three years of marriage with a short illness during which his father in law had been in 'almost constant attendance on him for 10 days in Jedburgh', some 30 odd miles from Berwick. Jane was responsible for collating and publishing 429 surviving letters in 1892, nearly 40 years after her father's death, as well as allowing the old family home to be used as a base for the Berwickshire Naturalists' Club until she died in 1903.

Patrick, their only son, joined the Royal Navy and died a bachelor in New Zealand; he caused his mother considerable anxiety in 1851 when he was shipwrecked and escaped with only his sword.

When Johnston published his *Flora of Berwick* in 1829 he offered a copy to any pupil at Edinburgh Royal High School who could find 20 plants not named in the book. Philip Maclagan found 26, claimed the prize, and later adorned it by marrying the donor's daughter, Margaret Johnston, and succeeding to Johnston's practice. The third generation Maclagan practised in Berwick until 1955 and died aged 91 as recently as 1978. Philip Maclagan came from a talented family and his father was Physician to HM Forces and was President successively of the Edinburgh Royal Colleges of Physicians and of Surgeons. One brother was the lecturer in forensic medicine in Edinburgh University, another was Archbishop of York.

Johnston's youngest daughter Catharine died shortly after her father, with cardiac compression due to gross kypho-scoliosis[6] and she was probably the dependant whose financial future he was anxious to secure after the Berwick bank failures.

Practice

So far as I know, Johnston ventured into print only once on a medical subject.[7] This was in a pamphlet on the 1832 cholera epidemic in Berwick, one of many issued in various parts of the North East at that time. It provided warnings and practical advice to the citizens of Berwick, describing four cases that had occurred in the town, but it was also largely directed against 'one, perhaps two, medical men' named as Dr WD How of Berwick and Mr J How, apothecary to the Dispensary, who claimed that all the other doctors were misdiagnosing other diseases as cholera. On the first page of the copy in the Robinson Library of the University of Newcastle upon Tyne is a manuscript note by Nathanial Winch, Secretary to the Newcastle Infirmary, reading 'Not published March 1832'; this may have been because of the potentially libellous statements it contains about Dr How.[8] The year before the two doctors had crossed swords; Johnston had visited a Dispensary patient at home, eight miles from Berwick, every day for 10 days and had then passed the patient on to Dr How, who was next in their 3-monthly rota,[9] prompting a subsequent complaint to the Dispensary Committee of 'Failure to visit'. Johnston lost when his opponent was supported by the rest of the medical men, but his distrust of How was proved right when the latter did a midnight flit the following year, causing some embarrassment to the Infirmary.

Johnston did not neglect post graduate education: he spent a day with Professor Sir James Young Simpson in 1847, learning how to use chloroform.[10]

Some flavours of the medical scene come across from Johnston's letters and the minutes of Berwick Dispensary. It may have been the excuse for late replies to letters, but practice seemed to be very busy — 'a loud ring summoned him away': 'overwhelmed with business': 'going to do his evening visits weary after being 7 hours in the country': 'just away to finish his evening calls'. Practice was stressful — 'I have had great anxiety of late for scarlet fever has been amongst us and people little know the anxiety that drags the poor doctor down': 'Four dangerous cases and all in the country, daily visits and long watchings' and 'Dull and out of spirits today having too much of a distressing nature on mind; two of my friends lost one child yesterday, are likely to lose another today, a third is in jeopardy ... I stopped writing to run to see my little patient, who expired as I entered the house'. Night calls were if anything more prevalent than 150 years later: 'I got home at 11 p.m. was summoned at 1 a.m. and did not get home until 6 a.m.' and 'Having been up all night waiting on a case attended with some anxiety, I felt weary'. A typical remark, familiar today, is that he 'should be astir and moving amongst real or imaginary invalids'. Travelling around the practice had its problems too – 'I have returned from a ride of 24 miles' and 'two horses scarcely suffice even with occasional use of rail'. He was summoned from a botanical meeting by telegraph on at least one occasion, which is at least different from our car phones. The coming of the railway to Berwick in 1846 made a great difference to life, and patients with serious illnesses could get to the Edinburgh Infirmary by rail and cab. Johnston's initial reaction to rail travel was that 'It was safe enough for one who had his life insured or who had no family'. The building of the Royal Border Bridge linking the Scottish and English railway systems brought much medical work to the district; eight fatal accidents were recorded by the Berwick Coroner in his inquest reports, and the Dispensary sent a bill for £2 to the railway company, the cost of two mattresses destroyed by 'the effusion of blood' when a railway worker had his leg amputated following an accident.[11]

After 1819 Johnston scarcely travelled away from Berwick further than Jedburgh. It is difficult to be sure whether this was the result of conscientiousness in his practice or a dislike of travel. Even his work as Secretary of the Ray Society was carried out entirely by correspondence from his home. He was an intensely serious man but his books do reveal flashes of humour. His *Introduction to conchology* opens wryly:

> There are not many inducements to become a conchologist: his pursuit has always been deemed one of an inferior character....Unless, therefore, you are prepared to forego all chance of literary fame, and to rest satisfied with a very moderate share of scientific reputation, you had better at once leave this private path, and betake yourself...[12]

He was human and he wrote of going to the circus, and that he was 'building in my yard a small greenhouse', even if the suspicion lingers that it was looked after by his long-suffering wife when not filled with specimens of one sort or another. He had his absent-minded moments too, as when he left someone's manuscript in his winter coat until the following autumn.

Final illness and death

At the age of 50 Johnston wrote that 'advancing years lessen the love of labour, what was once recreation is now taken up with reluctance', and that 'weariness felt after a day's business walk reminds me that my days for strolling far away are past'. Before about 1850 he made only occasional mention of having upper respiratory infections, but when he was 53 he began to write of being unwell, complaining for example that at a naturalists' meeting at Warkworth he was 'too ill to do anything'. He wrote 'I do not bear a doctor's business so well as I was wont' and 'I have been ill of late and cannot go out at night unless in very urgent cases'; although he does not say how he could avoid that, he presumably would not be accountable to a service committee in those pre-Lloyd George days. The next year he commented that he was not in working order and that he had headaches as the day wore on.

He had some six months of ill health in 1854, when he was unfit for work, and he convalesced by staying across the Tweed in Spittal when he could. He consulted Mr Syme in Edinburgh on several occcasions, and had a sore lip which only healed after 4 months. In 1855 he went to Bridge of Allan, near Stirling, on holiday but took a stroke there and died 10 days later aged 58, death being certified by his son in law, Philip Maclagan, as being due to 'softening of the brain'. This had the connotation of cerebrovascular accident rather than dementia, and he was certainly writing coherent letters six weeks before his death, and completed his *Catalogue of British worms* shortly before he died. My own conclusion is that he probably had a post-scarlatina nephritis with the insidious onset of renal failure causing chronic ill health, until the associated hypertension caused a terminal cerebrovascular accident.

By any standards Johnston was a remarkable man, but his lasting achievement was as the innovator of the field club in Britain, whose members would study natural history in its natural surroundings, and his lasting memorial is the Berwickshire Naturalists' Club, still going strong in 1993.

Further reading

Binnie GAC. George Johnston: 1797-1855. *Brit Med J* 1982; *285*: 1014-6.

Binnie GAC. Dr George Johnston (1797-1855). *Hist Berwickshire Naturalists' Club* 1981. *42*: 17-21.

Binnie GAC. Berwick Dispensary and Infirmary, 1814-1898. *Hist Berwickshire Naturalists' Club* 1980; *41*:243-59.

Craw JH. *Hist Berwickshire Naturalists' Club* 1932; Centenary Volume, pp 2-5.

Lunn AG (ed). *A History of Naturalists in North East England*. Newcastle upon Tyne: University of Newcastle Department of Adult Education, 1983; 46-49.

Notes and references

1. Hardy J (ed). *Selections from the correspondence of Dr George Johnston*...collected and arranged by his daughter Mrs Barwell-Carter. Edinburgh: David Douglas, 1892: 514.
2. Embleton R. Anniversary Address. *Hist Berwickshire Naturalists' Club* 1856; *3*: 201-8.
3. Hardy J (ed). *op cit* note 1: 387 & 447.
4. *ibid*: 283-284 note.
5. *ibid*: xiii.

6. Binnie GAC. Dr George Johnston (1797-1855). *Hist Berwickshire Naturalists' Club* 1981; *42*:20.

7. Johnston G. *An address to the inhabitants of Berwick- upon-Tweed.* No publisher, no date [1832]. A seven-page printed pamphlet.

8. Winch was a noted botanist of the day and was personally well acquainted with Johnston. The handwriting was identified in 1986, at an exhibition at the Pybus Society, by Mr Peter Davis, then the Deputy Curator of the Hancock Museum, an authority on Winch.
Despite the statement that it was not published, the pamphlet also appears in the British Library catalogue.

9. Binnie GAC. Berwick Dispensary and Infirmary, 1814-1898. *Hist Berwickshire Naturalists' Club* 1980; *41*:248. The six members of the medical staff of the Berwick Infirmary each did three months on duty with another member, and then were replaced with two others, handing over the patients to them.

10. Hardy J. *op cit* note 1: 384.

11. Binnie GAC. *op cit* note 9, 257.

12. Johnston G. *An introduction to conchology*. London: John van Voorst, 1850: 1.

Chapter 16

JOHN SNOW – VICTORIAN PHYSICIAN

Anthony Ashcroft

The School of Medicine in Newcastle upon Tyne dates its origin to 1832, when the first courses of lectures were given to a small group of students in rooms above a doctor's surgery in Bell's Court, Pilgrim Street. The building remains, in a dilapidated state, but the handsome original doorway was removed and is now in the new Medical School in Framlington Place.

John Snow was one of that first group and was destined to become the most celebrated. He is remembered both for his dramatic intervention in removing the handle of the Broad Street pump in Soho during the cholera epidemic of 1854, which brought the local outbreak to a speedy conclusion, and for his pioneer work on chloroform anæsthesia. The anæsthetists have an annual lecture in his name.

Original material relating to the life of John Snow is scanty and, like most accounts, this one is based largely on the Memoir published by Richardson in the year of Snow's death.[1] It is clear that he was both talented and industrious to a degree, and rose from humble beginnings to reach distinction in his relatively short life, only achieving due recognition some time after his death. Medical journals of the time tended to be verbose but the death notice in *The Lancet* of 26 June 1858 contained only the brief statement:

> Dr. John Snow — this well-known Physician died at noon on 16th inst. at his house in Sackville Street from an attack of apoplexy. His researches on Chloroform and other anæsthetics were appreciated by the Profession.

Such a brief notice may have been due to a difference of opinion with Thomas Wakley, the irascible and outspoken editor of *The Lancet* at that time. However, when his treatise on chloroform[2] was published later in the same year, it received very favourable reviews both in *The Lancet* and *British Medical Journal*, where it was noted as 'exhibiting the struggles of a poor man of sterling integrity and much merit, but destitute of those popular talents by which early success is sometimes attained'. 'Had the author survived a few years he would have reaped the desired fruits of his labour in seeing established a rational, safe and extended employment of anæsthetic agents.'

John Snow was born in North Street, York on 15 March 1813. The family had lived in North Street for many years and both his grandparents and father are buried in the tiny churchyard there. He was the eldest of eight children and the others followed diverse occupations; for example, his brother Charles became an hotel keeper in York but later emigrated to Australia; another brother became a colliery manager in Yorkshire; and yet another took Holy Orders, whilst two of his sisters opened a private college for young ladies at The Mount, York.[3] At the time of John's birth, his father's occupation was recorded as "labourer" and he later became the driver of a horse drawn bus; it was only some time after John had left home in 1827 that his father acquired a small farm near York and became rather more prosperous, but at the time of John's birth and early childhood the family was not at all affluent and it is a source of some mystery where the means were derived for his education. We know that he was privately educated in York, possibly at St Peter's, although no records remain to confirm or deny this possibility. Little is known about his schooldays except that he was very proficient in arithmetic and interested in natural history, a fondness for which continued all his life.[4]

A possible source of means for his education, both at York and later at Newcastle, lies with his close life-long relationship to the Empson family. We know that his mother Frances Askham had adopted the name of Empson and it is probable that she was the illegitimate daughter of Mary Askham, who subsequently married John Empson. John Empson went to live in Bath and was probably well-to-do and well-connected because we find that in 1856 he took John Snow on a visit to Paris, meeting the Emperor Napoleon. The young John Snow was particularly industrious at school, being fond of mathematics, but we know little of his life there and at the age of fourteen he was apprenticed to William Hardcastle, a General Practitioner Surgeon in Newcastle.[4] At that time William Hardcastle was living and practising in Westgate Street opposite St John's Church, although after John Snow left Newcastle he removed to one of the elegant houses in Greenfield Place.

Apprenticeship to a General Practitioner Surgeon in those days was usually for a period of five years and would have cost about 100 guineas, quite a substantial sum in 1827. The apprentice would have spent the first years living with his master and assisting in the day to day duties of the practice, including the preparation of drugs and dressings, writing up the day book and acting as general dog's body, observing over his master's shoulder, as it were, the practical application of the healing art. It was a well tried method of medical education, although poles apart from the highly structured vocational schemes of today. In the last two years of the apprenticeship it was customary to obtain hospital practice by walking the wards at the infirmary.

William Hardcastle was well established and highly thought of in the Parish of St John's. We find that he was surgeon and secretary to the lying-in hospital in Rosemary Lane and, after he died in 1860, a stained glass window was placed to his memory in St John's Church. In the autumn of 1831 cholera appeared in Sunderland and quickly spread over the north east of England and other parts of the country. William Hardcastle was appointed by St John's parochial council to minister to the sick in that parish and, because there were violent outbreaks in neighbouring villages, he sent his apprentice to cope with the epidemic at Killingworth Colliery. So in 1832 at the tender age of nineteen John Snow achieved the responsibility of independent and as yet unqualified medical practice.[5]

Little of the old Killingworth remains. Dial Cottage, half a mile away in Forest Hall, was for many years the home of Robert Stephenson, the railway pioneer and inventor. Killingworth High Pit, where he was the engineer, has long since been worked out and filled in. It is now such a picturesque village that it is difficult to visualise the squalid, overcrowded and unhygienic pit rows of the mid 19th century, and of course the pattern of a collier's life contributed greatly to the rapid spread of infection. John Snow wrote subsequently of the colliers, who descended the pit with food and drink for a shift of eight or nine hours:

> The pit is one huge privy, and of course the men always take their victuals with unwashed hands..... That the men are occasionally attacked while at work I know, from having seen them brought up from some of the coal-pits in Northumberland in 1831-32, after having had profuse discharges from the stomach and bowels, and while fast approaching to a state of collapse.[6]

With the benefit of hindsight and our knowledge today, it is hardly surprising that cholera spread like wildfire in such conditions. In 1832 doctors were only just beginning to understand the infectious nature of cholera and the remedies available were limited, being confined to the prevention of dehydration, together with the use of opium derivatives and other simple drugs; nevertheless John Snow's efforts appear to have been much appreciated. Persons who died in the parish were buried at Longbenton churchyard, the average number of deaths per annum being seldom more than 100 but in the year 1832 there were no fewer than 235. Unfortunately for our researches the cause of death was not recorded prior to 1837. The attractive church at Longbenton is surrounded by serried rows of tombstones, apart from the large area where cholera victims were hastily buried in unmarked graves. Within a short space of time, the usual funeral observances were abandoned. Coffins were smeared on the inside with coal tar and the dead were buried within nine hours of death, the pall being dispensed with and frequently the hearse abandoned in favour of a cart, a single attendant leading the horse at arm's length. The coffin was tipped into the grave and speedily covered with quicklime.[7]

The epidemic lasted several months and his first impression of medicine in the raw must have made a profound impression on the young John Snow, but the practice of medicine alone was not enough and in October 1832 he returned to Newcastle to pursue his studies. Whilst still an apprentice in Newcastle, John Snow became interested in his own health, becoming a vegetarian and teetotaller, a regime which he preached and practised for almost the whole of his life, and may have carried to absurd extremes, because we learn that he developed phthisis, renal disease and a duodenal ulcer – evidence of which was ultimately found at post-mortem.[5]

The population of Newcastle at that time was about 40 000 and there were only 10 physicians and 28 surgeons, most of whom would be in General Practice. A small group of them decided to commence instruction in medicine and surgery and a course of lectures was advertised in 1832, the modest premises over the entrance to Bell's Court being acquired for the purpose.

There were only eight students in the first session, who paid two guineas for the course of lectures and five guineas for hospital practice in the Newcastle Infirmary. After two sessions the premises proved inadequate and in 1834 the embryonic school was transferred to the Hall of the Barber Surgeons at Manors. Following this brief course of lectures and hospital practice, coming at the end of five years' apprenticeship, most students would take the LSA or MRCS, but it was not until the Medical Act of 1858 that registration became compulsory.[8]

When John Snow reached the end of his apprenticeship he must have wondered, like so many young doctors, what should be the next step in his professional life. He did not come from a wealthy or medical background and had his own way to make in the world, so perhaps his intention was to earn a little money as well as to broaden his experience, because in 1833 at the age of twenty we find him as an assistant to Mr Watson of Burnopfield, where he stayed for about twelve months, following which he returned to his native York for a brief visit. He then moved on to Pateley Bridge in Nidderdale, becoming assistant to Mr Warburton, where he stayed for about eighteen months. He seems to have found his work there very rewarding, but it must have been a hard life and he speaks of many rough rides and a fair share of night work; those who know the dale with its scattered farms will appreciate that the life of a country doctor in those times must indeed have been hard. We do not know the house where he stayed at that time but perhaps it was the apothecary's shop in the High Street, now a delightful tea room. In later years he spoke with great affection of Mr Warburton 'his old master', who must have been well thought of in the neighbourhood. Perhaps he was getting itchy feet again, because he then returned to the family home at York, engaging himself in the formation of Temperance Societies and taking long walks into the country, pursuing his study of natural history.[9]

It was in 1836 at the age of twenty-three that the great change in direction was made, when he decided to become a student in London. This involved quite an adventure and he made a long pilgrimage on foot from York, via Liverpool, and through North and South Wales, staying at Bath with his uncle, John Empson, and thence to London, where he attended the Hunterian School of Medicine in Windmill Street. In 1837 he enrolled at Westminster Hospital and in the following year became MRCS and LSA. He was then in a position to engage in independent practice and, to use his own phrase, he 'nailed up his colours' at 54 Frith Street, Soho, and, although he subsequently moved to Sackville Street, he spent the remainder of his professional life living and working in Soho.[10]

By the year 1837, when he was only twenty-four years of age, John Snow had already laid a very firm foundation for his distinguished life. He had spent five years in apprenticeship to an established General Practitioner, with hospital practice in a well respected provincial hospital; he had spent two years assisting in very different practices; he had coped with the desperate extremes of a cholera outbreak whilst still a student and had then made his way to London, where he had taken the two most necessary basic medical qualifications, which would enable him to set up in practice. I wonder if he paused at this point and came to a conscious decision as to the ways in which his energy should be directed – we will probably never know but several strands of his life seem to begin simultaneously at this point. Firstly, he seems to have sought experience and clinical practice wherever the opportunity presented itself and we find him visiting the out-patients of Charing Cross Hospital on a purely honorary basis, hoping no doubt that his name would become known and that a procession of patients would soon begin to roll up to his rooms in Frith Street, Soho Square. I expect that, as for so many of his generation who were lacking in influence or private means, this was a long slow business and it was some years before he was properly established in practice but he lived a simple quiet life until his practice increased. Perhaps he worked off excess energy in violent exercise; for example, on Easter Monday 1837 he walked to St Albans and back, a distance of fifty miles, with his friend Joshua Parsons but he needed to take the horse bus the last mile or so down the Edgeware Road.[10]

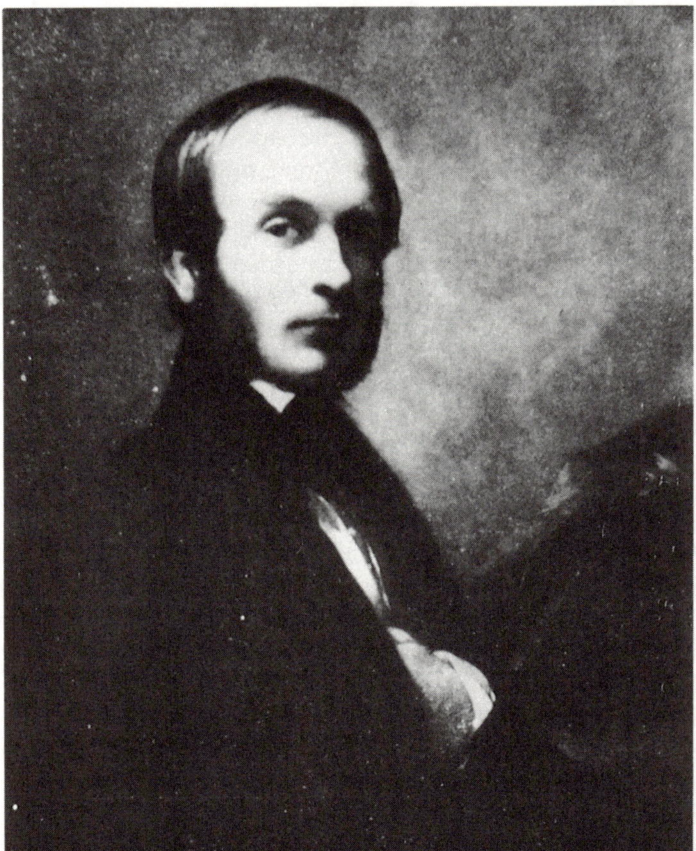

Figure 1. Snow – early in his career.

The second strand in his medical progress was the pursuit of further academic honours. Now, whilst it was not entirely necessary to possess a University degree, it was certainly a pre-requisite for one who aimed at consultant practice and so we find him taking the MB of the University of London in 1843 and proceeding MD with Honours in 1844 at the age of thirty-three.[11]

The third strand in his medical life was his involvement with the Westminster Medical Society.[12] I suspect that, being of a shy and retiring nature, both a vegetarian and teetotaller, of slender means, living very plainly and keeping no company, he must have found this a somewhat painful experience. Most medical societies in those days were no less convivial than they are today. Nevertheless he persevered and his efforts achieved recognition. It is recorded that, when he first attended the meetings, he was very timid and, although he spoke to the point, his contributions seemed largely ignored,[12] but he continued to attend the meetings[13] and reported in *The Medical Gazette* the results of his researches into a wide variety of medical topics.[14] Research, then, was the fourth strand in his medical life. The research and the publication of his findings must have occupied a considerable proportion of his time, because the experimental work was carried out with tremendous application and in great detail, the two most famous examples being, of course, his work on anæsthetic agents and the epidemiological study of cholera, to which we shall turn shortly.[15]

John Snow's experimental work in anæsthesia probably began about 1846 but ether anæsthesia dates back to 1842, when it was used by Long on a small scale; it was later used by Morton for dental extractions in 1846 and its popularity really began at that time. With his by now accustomed thoroughness, he investigated all the physical properties and physiological effects of ether[16] and various other similar chemical compounds and experimented on a considerable scale first with animals, before applying for permission to use it in the out-patients' dental department at St George's Hospital. There he acquired a reputation as an anæsthetist of great skill. He soon progressed to general surgery and made a great impression on Robert Liston of University College Hospital, who was responsible for his introduction to that hospital. Unfortunately Robert Liston died in 1847 but by this time John Snow's reputation was advancing. Like so many anæsthetists, then and now, he designed and made his own apparatus, but with his ether apparatus the main difficulty lay in producing quantities of anæsthetic vapour at the right temperature, a problem which he soon overcame by the use of a copper spiral placed in a water bath.[17]

The use of ether was, however, soon superseded by chloroform, which James Young Simpson had used for midwifery in November 1847; Snow turned his attention to this and characteristically designed a special inhaler with face piece, which, with only minor modifications, became used in many London hospitals and elsewhere. In Newcastle the Infirmary report for 1850 records that the use of chloroform was most general, being administered in all severe operations and being universally successful and perfectly safe – the patients indeed insisting on its use – 'they should first of all have the chloroform and be set fast asleep'. Snow was, of course, quick to publish the results of his work[18] but unfortunately it was not until after his death that his major work on chloroform and other anæsthetics was published. Not only was Snow most careful in all his experimental work, but he meticulously recorded, in the three volumes of his diary, the clinical details of all his patients.[19] These diaries are now in the possession of the Royal College of Physicians and make fascinating reading, being as legible today as they were at the time when they were written. Two representative pages, not entirely chosen at random, include the accounts of the administration of chloroform to his most famous patient, Queen Victoria.[20] John Snow had been consulted at the birth of Prince Arthur in 1850 but did not actually administer the anæsthetic then; however, he was called in attendance on 7 April 1853, when Prince Leopold was born. The extract from his diary reads as follows:

> Thursday 7th April:
>
> Administered chloroform to the Queen in her confinement. Slight pains had been experienced since Sunday. Dr. Locock was sent for about nine o'clock this morning, stronger pains having commenced, and he found the os uterus had commenced to dilate a very little. I received a note from Sir James Clark a little after ten asking me to go to the Palace. I remained in an appartment near that of the Queen along with Sir J. Clark, Dr. Fergusson and (for most part of the time) Dr. Locock till a little after twelve. At twenty minutes past twelve by a clock in the Queen's apartment [*sic*] I commenced to give a little chloroform with each pain, by pouring about 15 minims by measure on a folded handkerchief. The first stage of the labour was nearly over when the chloroform was commenced. Her Majesty expressed great relief from the application, the pain being very trifling during the uterine contractions, whilst between the periods of contraction there was complete ease. The effect of the chloroform was not at any time carried to the extent of quite removing consciousness. Dr Locock thought the chloroform prolonged the interval between the pains and retarded the labour somewhat. The infant was born at thirteen minutes past one by the clock in the room (which was three minutes before the right time) consequently the chloroform was inhaled for 53 minutes. The placenta was expelled in a very few minutes and the Queen appeared very cheerful and well, expressing herself much gratified with the effect of the chloroform.[21]

This of course was his own account but Queen Victoria herself recorded in her diary:

> Dr. Snow gave that blessed chloroform and the effect was soothing, quieting and delightful beyond measure.

One could hardly be more appreciative than that!

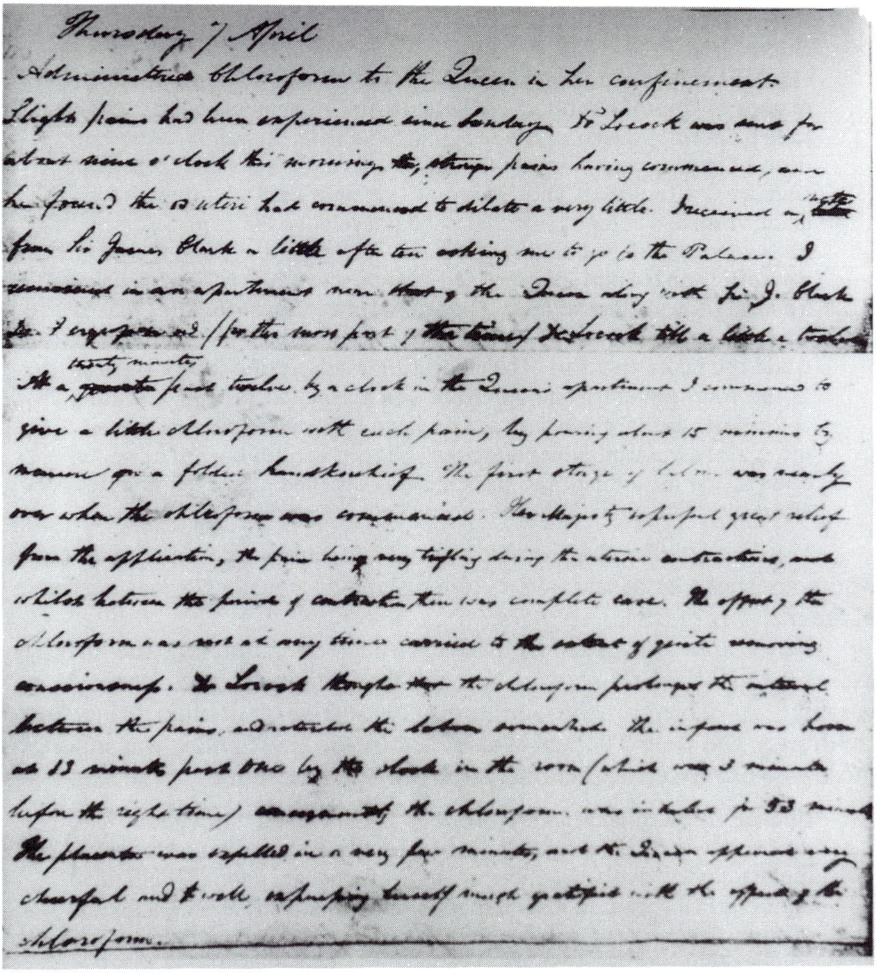
Thursday 7 April
Administered chloroform to the Queen in her confinement. Slight pains had been experienced since Sunday. Dr Locock was sent for about nine o'clock this morning, stronger pains having commenced, and he found the os uteri had commenced to dilate a very little. I received a note from Sir James Clark a little after ten asking me to go to the Palace. I remained in an apartment near that of the Queen along with Sir J. Clark, Dr Ferguson and (for the most part of the time) Dr Locock till a little after twelve. At twenty minutes past twelve by a clock in the Queen's apartment I commenced to give a little chloroform with each pain, by pouring about 15 minims by measure on a folded handkerchief. The first stage of labour was nearly over when the chloroform was commenced. Her Majesty expressed great relief from the application, the pains being very trifling during the uterine contractions, and whilst between the periods of contraction there was complete ease. The effect of the chloroform was not at any time carried to the extent of quite removing consciousness. Dr Locock thought that the chloroform prolonged the intervals between the pains, and retarded the labour somewhat. The infant was born at 13 minutes past one by the clock in the room (which was 3 minutes before the right time); consequently the chloroform was inhaled for 53 minutes. The placenta was expelled in a very few minutes, and the Queen appeared very cheerful and well, expressing herself much gratified with the effect of the chloroform.

Figure 2. Snow's diary entry for 7 April 1853.

Some four years later on 14 April 1857, he was again called to administer chloroform to the Queen in her ninth confinement; clearly this was not quite so straight forward as last time. His account of the confinement reads as follows:

> Tuesday 14th April
>
> Administered chloroform to her Majesty the Queen in her ninth confinement. The labour commenced about a fortnight later than was expected. It commenced about 2.00 a.m. of this day when the medical men were sent for. The labour was lingering and a little after 10 Dr. Locock administered half a drachm of powdered ergot, which produced

> some effect in increasing the pains. At 11 o'clock I began to administer chloroform. Prince Albert had previously administered a very little chloroform on a handkerchief about 9 or 10 o'clock. I poured about 10 minims of chloroform on a handkerchief folded in a conical shape for each pain. Her Majesty expressed great relief from the vapour. Another dose of ergot was given about 12 o'clock and the pains increased somewhat afterwards. The Queen at this time kept asking for more chloroform and complaining that it did not remove the pain. She slept, however, sometimes between the pains. Before one o'clock the head was resting on the perineum and Dr. Locock wished the patient to make a bearing down effort, as he said this would effect the birth. The Queen, however, when not unconscious of what was said, complained that she could not make an effort. The chloroform was left off for 3 or 4 pains as the royal patient made an effort which expelled the head, a little chloroform being given just as the head was passed. There was an interval of several minutes before the child was entirely born; it however cried in the meantime. The placenta was expelled about ten minutes afterwards. The Queen's recovery was very favourable.[21]

It is noteworthy that he did not use his vaporiser in obstetric cases where analgesia, or at any rate a lighter plane of anæsthesia, was desirable in the majority of cases.

Royal approval of chloroform did much to counteract the strongly expressed views of those who thought that childbirth was meant to be painful.[22] As it says in the Scriptures, 'In sorrow shalt thou bring forth children'. The fiery Thomas Wakley, editor of *The Lancet*, was amongst those who expressed a reactionary opinion, when he wrote:

> Intense astonishment, therefore, has been excited throughout the profession by the rumour that Her Majesty during her last labour was placed under the influence of chloroform, an agent which has unquestionably caused instantaneous death in a considerable number of cases..... We could not imagine that anyone had incurred the awful responsibility of advising the administration of chloroform to Her Majesty during a perfectly natural labour with a seventh child.[23,24]

As we have seen, the antagonism between Snow and Wakley continued until Snow's death.

It is perhaps somewhat surprising that John Snow does not appear to have received any honour following his attendance on the Queen but then anæsthesia hardly achieved the respectability that it enjoys today. The administration of anæsthesia seems to have been a major activity of his, although it cannot exactly have been a moneyspinner, because his income from all sources never exceeded £1000 per annum, even at the height of his career.[25]

We now turn from John Snow's contribution to anæsthetic science to his work on cholera. The cholera epidemic of 1832, of which he had experience at Killingworth, was part of a widespread outbreak but was nothing like so severe as the succeeding epidemics of 1848 and 1853. The problem of the transmission of cholera, and indeed its very nature, was quite unknown in 1832 although a Newcastle practitioner, TM Greenhow, and Dr WR Clanny of Sunderland, both published small volumes on its treatment at that time.[26] It is of interest that William Hardcastle, John Snow's principal, and Greenhow had applied for the same surgical post at Newcastle Infirmary, but Hardcastle withdrew his application and Greenhow was appointed, and by the year 1848 Greenhow was the senior surgeon to the Infirmary. I wonder whether getting into print was as important then as it appears to be today in securing advancement. Be that as it may, the treatment for cholera advocated by Greenhow seems to have depended on the use of mustard emetics, tobacco enemas and the liberal use of opium tincture, calomel and brandy. England was virtually free of cholera between 1832 and 1848 but Snow's experiences in the earlier epidemic were not forgotten and, when he spoke to the Westminster Medical Society in 1849[27] and also at greater length in his book *On the mode of communication of cholera*,[28] he emphasized the importance of personal cleanliness and also incriminated contaminated drinking water as the medium for communicating the infection. There were others who felt that the disease was airborne or spread by fomites but Snow's observations, that in areas of outbreaks the water itself was offensive, proved to be the clue from which all else followed. It became clear that the water supply was frequently contaminated from adjacent sewers, house drains or cess pools. He presented these observations and advanced his theory as to the likely mode of infection, recommending a few simple measures by which the disease could be avoided:

1) the washing of hands after touching patients:
2) the washing of hands before touching food:
3) that one should drink only pure water or water which had been filtered or boiled.

He hastened into print in 1849[15,27] because, as we have seen, he was simultaneously deeply involved with his work on chloroform. There was a great deal of argument and discussion about cholera in both the lay and medical press of the time but it was not until the next outbreak in 1854 that his views were accepted. Having implicated an impure water supply as the likely cause of cholera, he devised a simple test with silver nitrate, which readily confirmed the presence of impurities, visiting each house for the purpose. He noted that in Southwark and Lambeth the population derived their water supply from two companies; the Lambeth Water Company supplied pure water drawn from Thames Ditton and the Southwark and Vauxhall Company supplied water from the river at Battersea, which was contaminated. In the Southwark and Vauxhall area twelve times as many cases of cholera occurred as in the Lambeth area. He published his findings and supported them with evidence in incredible detail so that there remained no doubt of the truth of his assertions.[29]

It was, however, the catastrophic outbreak in his own practice area which supplied the final proof and by which he is remembered. This is the episode of the Broad Street pump; Broad Street lies in Soho between Frith Street, where he originally set up in practice, and Sackville Street where he then lived. At the end of August 1854 an explosive outbreak of cholera occurred in the area of Broad Street and Golden Square and there were more than five hundred fatal cases of cholera in ten days. He would have attended many of these patients himself and numbers were admitted to hospital, but of course the majority would die at home. Snow had noted where the deaths occurred and subsequently published, in the second edition of his book, a map showing the situation of each death. Although there were several other pumps in the district, the majority of deaths were in the immediate vicinity of the Broad Street pump. It is difficult for us in these healthy times to visualise the horror of such an epidemic – five hundred deaths in an area of a quarter square mile over a period of ten days; Snow recorded every one.[30]

Not since the Great Plague had there been such an outbreak and the population of the area was on the verge of panic, ready to leave homes and possessions to escape to healthier areas. The parochial church council or Board of Guardians was responsible for the health of the community and, on the evening of Thursday 7th September, the vestrymen of St James Church met to discuss the cause of the outbreak and what might be done to contain it.[31]

Dr Snow requested a hearing and, with brief but cogent argument, persuaded the vestrymen that the Broad Street pump was the source and centre of the outbreak.[32] The vestry was incredulous but, fortunately for history, heeded his advice and followed his prescription – to remove forthwith the handle of the pump.[31] Within days the epidemic waned. There are those who have suggested that the epidemic was already past its peak at this point but there can be little doubt that this simple but striking prescription rapidly brought the epidemic in that area to an end.[33] The site of the pump is still marked and the public house, which used to be named the City of Newcastle, has been renamed the John Snow in his memory. Professor Bradford Hill was invited by Watneys to dedicate it to his memory in 1955, although JF Fulton commenting on the address by Professor Mackintosh, Professor of Public Health at the London School of Hygiene and Tropical Medicine, felt that it was somewhat inappropriate that John Snow, who remained a bachelor, a teetotaller and a vegetarian[34] all his life, should have a Soho public house as his chief memorial.[35] Snow himself, however, noted that the brewery workers themselves appeared immune to cholera – their fluid requirements were met exclusively from the barrel. Snow published the whole of this research in 1855 in the second edition of his work *On the mode of communication of cholera* and in 1856 he visited Paris with his uncle, Mr Empson, who had known the Emperor Napoleon for many years. During this visit he entered a copy of his treatise in competition for a prize of £1200, offered for the discovery of a means of preventing or curing the disease but he was not successful.[31] With the advance in public health and the provision of a pure water supply, cholera soon became a thing of the past so far as this country is concerned and John Snow returned to devoting his energies to the development of anæsthesia. His treatise on chloroform was an immense labour of love running to over 400 pages, representing the culmination of his life's work, but unfortunately his health was beginning to deteriorate. Whilst still in his thirties he suffered from pulmonary tuberculosis and probably nephritis also. His friends managed to induce him to relax his strict vegetarian ways and to take a more varied diet.[35]

More recently he had suffered a hæmatemesis and in December 1857 he had a slight stroke but continued with his writing and all his other professional activities until the last.[36]

He had just completed the last sentence of his treatise when he sustained a cerebral infarction from which he eventually succumbed on 16 June. The following Monday he was buried in Brompton Cemetery,[37] where his grave is marked by a distinctive memorial. His was a short life of considerable activity in a wide range of general and special interests and we can be proud that the Newcastle School of Medicine influenced him in this to some considerable extent.

Acknowledgements

I am grateful to Elizabeth Lazenby for providing the notes and references, and to the Royal College of Physicians for permission to reproduce Figure 2.

Selected bibliography

Armstrong Davison M H. John Snow and the Enlightenment. *Proc Roy Soc Med* 1958; *51*: 834-5.

Barrett N R. Tribute to John Snow. *Bull Hist Med* 1946; *19*: 517-535.

Bradford Hill A. Snow – An appreciation. *Proc Roy Soc Med* 1955; *48*: 1008-12.

Cohen, Lord. John Snow – 'The Autumn Loiterer'. *Proc Roy Soc Med* 1969; *62*: 99-106.

De S N. *Cholera*. Oliver and Boyd, 1961.

Duncum B. *Development of Inhalation Anæsthesia*. Wellcome Historical Medical Museum, Oxford 1947.

Fraser I. John Snow and his surgical friends. *Anæsthesia* 1968; *23*: 501-14.

Fulton J F. Editorial. A Snow Centenary. *Lancet* 1955; *1*: 1113-4.

Hume G H. *History of the Newcastle Infirmary*. Andrew Reid: Newcastle, 1906.

Keys T E. John Snow, M.D., Anesthetist. *J Hist Med* 1946; *1*: 551- 566.

Longmate N. *King Cholera*. Hamish Hamilton: London, 1966.

Mackintosh J M. Snow – the man and his times. *Proc Roy Soc Med* 1955; *48*: 1004-07.

Snow J. *On the mode of communication of cholera*. First edition, London 1849; second edition enlarged, London 1855; reprinted with introduction by Wade Hampton Frost, New York, 1936.

Snow J. *On narcotism by the inhalation of vapours*. (1849-52). Facsimile edition with an introductory essay by R H Ellis. London: Roy Soc Med, 1991.

Snow J. *On Chloroform and other Anæsthetics*. London 1858. (Ed. Richardson B W).

Turner G G, Arnison W D. *The Newcastle School of Medicine*. Andrew Reid: Newcastle, 1934.

Notes and references.

1. Richardson B W. Memoir of John Snow: appended as an introduction to Snow J., *On Chloroform and other Anæsthetics*, London: John Churchill, 1858: pp i-xliv. In the following notes, where the memoir is indicated, as opposed to Snow's actual text, the references given are to Richardson, but with arabic numerals substituted for the original roman.
2. Snow *op cit* note 1.
3. NB. This is not the present-day Mount School run by the Society of Friends.
4. Richardson *op cit*: 2.
5. Richardson *op cit*: 3-4.
6. Snow J. On the prevention of cholera. *Med Times Gaz* 1853; *ns7*: 367-9.
7. See for example: [Sykes J] *An account of the disease termed cholera morbus, from its first appearance at Sunderland, to its final departure from Northumberland and Durham....* Newcastle: John Sykes, 1832.
8. Newman C. *The Evolution of Medical Education in the Nineteenth Century*. London: Oxford University Press, 1957: 186-193.

   O'Malley C D. *The History of Medical Education*. Los Angeles: University of California Press, 1970: 243-244.

   See also the chapter and references concerning Education and the General Medical Council in F N L Poynter: *The Evolution of Medical Education in Britain*, London, 1966.
9. Richardson *op cit*: 4.
10. Richardson *op cit*: 6-9.
11. Richardson *op cit*: 12.
12. Richardson *op cit*: 8-9.
13. John Snow's contributions to the Westminster Medical Society were recognised when, after its amalgamation with the Medical Society of London in 1849-1850, he became Orator and in 1855 President of this re-formed Society.
14. Snow published more than thirty papers on cholera and public health and a similar number on ether, chloroform, other anæsthetics and respiratory physiology. Many were read to the Westminster Medical Society and later published in the *London Medical Gazette*. Among the most important of these papers in chronological order are:

    Asphyxia and the Resuscitation of New-born Children. 1842; *ns1*: 222-227.
    On the Use of Ether as an Anæsthetic. 1847; *ns4*: 156- 157.
    On the Pathology and Mode of Communication of Cholera. 1849; *44*: 730, 745, 923.
    On the Communication of Cholera by Impure Thames Water. 1854; *ns9*: 365-366.
    On the Chief Cause of the Recent Sickness and Mortality in the Crimea. 1855; *ns10*: 457-458.
    Drainage and Water Supply in Connection With the Public Health. 1858; *ns16*: 161, 189.

See also *Dictionary of Scientific Biography*, volume 12, 502-503, and Youngson A J. *The Scientific Revolution in Victorian Medicine*. New York: Holmes and Meier, 1979: 76.

Snow J. *On narcotism by the inhalation of vapours*. London: Wilson and Ogilvy, 3 volumes, 1848, 1851, 1852. Facsimile edition, edit Ellis R H; London: Roy Soc Med, 1991.

15. Snow J. *On the mode of communication of cholera*. First edition, London 1849; Second edition enlarged, London 1855; Reprinted with introduction by Wade Hampton Frost, New York, 1936.

Snow J. *On Chloroform and other Anæsthetics*. London: John Churchill, 1858. (Edited by B W Richardson).

16. Snow J. *On the Inhalation of the Vapour of Ether in Surgical Operations*. London: Churchill, 1847;
Snow J. *On narcotism by the inhalation of vapours*. *op cit* note 14.

17. Richardson *op cit* note 1: 14-15.

18. Some of Snow's papers on chloroform are:

On the Inhalation of Chloroform and Ether, with description of an apparatus. *Lancet*, 1848; *1*: 177-180.
On the Administration of Chloroform During Parturition. *Assoc Med J* 1853; *1*: 500-502.

19. Richardson *op cit*: 32.

20. Richardson *op cit*: 31.

21. Snow's diary is in the library of the Royal College of Physicians, London.

22. Snow, in 1853, showed that chloroform could hardly be refused to mothers on the grounds of safety, when he stated in *The Lancet*, 1853; *2*: 609-10, 'It should be remembered that no death from chloroform had occurred in midwifery, and he only knew of one case where the patient was in danger, and that arose from gross mismanagement, for the husband was giving the chloroform, and looking another way.' Prince Albert was obviously more adept!

23. Editorial in *The Lancet*, 1853; *1*:452.

24. Twenty five deaths from chloroform anæsthesia were reviewed in the *Assoc Med J* 1853; *1*:134-6. The very first was recorded in 1848 in the practice of Dr TN Meggison of Winlaton (near Gateshead) and the post-mortem examination of the case was made by Sir John Fife.

Fatal application of chloroform. *Lancet* 1848; *1*:161-2.

Simpson JY. Remarks on the alleged case of death from the action of chloroform. *Lancet* 1848; *1*:175-6.

Snow J. The fatal chloroform case at Newcastle. *Lancet* 1848; *1*:239.

25. Richardson *op cit*: 40.

26. Greenhow T M. *Cholera: its non-contagious nature, and the best means of arresting its progress shortly examined. In a letter addressed to the Right Worshipful Mayor of Newcastle*. Newcastle: E. Charnley, 1831.

Clanny W R. *Hyperanthraxis or the cholera at Sunderland*. London: Whittaker, Treacher and Arnott, 1832.

27. Snow J. On the mode of communication of cholera. *Lond Med Gaz* 1849; *ns9*: 466-470.

28. First published in London in 1849; see note 15 above.

29. Richardson *op cit*: 20.

Also: On the Communication of Cholera by Impure Thames Water. *Medical Times and Gazette*, 1854; *ns9*: 365-366.

Snow, on page 88 of the second edition of *On the mode of communication of cholera* (see note 15 above), gives the following table as proof of these findings:

	Population 1851	Cholera deaths in 14 weeks ending 14 Oct.	Deaths per 10,000 living
Houses supplied by Southwark and Vauxhall Water Company	266,516	4,093	153
Houses supplied by Lambeth Water Company	173,748	461	26

30. Richardson *op cit*: note 1:20-22.

Snow J. Communication of cholera. *Med Times Gaz* 23 September 1854, 39-54.

Report on the Cholera outbreak in the parish of St James, Westminster, during the autumn of 1854, presented to the vestry by the Cholera Inquiry Committee. London: July 1855.

31. Richardson *op cit*: 20-22.

32. Rawnsley states that Snow found the source of the outbreak with the help of the local curate, Rev Henry Whitehead, who had discovered that, just before the outbreak, a child had died at 40 Broad Street from exhaustion following diarrhoea, but that the symptoms were those of cholera. The child's napkins had been soaked in water, which was then thrown down a sink and thence into a cesspool which seeped into the pump well. Rawnsley H D. *Henry Whitehead, 1825-1896*. Glasgow: 1898: 29-42 and 206.

33. Chave S P W. Henry Whitehead and Cholera in Broad Street. *Med Hist* 1958; *2*: 92-108.

Chave S P W. The Broad Street pump and after. *Medical Officer* 1958; *99*.

Bailey W and Gull W. *Reports on the epidemic cholera drawn up at the desire of the Royal College of Physicians*. London: 1854.

34. Richardson *op cit* 2-3; Richardson states here that, 'During the third year of his apprenticeship, viz., when he was seventeen years old, he formed an idea that the vegetarian body-feeding faith was the true and the old; and with that consistency, which throughout life attended him, tried the system rigidly for more than eight years.'

See also Richardson *op cit* 13.

35. Richardson *op cit*: 2-3.

Richardson, *op cit*: 13, says that he relaxed his strict vegetarian diet in 1845.

Fulton J F. John Snow – Epidemiologist. *J Hist Med* 1955; *10*: 428-9.

Mackintosh J M. Snow, the man and his times. *Proc Roy Soc Med* 1955; *48*: 1004-07.

36. Richardson *op cit*: 41.

37. Richardson *op cit*: 42-44.

Chapter 17

ROBERT SEPTIMUS PEART MD, EPIDEMIOLOGIST

Ralph Wales Gould

It was 1869. Bacilli were beginning to be seen and discussed by the elect, but miasmata or odours were still generally considered to be the mechanism of spread of cholera and typhoid. Koch's paper on anthrax, which was the first to prove that bacilli are the cause of an infection, was still seven years away,[1] and a *Lancet* editorial of 1873 would still be suggesting that Pasteur and Lister were wrong in postulating tiny living particles, settling out of the air, as the causes of wound inflamation and fermentation.[2] The postulates of Pasteur, Lister and Koch were going to take quite a while to become the accepted beliefs.

John Snow (who had studied medicine at Newcastle in the 1830s) had removed the handle of the Broad Street pump to halt a cholera epidemic 15 years earlier,[3,4] but had failed to convince all his fellows. The *Lancet* leader-writer of 1855 went so far as:

> But Dr. SNOW claims to have discovered that the law of the propagation of cholera is the drinking of sewage-water. His theory, of course, displaces all other theories. Other theories attribute great efficacy in the spread of cholera to bad drainage and atmospheric impurities .... The fact is, that the well whence Dr. SNOW draws all sanitary truth is the main sewer. ... he has fallen down through a gully-hole and has never since been able to get out again.[5]

William Budd, whose father and six of his eight brothers were (mostly prominent) medical men, had had a top-flight medical education in Europe, where he learned to digest French and German medical publications, which he continued to follow in later years. After returning to England, he had nearly died of typhoid, acquired while working at the *Dreadnought* seamen's floating hospital at Greenwich.[6,7] Ever since, he had taken a close interest, both bedside and scientific (for example by post-mortem and microscopic examination) in 'zymotic' or epidemic diseases, especially typhoid, including its differentiation from typhus;[8] he was also interested in cholera,[9] yellow fever,[10] phthisis (which he understood as a transmissible disease as early as 1856),[11] and typhoid equivalents in pigs[12] and cattle.[13]

He had also laboured long and hard to spread the gospel that country practice in Devon had taught him that 'intestinal fever' (our 'enteric fever' or typhoid) was due to a living 'morbid poison' that passed from person to person, and grew inside the body until it could cause disease;[14] that it was then shed from the sick person, mainly in the faeces; that it could infect the privy, or bed-linen; that enthusiastic and consistent disinfection of discharges with lime or zinc chloride, with isolation of sufferers, would do much to cut or abolish transmission,[15] coupling this, in the case of animal outbreaks, with the policy (still in use) of slaughtering infected animals and burying them in

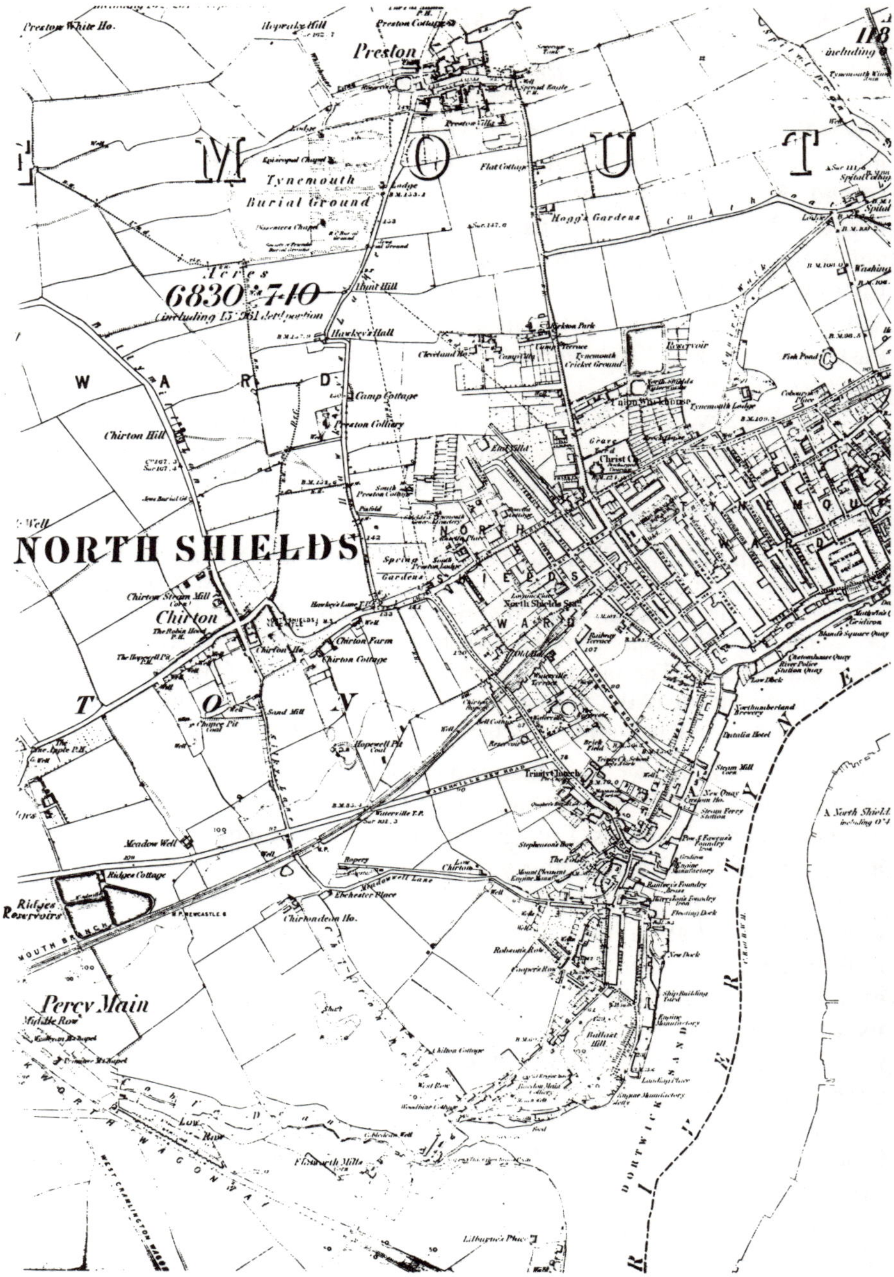

Figure 1. Ordnance Survey (6") map of North Shields in 1858. Note Dockwray Square near the middle of the eastern edge and the two reservoirs, *The Ridges*, near Percy Main to the west, and *Brock Farm*, just north of the town.

quicklime.[6,13] Budd published a number of papers and books,[9,16] but he had not managed to convince the whole profession.

In 1869, Dr Robert Septimus Peart was 32 years old. Born into a North Shields seafaring family, a trip in a wind-jammer drove him to forsake the family tradition and serve an apprenticeship with the town's leading general practitioner, Samuel Fenwick, of the most fashionable Dockwray Square. Peart also enrolled in Newcastle Medical School's 1853-4 session for their two and a half-year course during that apprenticeship; there he acquired a lasting keenness for microscopy and post-mortems. Peart had then succeeded to the practice in 1863, when Fenwick left to become a physician at the London Hospital.[17]

A member of the Northumberland and Durham Medical Society, he gave a paper to the January 1869 meeting:[18]

> At the end of September [1868] ... cases of typhoid fever became more numerous; but its height was arrived at suddenly in the middle of October, when, speaking for myself, fresh seizures came under observation often at the rate of ten to twenty per day up to the end of the month, after which a rapid decline took place to the middle of November, and then comparatively few ... till the beginning of December.

He went on to enlarge on the aspect touched upon in the *Lancet* note about the North Shields outbreak,[19] that the higher part of the town had been hit badly, whereas the lower, crowded, insanitary part of the town had only had a handful of cases – and they had some connection with the more prosperous, higher area, such as attending school there, and drinking from their fountain. The poorer folk received their water from wells and reservoirs at 'The Ridges', which gave an ample supply of acceptable water, and where the supply pipes were in good condition, whereas the higher area drew from an inadequate and dubious reservoir at 'Brock Farm'. The water at Brock Farm came from several sources, including one at Whitley Quarry 1½ miles to the north, where the supply had to be supplemented at times from a nearby partially disused and flooded coal mine. There open water-courses ran close to open cess-pools underground. By one of the cess-pools a pony and boy were on constant duty to operate the force-pump which drained the seams that were still in use towards the flooded workings. Contamination was only to be expected, and the water from this source usually needed filtering to remove the obvious 'large quantities of suspended mud, besides water-animals of various kinds and sizes'. Peart could not convince himself that any of the other theories then prevalent explained the distribution of the outbreak.

A month later however, Dr JB Bramwell, also of North Shields, firmly contradicted Peart, stating that the drains and the emanations from them were the causes of the typhoid.[20] He took pains to point out that only 20 houses in the lower part of the town, supplied from 'The Ridges', had water-closets inside the houses, and that very few of them had any other opening to the drains, inside the houses. In contrast, about 350 houses in the upper part had inside water-closets, and, he believed, the house drains were 'very imperfectly laid, built, in most cases, by small builders and without inspection'. Also:

> very many have sinks on the lower flat, even if the w.c. is outside. The water closets in the higher levels of the town were often, for days together, unsupplied with water, and also many of them, for weeks together, when they were on the second or upper storey of the house.

The numbers of water-closets in the two portions of town were as seventeen to one, and Dr Peart had said that the deaths in the two areas were also as seventeen to one. Furthermore, the drains ran downwards to the sea; their outlet was, twice a day, stopped up by the tide and there were no vents supplied for sewer gases to escape. So each water flush would drive air out of the sewer into the house, or into the town from any little crack it could find, thus in either case leading to disease. Also, the drains would be sedimented due to the excessive drought last summer; then on the two days when 0.75 inches and 0.96 inches of rain fell, the 'excrementous matter' would be stirred up, thus causing unusually severe exhalations. Besides, he much doubted the illness was really typhoid!

Professor Dennis Embleton (holder of the Chair of the Practice of Physic and shortly to become the first Professor in Medicine after the integration of the College of Medicine with the University of Durham), who was at the lecture, seems to have shown the British genius for compromise, almost at the end of the discussion after Bramwell's paper, by suggesting that perhaps contaminated water and sewage exhalations were about equally involved. Nevertheless Bramwell's view was backed up by a report that had recently appeared in the *Lancet*, of a family outbreak of typhoid, allegedly due to emanations from a gutter (contaminated from a drain), smelled via the window beneath which it passed.[21]

The scientist commissioned by the Corporation to analyse the North Shields water supplies stuck to the chemistry.[22] He did not seem to have a 'germ' or a 'virus' in mind, although he took the trouble to find the weight of oxygen needed to oxidise the organic matter in each sample submitted to him.

Robert Peart was not only in the vanguard of thought but achieved eminence in medical society, helping and inspiring many, including the Newcastle surgeon, Grey Turner, who was eventually to supply his obituary. Peart was also resourceful, catheterising himself for 15 years, before submitting to prostatectomy by Rutherford Morrison. As late as the influenza pandemic of 1918, when he was 83 years old, he said he was working harder than he had ever worked in his life.[17] He died on 23 Jan 1922, in his 86th year.

Acknowledgements

I have to thank Dr D Gardner-Medwin, Mr Eric Hollerton, Dr SWS Menzies and Elspeth Gould, for much help.

References

1. Koch R. In: *Cohn's Beitr z Biol d Pflanzen* 1876-7; *2*:277-310. See also *Webster's Biog Dict.*
2. Editorial. *Lancet* 1873; *ii*:529-30 & 600-2.
3. Snow J. Propagation of cholera. *Lancet* 1855; *i*:456.
4. Davison MHA. John Snow. *Univ Durham Coll of Med Gaz* 1959; *54*:3.
5. Editorial. *Lancet* 1855; *i*:635.
6. *DNB*.
7. [Obituary] William Budd MD. *Lancet* 1880; *i*:148-9.
8. Budd W. On intestinal fever: its mode of propagation. *Lancet* 1856; *ii*:694-5; Budd W. On intestinal fever. *Lancet* 1859; *ii*:131-3.
9. Budd W. *Malignant cholera: its propagation and its prevention*. London: Churchill, 1849; *Cholera and disinfection, or asiatic cholera in Bristol in 1866*. (1871), cited in *DNB*.
10. Budd W. On the contagion of yellow fever. *Lancet* 1861; *i*:337-8.
11. Budd W. Memorandum on the nature and the mode of propagation of phthisis. *Lancet* 1867; *ii*:451-2 (in which Budd dates to 1856 his opinion that phthisis in infectious).
12. Budd W. Observations on typhoid (intestinal) fever in the pig. *Brit Med J* 1865; *ii*:81-7.
13. Budd W. The Siberian cattle plague; or, the typhoid fever of the ox. *Brit Med J* 1865; *ii*:169-79.
14. Budd W. Intestinal fever essentially contagious. *Lancet* 1859; *ii*:4- 5, 28-30, 55-6, 80-2.
15. Budd W. On the fever at the clergy orphan asylum. *Lancet* 1856; *ii*:617-9.
16. Budd W. *Typhoid fever: its nature, mode of spreading, and prevention*. London: Longmans & Co, 1873.
17. Turner GG. The late Dr. R. S. Peart of North Shields. *Univ Durham Coll of Med Gaz* 1926; *27*:13.
18. Peart RS. Remarks on the late epidemic of typhoid fever in North Shields. *Proc Northumb & Durham Med Soc* 1868-9: 62-7.
19. Editorial. Outbreak of fever at North Shields. *Lancet* 1868; *ii*:581.
20. Bramwell JB. The typhoid epidemic of North Shields, of October, 1868. Its Cause or Causes. *Proc Northumb & Durham Med Soc* 1868-9:77-83.
21. Buzzard T. How an outbreak of typhoid was produced. *Lancet* 1868; *ii*:597.
22. Mr. Hawksley's report on the water supplied to North Shields. *The Shields Daily News* 11 Jan 1869.

Chapter 18

PHARMACY IN OLD NEWCASTLE

WA Campbell

There were two strands to the practice of pharmacy in 18th and 19th century Britain: the first was the sale of drugs, an activity taken over from the ancient Companies of Grocers and Spicers, while the second, the dispensing of prescriptions, was inherited from the Apothecaries, who had been permitted to charge for the medicines which they prescribed but not for medical advice.

The trade of chemist and druggist first emerged in the early 18th century, when several famous firms were founded; Sylvanus Bevan, for example, opened the Plough Court Pharmacy in Lombard Street, London, in 1715, this enterprise later becoming Allen and Hanbury, now part of Glaxo.[1] The unwieldy title of 'chemist and druggist' stems from another fusion of two functions. The druggist (or drugger) sold galenicals or drugs of mainly plant origin, and was skilled in the recognition, gathering and preparation of these materials; the chemist (or chymist) prepared the acids, bases and metallic salts which formed the backbone of iatrochemistry or Paracelsian medicine. By the beginning of the 18th century both kinds of skill were necessary in order to cope with the expanding materia medica.

The medicaments of this period were divided into four main categories: laxatives, opium preparations, metallic remedies and herbal mixtures. Foremost amongst the vegetable cathartics were aloes, scammony, jalap, senna and rhubarb; gamboge, a bright yellow gum-resin, served both as an artist's pigment and a violent purge. Opium was widely prescribed as a cough cure, for the relief of pain, and in the treatment of diarrhoea, while laudanum, paregoric, Venice treacle and black drop (invented by Dr Edmund Tunstall of Bishop Auckland, and containing spiced opium in fermented crab-apple juice) were equally popular products. There was also a brisk trade in the former proprietary Godfrey's Cordial (also containing opium), often used to send fractious children to sleep.

The Paracelsian remedies based on arsenic, antimony and mercury still found favour. Mercury was used both as an antisyphilitic and as a vermifuge in the form of 'worm lozenges', whilst an ointment of mercury oxide was sold as Singleton's Golden Eye Ointment. The fourth category drew on such wild plants as dandelion, burdock, waterdock, agrimony, gentian, horehound and fennel, all of which had been made popular by the horticulturist 'Sir' John Hill. Also of vegetable origin were cinchona bark, ipecacuanha (widely used in Dover's Powder) and, towards the end of the century, the leaves of purple foxglove.

Whilst many of the operations of early pharmacy were merely those of general chemistry, such as solution, crystallization, filtration, decantation and distillation, some processes were peculiar to pharmacy. Drugs frequently had to be reduced to the finest of powders, often by means of a spring-loaded pestle of considerable weight. Towards the end of the 19th century Sir Joseph Wilson Swan recalled with disgust 'the days when I first smelt powder' and the tedious hours which he had spent as a young apprentice in grinding drugs. Camphor in particular presented difficulties in powdering, and was often ground with a few drops of alcohol to prevent the formation of lumps. The processes of maceration, percolation and infusion sometimes took days or even weeks to accomplish.

Although wholesale houses began to appear in the provinces early in the 19th century, in general the pharmacist would make the lotions, emulsions, ointments, tablets and pills which he sold. Perhaps the most irksome task, apart from pounding the drugs, was the making of pills. The physical properties of the pill mass had to be just right in order that the pill might be shaped without crumbling and preserve its shape over a period of time. The excipient might be treacle, wax, gum tragacanth or glycerine, but the commonest was simply soap; thus a very popular laxative pill contained equal parts of aloes, ginger and soap.

The household pharmacist: Taylor Gibson

Newcastle did not begin to break out from the confines of the mediaeval walls until about the middle of the 18th century. In the 1760s Northumberland Street and Percy Street were built and named in honour of the return of the Percy family to the Dukedom of Northumberland. In 1784 Dean Street and Moseley Street were laid out, the one to connect the ancient *Vicus Peregrinorum* or Pilgrim Street with the market area around the parish church of St Nicholas, the other to provide an easier route from the Quayside to the developing upper town. Trade and industry were still concentrated in the riverside districts, so Sandhill, Side, and Dean Street remained good addresses for a chemist and druggist. However, after the speculative builder Richard Grainger built the upper town in the Classical style in the 1830s, the commercial centre began to shift away from the riverside, a process accelerated by the opening of the Central Station in 1850. Many of the older pharmacies moved into new premises in Grey Street, Clayton Street, Newgate Street or Grainger Street, or into modernized older buildings in the Bigg Market area.

One pharmacy business in the Bigg Market had already started trading in 1800, when Taylor Gibson, chemist and druggist, entered into partnership with Christopher Myers, a chemist; much insight into their trade is offered by the survival of two books of pharmaceutical recipes from 1887 and 1914.[2] By the second half of the 19th century the pharmacist had become the wise man of the neighbourhood, being consulted on all manner of problems, embracing first-aid, the removal of stains from fabrics, the extermination of vermin, the restoration of leather and woodwork, and the colouring and flavouring of food. Many pharmacists made their own brands of stains, polishes, cleansing fluids and insect powders, as well as hair-oil and cold cream; these were usually standard formulations but carrying the pharmacist's own label. The Taylor Gibson notebooks show a great deal of this kind of trade. The firm made red and green ink, marking ink, French polish, baking powder, perfumed hair oil, knotting varnish, violet dusting powder and curry powder, all sold as Taylor Gibson products. Nor was veterinary medicine eschewed, for two horse powders were produced, one containing potassium nitrate, fenugreek and flowers of sulphur (a potentially incendiary mixture!), and the other consisting of ginger, aniseed, caraway, quassia and Epsom salt.

Another interesting line was the preparation of dye-baths, magenta, maroon and violet; since these were made up in several gallons of boiling water, it seems likely that goods were accepted for dyeing on the premises. Liquid blue was also supplied to a local manufacturer of paint, Holmes of Westgate Street, who was later to become one of the founders of British Paints Ltd. All this was undertaken in addition to the ordinary dispensing work and the making of pharmaceutical products on a considerable scale. Laudanum or tincture of opium was made in 16-gallon lots, and tincture of hyoscyamine in three gallons. They produced their own Godfrey's Cordial from treacle, potassium tartrate, oil of aniseed, caraway and sassafras, made up in aqueous alcohol; unlike the original and most of the imitations this Godfrey contained no opium, being merely a warming drink. Similar in nature and effects was their Compo powder made from bayberry bark, ginger, Canada tar, capsicum and caryophyllene. Inevitably, the firm had its own effervescing salts made from Epsom salt, sugar, cream of tartar, soda and tartaric acid. By 1914 they were also making a tincture of absinthe and a sulphur lotion for ringworm.

The breadth of the Taylor Gibson business was by no means unusual and has been selected here merely as an example of a type. In the 1850s John Parkinson, a wholesale druggist in the Close, announced that in addition to supplying every kind of drug he also sold paint, seeds, vinegar and blacking of his own manufacture. He was also an importer of German and Dutch yeast, and a dealer in anti-friction grease, black beer, British wines and Congreve matches, all of which he was prepared to supply to ships at the shortest notice.[3] A few years later Alfred Hume of 18 Grey Street was advertising his Celebrated Northumbrian Sauce, pickling vinegar, paints, oils, colours, horse and cattle medicines, soda and sedlitz powders, perfumery of every description, Hume's Rifle Jet for blacking, rifle sights and patent linen markers. He was also an agent for the Himalayan Tea Company.[4]

The mineral water pharmacists: J Gilpin and W Owen

In 1767 Joseph Priestley, the discoverer of oxygen, moved into a house in Leeds which was next door to a brewery, which gave him the opportunity to carry out experiments in 'fixed air' or carbon dioxide. He suspended a shallow dish of water in the layer of carbon dioxide which hung over the surface of the fermenting liquor and discovered next morning that the water had acquired a pleasantly sharp taste. The same effect could be produced by pouring water back and forth between two vessels held in the carbon dioxide layer. The resulting liquid was very similar to Pyrmont or Seltzer water.[5]

During the next twenty years, impregnation of water with carbon dioxide was suggested as a cure for scurvy, for making putrid water palatable on long sea voyages, and for revivifying flat beer. These, together with the recent revival of interest in the watering places, turned the attention of pharmacists to soda water manufacture. The name 'soda water', dating from 1802, arose from the observation by Richard Bewley, a Norfolk apothecary, that the addition of a little sodium carbonate to the water greatly facilitated the absorption of carbon dioxide.[6]

Many pieces of apparatus were devised for impregnating liquids with gases, but these operated only on a small scale. For the industrial production of soda water, Thomas Henry of Manchester invented suitable pumping equipment,[7] modified and improved by WH Pepys. Soda water factories soon sprang up in Bristol, Manchester and Birmingham. In 1792 a Swiss jeweller named Jacob Schweppe, who had received instruction in handling gases on a large scale from the balloonist James Sadler (himself a chemist), opened a soda water factory in London, followed by another in Bristol. Soon Schweppe had agencies in all the major towns of this country.

Most retail pharmacists, including those in Newcastle, prepared only small quantities of soda water, often for drinking on the premises when a customer came in for a pick-me-up. Among these small-scale manufacturers, many held agencies from the national firms to supply bottled waters. Thus George Currie, chemist and druggist at 19 Sandhill, advertised Harrogate water direct from the spa, and Hamilton's London Soda Water; Hamiltons gave their name to the egg-shaped bottle designed to withstand pressure.[8] Similarly W Proctor & Son were described as agents for Schweppes & Co.

There were a few however who engaged in mineral water manufacture on a considerable scale, one of these being J Gilpin, chemist and druggist of 56 Pilgrim Street, who also described himself in the directories as 'mineral water manufacturer'. Gilpin's pharmacy was opened in 1790, and by 1814 he had begun the secondary business of London porter merchants.[9] Both Gilpin and his partner Brumell came from long-established Quaker families in Newcastle. The business passed into the hands of Bartleman and Creighton, and then to Turnbull and Wilson; finally Richard Thomas Wilson became the sole proprietor, though still preserving the name of Gilpin & Co. The Pilgrim Street shop, originally 95 but renumbered to 137, was an 18th-century alderman's house which had served as a lodging for the Assize judges on their visits to the town. The aerated water factory, the first in the north-east, began by generating its own carbon dioxide from chalk and sulphuric acid; the resulting by-product of calcium sulphate was used as a filler in the manufacture of paper. The factory extended as far back as Manors, where there was a delivery bay. In 1842 the firm introduced the bitter beers of Burton-on-Trent to drinkers in the north-east by taking an agency for Allsopps and for

Bass. They also cut their own corks, and soon were supplying chemists, brewers, pickle manufacturers, and the wine and spirit trade.[10]

W Owen's business was founded in 1847 in Collingwood Street.[11] Here he made an anodyne liniment, 'an effective cure for croup, bronchitis, whooping cough, rheumatism and lumbago', all for 1s 6d a bottle. He also made balsam of honey, a remedy popularised by the earlier-mentioned 'Sir' John Hill, and featured in his rhyming response to a suggestion that he should take his own medicine:[12]

> I'll take neither essence nor balsam of honey,
> Do you take the physic, and I'll take the money.

In the 1880s Owen opened a second shop at 151 Barras Bridge. These premises were rebuilt to a palatial standard in 1894, a prominent feature being an elaborately moulded ceiling; showcases and cabinets abounded, and a general air of opulence prevailed. Behind the shop was the mineral water factory, marked on some maps simply as 'Lemonade Factory'. Here soda, potash, lithia, and seltzer waters were made, along with lemonade, ginger ale, lemon squash and a sparkling tonic water claimed to be of value in treating liver complaints. All the waters were supplied both in bottles and syphons. The firm was also an agent for Schweppes, Appolinaris and other table waters including Vichy and Carlsbad.

In the 1920s, Professor FC Pybus, then making his way as a young surgeon, had patients in the private nursing homes which abounded in Jesmond and Gosforth. For those recovering from operations he provided a pleasant energy-giving drink containing glucose, with a citrus flavour and an engaging sparkle; this mixture was made up at Owen's pharmacy nearby. On discharge from the nursing homes, many patients came to Owen with requests for further supplies of the drink. The chief assistant, Mr Hunter, realised that there was money to be made from this formulation and began to manufacture it in the firm's factory. The drink was called 'Lucozade'.[13] The position of Owen's pharmacy is now marked only by an air shaft for the Metro rail system, and the factory which saw the birth of Lucozade is now a University car-park.

The popular pharmacy: 'Dirty Dick'

This Clayton Street business had for several decades an extraordinary reputation for what is described as 'counter prescribing'. Such was the extent of its fame that people would queue for hours, often in bad weather, for a consultation and the opportunity to buy a jar of ointment or a bottle of lotion. The shop windows were encased in wooden shutters which bore the name of Forster & Co Ltd and the legend in gothic script 'Ye Olde Chymists Shoppe'.

Clayton Street was completed in 1837, and from the start No 105 had medical and pharmaceutical connections. For twenty years it was occupied by Francis Marshall, grocer and druggist; for three years it was a 'Doctor's shop' under John Samuel Pearce MD, and then it reverted to a pharmacy run by Thomas Herring, until it was acquired in 1867 by James Crozer.

James Crozer was born in Alnwick in 1813, the youngest of nine children. He was apprenticed to a druggist, Mr Sharp in High Street, Berwick, and after completing his apprenticeship joined Cornelius Garbutt at 21 Bridge Street, Gateshead. Three years later he set up his own business in Denton Chare near to St Nicholas' church, not as a druggist but as an agent for the carriage of goods. Unable to settle in one place for long, he soon set sail for America, where he opened a pharmacy in a small town. His restless nature took him to Cuba and then to Jamaica, where he worked as a schoolmaster. Returning to America, he speculated unwisely and suffered financial ruin, so that he was forced to work as a labourer, first on road-making and then on the railways.

Once he had scraped up sufficient money for his passage, he returned to Tyneside, where he joined his father in a seedsman's business at Wallsend. Wanderlust gripped him once more, and in 1858 he was working as a pharmacist in Benares, leaving just before the Mutiny. He next appeared in Shanghai, where he worked as a hospital pharmacist for three years, before signing on as a ship's surgeon in the *Rajah*, which traded between Shanghai and the islands in the Indian Ocean. At the age of 54, Crozer abandoned his wandering life, returned to Newcastle, and opened a pharmacy at 105 Clayton Street.

His tall, bearded figure, clothed in what was apparently his only suit, and that more fitted to the Indian climate than to the rigours of Tyneside weather, soon became familiar in the town. He slept on the floor at the back of the shop, and this fact, coupled with his disregard for his personal appearance, gave rise to the nickname of 'Dirty Dick'. He adjusted the price of his medicines to the pockets of his customers, giving free treatment to the poor. Prosperous persons sometimes put on old clothes or sent their servants, but Crozer, wise from his rich experience of the world, always saw through the ruse and charged accordingly.

Despite his image, Crozer was well-connected in the town. Henry Watson, the engineer and brass-founder who assisted, encouraged and advised the future Lord Armstrong in his early ventures into hydraulic engineering, was his brother-in-law, while William Newton, the parish surgeon for All Saints district, whose heroism during the cholera outbreak of 1853 earned him a public banquet and a presentation from his fellow townsfolk, was his nephew.[14]

One day in 1869, Crozer left his shop at mid-day and returned to find that it had been broken into and his money stolen. Deciding that the thieves had watched him through the window in order to see where he kept the money, he ordered wooden shutters to be fitted to the windows; these were never taken down during his tenancy.

In 1885 Crozer retired from business and went to live in a one-roomed cottage in Brandling Village, to the immediate north of Newcastle. His furniture matched his frugal life-style: a bed consisting of a board supported on two wooden boxes, three chairs, an iron safe, a nest of pharmacy drawers and a harmonium; lying about were several jars and bottles of medicinals, a musical box and two tin whistles. Here he died on 16 June 1888. It was widely believed that he was penniless, but in fact he had nearly £4000 in a bank in China.[15]

The Clayton Street business was taken over by John Robert Forster and continued as a pharmacy of no particular distinction until 1900. In that year Alfred Conroy became the managing chemist, and in 1913 was appointed managing director of the company. Conroy, a tall man of striking appearance, saw the publicity value of Crozer's reputation and put about the story that the shop windows (hidden by the shutters) had not been washed for 50 years. On this legend the name of 'Dirty Dick' was revived, and with it a reputation for successful counter prescribing. In 1931 Conroy celebrated 50 years as a qualified pharmacist, and it was said on that occasion that he had never lost a day through illness and had never taken a holiday.[16] The motto of the shop was 'Not to fit the case to a particular bottle but to fit the bottle to a particular case', with the result that for a period the telephone was taken out, as its constant ringing distracted the chemists from what they saw as their main business, ie taking case histories. Conroy died in 1932 and was succeeded by his son. The firm was latterly managed by Mansfield Todd; it closed in the late 1970s.[17]

The scientific pharmacy: Mawson, Proctor, Swan and Weddell

Two lines of descent coalesce to form this important business which was to influence pharmacy on a national level. The earlier of these began when John Proctor opened a druggist's shop at the head of the Side in the autumn of 1768. Proctor was joined by his son William, and in the 1840s the business was transferred to impressive premises at 11 Grey Street. This was a double-fronted shop in a fashionable area, with a laboratory and dispensing rooms above, and warehouse accommodation at the rear. Here the firm made their own lavender water, toilet essence, myrrh tooth-paste, areca nut paste, antiseptic mouthwash (from the newly-isolated carbolic acid) and preparations for the hair.

John Proctor's grandson, Barnard Simpson Proctor, born in 1829, was a nephew by marriage of Michael Faraday. The first Newcastle chemist to qualify by examination, he became a member of council of the Pharmaceutical Society, and an examiner from 1867 to 1869. With NH Martin (of Brady & Martin) he founded the British Pharmaceutical Conference. BS Proctor became Reader in Pharmacy at the College of Medicine in Newcastle, and published two books which became standard texts, *Lectures on Practical Pharmacy* and *A Manual of Pharmaceutical Testing*. In 1885 he joined NH Martin in setting up the North of England School of Pharmacy at the corner of Northumberland Street and Northumberland Road.[18] Through all these varied activities Proctor continued to run the Grey Street pharmacy single-handed until 1885, when he was joined by Thomas Maltby Clague as a partner. Clague was interested in industrial health and collaborated with Sir Thomas Oliver in research on lead poisoning and 'phossy jaw' among phosphorus workers, especially in match factories.

In 1912 Proctor and Clague amalgamated with Mawson and Swan to form a new company styled Mawson & Proctor. John Mawson had opened his druggist's shop in Newcastle in 1828 and very soon established a reputation for probity. He had stood surety for a friend who absconded leaving large debts. Mawson could not immediately meet the unexpected drain on his resources and became bankrupt. At great self-sacrifice he gradually paid off all the creditors, who responded by presenting him with a mahogany bookcase containing 21 volumes of *Encyclopaedia Britannica*, 20 volumes of *Allison's History of Europe* and a silver tea service inscribed 'A testimonial to the exemplary honour and rectitude of Mr John Mawson'.[19]

Owing to the unlikely concatenation of a series of bizarre events, a large deposit of nitroglycerine for blasting purposes was found in a stable in the White Hart Yard, Cloth Market, in December 1867. In that year Mawson had been elected Sheriff of Newcastle, and in that capacity he offered to superintend the removal and safe disposal of the explosive liquid. Exactly what happened will probably never be known, but during the act of pouring the liquid into disused pit workings on the Town Moor an explosion occurred which killed him.[20]

In 1846 Mawson had been joined by Joseph Wilson Swan, a young pharmacist from Sunderland, who was later to become his brother-in-law. Swan's interests ranged far beyond the everyday business of a pharmacy; he made friends with other scientifically-minded young men, particularly Barnard Simpson Proctor and John Pattinson, the Public Analyst. Known as the 'Three Philosophers', they met in each other's houses to discuss scientific problems. Mawson grasped the calibre of his young partner and wisely gave him his head, with the result that a great deal of fruitful research into photographic processes and materials was carried out and the firm was admirably placed to take advantage of the coming boom in photography. After Mawson's death, Swan carried on the business but took Mawson's widow as a business partner, to ensure for her a continuing income.

One of the specialties of Mawson & Swan was the preparation of oxygen, which was supplied to theatres for use in lime lights. Under Swan, the firm also turned to the supply of scientific instruments, chiefly optical and electrical; altogether four richly illustrated catalogues were issued to cover the various aspects of the firm's output. In December 1878 Swan was able to show his incandescent filament electric light bulb to a meeting of the Newcastle Chemical Society, of which he was president, and in the following February he gave a demonstration lecture under the chairmanship of Sir WG Armstrong to an audience of 700 at the Newcastle Literary and Philosophical Society. The development of electric lighting was to take Swan away from

Newcastle.[21] He was however able to hand over to a gifted Scottish pharmacist named George Weddell.

Weddell's interests were also very broad. He had acquired Gilpin's pharmacy in Pilgrim Street, where he discovered in an attic an ancient chemical manuscript which he edited and published as *Arcana Fairfaxiana*. On joining the Mawson & Swan enterprise, he developed the firm's earlier interest in water filters; these he manufactured in five sizes, from portable miniatures for travellers to 6-gallon family models. Weddell's third achievement was to take him out of the business. He had discovered a way to make free-running table salt by the addition of small amounts of calcium phosphate. The salt was manufactured as 'Cerebos Salt', initially in a building in Ellison Place, but later on Teeside which was nearer to the salt deposits. His departure led to the amalgamation with Proctor & Clague.[22]

There were other Mawson & Swan businesses. They had joined Thomas Morgan in a stationery and bookselling shop in Grey Street and an art shop in Grainger Street, both under the name of Mawson, Swan & Morgan.[23] In the district on the west side of the Ouseburn known as Red Barns, Mawson & Swan had an egg and yeast importing establishment; this was long known as the 'Egg Factory' amongst poor people, who could buy cracked eggs there very cheaply.

Until 1928 the Mawson & Proctor pharmacy was managed by Clague. The wholesale side was becoming more important, and in 1948 that department was moved to Low Friar Street; it subsequently moved to the Team Valley Trading estate under the name of Mawson & Proctor Pharmaceuticals Ltd. The Grainger Street pharmacy was re-organized as Mawson Proctor Group Pharmacy in collaboration with 45 Newcastle pharmacists; it is now owned by Vantage Chemists.

The effervescent pharmacy: JC Eno

James Crossley Eno was born in the Barrack Square, Newcastle, in 1820. His parents kept a general dealer's shop set amongst housing of low quality; their neighbours were mainly carters and cowmen tending herds on the Castle Leazes moor across the road. At the age of 14, young Eno was apprenticed to a chemist and druggist in the Side, probably Joseph Garnett who can be seen (with his shop in the background) in the 'Chemist's Window' in St Nicholas' Cathedral. When his time was served, Eno was engaged as a Dispenser at Newcastle Infirmary near the top of the Forth Bank. His salary was £60 a year, compared with £40 for the Matron and £100 for the Surgeon. Here he came into contact with many of the leaders of Newcastle's medical community, including several who played an important part in the government of the town. In addition to dispensing prescriptions, and apparently without any special training, Eno undertook dental work, drawing teeth and inserting gold fillings.[24]

In 1852 Eno left the Infirmary and took over John Burrell's pharmacy at 57 (re-numbered as 5) Groat Market. He described himself as 'Dispensing

Chemist and Surgeon Dentist' and for several years practised both professions. Like many other pharmacists mentioned in this chapter, Eno made products under his own brand-name; here his originality (or eccentricity) began to show, for one of the preparations was a tooth enamel with which the sufferer could make his own fillings. He also made a hair restorer and a special variety of linseed oil for poultices.

A year or two later he began the preparation of Eno's Fruit Salt, a mixture of citric and tartaric acids with sodium bicarbonate. The story that Eno stole the formulation from a visiting physician at the Infirmary is probably untrue; there was little to steal, for the reaction between acids and bicarbonate was well-known. Eno may nevertheless have been the first to use it in a popular medicine. 'Effervescent Granules' were introduced into pharmacy by Alfred Bishop in 1857, though here the aim was to make the unpleasant medicines more palatable.

Drawing on his experience as an apprentice in the riverside area, Eno packed his Fruit Salt into boxes of one- and two-dozen and distributed them freely to the captains of ships which traded from Newcastle. The policy was successful, for he soon began to receive orders from distant parts of the world. In 1868 he became MPS, not by examination but under a clause which admitted those who had been in business for some time. Six years later he wrote a little book, *A Treatise on the Stomach and its Trials*, published like many more important medical works by Francis Newbery of Amen Corner, London.[25]

In 1876 Eno found the Groat Market premises too small for the burgeoning Fruit Salt business, and so set up a large factory at New Cross, London. He took whole-page advertising space in such journals as *The Graphic* and *Illustrated London News*, writing the somewhat turgid text himself. One of his keenest supporters was a retired general aged 67 and living in Ascot: 'Here stands the cherished bottle on the chimney-piece of my sanctum, at home my household god, abroad my vade-mecum' wrote the old soldier, adding a touching rhyme by way of reinforcing his message:[26]

When Eno's salt betimes you take
No waste of this elixir make,
But drain the dregs and lick the cup
Of this, the perfect pick-me-up.

For much of his life Eno was troubled by deafness, but he seems to have suffered in no other way. He died at the age of 95, convinced that his own remedy had prolonged his life. He had given generously to the new Royal Victoria Infirmary, yet was still able to leave the sum of £1 611 707.

The Groat Market pharmacy passed into the hands of John Walton and George Heslop, who continued to act as agents for Eno. This firm made a Balsam of Liquorice and a Golden Balm for sprains, stiffness, bronchitis and rheumatism, supported by testimonials from doctors, nurses, ships' captains, and ministers of religion.[27] The building, erected in 1607 and a pharmacy since 1820, was demolished to make way for the Northern Assurance Building at the close of the last century, but by way of compensation, 5 Collingwood Street was named Eno Chambers. No longer described as a fruit salt, 'Eno' was taken over by Beecham.

References

1. Morris PJ, Russell CA. *Archives of the British chemical industry* 1750-1914. BSHS Monograph *6*, Stanford-in-the-Vale; BSHS, 1988:4.
2. Taylor Gibson. *Pharmaceutical preparations* (notebooks for 1887 & 1914). Tyne Wear Rec Off:113R2, 113R3.
3. Ward's *Directory of Newcastle upon Tyne* 1851. Advertisement directory: 51.
4. Ward's *Directory of Newcastle upon Tyne* 1865-6. Advertisement directory: 43.
5. Campbell WA. Joseph Priestley and his soda water. *Endeavour* 1983; ns *7*:141.
6. Musson AE, Robinson E. *Science and technology in the industrial revolution*. Manchester: U Press, 1969:177.
7. Farrar WV, Farrar KR, Scott EL. The Henrys of Manchester. *Ambix* 1977; *24*:1.
8. Hamilton WH. British patent 3232 of 1809.
9. *Newcastle Courant* 8 March 1814.
10. *Tyneside industries*. London & Newcastle: Historical Publishing Co, nd (?1809):137.
11. *Review of Newcastle and District*. Nottingham: Thos Forman, 1896:68.
12. *Notes and Queries* Ser 2 1857; *3*:55; 1861; *11*:52; Ser 4 1871; *8*:206.
13. *Newcastle Journal* 12 March 1975; personal communication from the late Professor Pybus.
14. Welford R. *Men of mark 'twixt Tyne and Tweed*. Newcastle upon Tyne: Walter Scott, 1895; 3:220-3.
15. *Newcastle Journal* 16 June 1888; *The Leader* 18 June 1888.
16. *Newcastle Journal* 1 Aug 1932.
17. Personal communication from Mrs Alice Todd.
18. *Chemist & Druggist* 16 Nov 1968.
19. Fordyce T. *Local records*. Newcastle upon Tyne: Fordyce, 1867; II:258.
20. *Proceedings of the Town Council of the Borough of Newcastle* 1867-68; xi-xiv, 68, 202, 375-6, 426.
21. Swan ME, Swan KR. *Sir Joseph Wilson Swan FRS*. Newcastle upon Tyne: Oriel Press, 1968; Chirnside RC. *Sir Joseph Wilson Swan FRS*. Newcastle upon Tyne: Lit & Phil, 1979; Campbell WA. Newcastle Chemical Society and its illustrious child. *Chem & Industry* 1968:1463; *Trans Newc Chem Soc* 1877-80; *IV*:190.
22. *Pharmac J* 1968; *201*:523; *Border Magazine* 1916; *21*:58.
23. *Newcastle Life* Nov 1976:26.
24. Campbell WA. James Crossley Eno and the rise of the health salt trade. *Univ Newc upon Tyne Med Gaz* 1966; *LX*:106; *Newcastle Daily Chronicle* 17 May 1915.
25. Campbell WA. James Crossley Eno. In *Dictionary of Business Biography*. London: LSE, 1984; *I*:293.
26. *The Graphic* 17 March 1888:283.
27. *Tyneside industries. op cit* note 10:203.

Chapter 19

HISTORY OF PSYCHIATRY ON TYNESIDE

John Le Gassicke

Introduction

Organised care for the mentally ill in England did not really start until the 18th century. Gradually public concern developed and it led to the establishment of public subscription hospitals, of which Bethel, Norwich (1725), St Luke's, London (1751), the Manchester Lunatic Hospital (1766), and The Retreat, York (1792), are the most notable.[1] For affluent patients there were a number of private mad houses, later officially called Licensed Houses, scattered about the country. They changed their names to private asylums and by 1880 there were forty outside the metropolitan area. Because of irregularities in their management, a Private Mad House Act (1774) provided for the provincial houses to be inspected by local Justices. In practice this Act was not very effective, but it is of interest because it was the first formal legislation for the mentally ill.[2]

As time went on, the plight of the so-called pauper lunatics and idiots caused increasing concern. In practice, they ended up in work-houses. Conditions in some of these were appalling, although larger ones tended to provide separate wings for this type of patient. As the 19th century went on, where there was no public provision the private asylums admitted pauper patients, financial provision coming from the Poor Law Guardians. They remained in use until the county asylums were built.

In 1808, a County Asylum Act was passed, which enabled local authorities to provide for the mentally ill. It was not until 1845 that there was comprehensive lunacy legislation which laid down the policy of the following hundred years. The mentally ill were segregated into large asylums, often several miles from the patient's home. These institutions increased in number as the 19th century progressed and many of them are still in active use. The term 'asylum' was replaced in the early 20th century by the name 'hospital'. The mentally handicapped and the mentally ill were cared for together until the early part of this century, when they were separated under special legislation.

After the Second World War, the Mental Health Commission was set up under the chairmanship of the Duke of Northumberland which led to the 1959 Mental Health Act and a fundamental change in public policy. In one word it could be described as desegregation. It meant that mentally ill patients could be admitted informally into hospital beds. Prior to 1959, the vast majority of places for the mentally ill were designated and the patients were detained by legal procedures, which were sometimes quite complicated. Of course, the development of electric convulsive therapy from about 1940 and the major tranquillising drugs from about 1950, made the management of seriously disturbed mentally ill patients much easier, which in turn increased the confidence of those who cared for them. The 1959 Act and the development of physical treatment enabled the establishment of the care of the mentally ill in General Hospital Psychiatric Units with increasing emphasis on community care. The policy is to close the large Mental Hospitals and most of them will be gone by the year 2000.

The evolution of the Mental Health Service on Tyneside to the opening of the county asylums can now be considered in more detail.[3] In Newcastle, a public subscription hospital and a private licensed house were established in the 18th century and there was a number of flourishing private asylums in Gateshead.

Early history of psychiatry on Tyneside

For most of the 18th century, Newcastle had a truly medieval appearance with a huge Norman castle and an enormous defensive city wall built in the reign of Edward I (1239-1307). There were a number of hospitals of charitable and religious foundation, of which the Holy Jesus was the most notable. The General Infirmary, which was the first public subscription hospital, was opened on the Forth Banks in 1753 and remained in use until 1906, when the present Royal Victoria Infirmary replaced it.

In the City Archives of Newcastle upon Tyne, there is record of a conveyance of 1686 between Dr William Luck and Newcastle Corporation for a room in a place called Shoulder of Mutton Close, close to where the Lunatic Hospital came to be built in 1767.[4] Although the details of the conveyance do not specify the proposed use of the room, it is possible that it was for the care of lunatics from the neighbouring work-houses. Shoulder of Mutton Close subsequently became known as Luck's Close. The first definite record of public provision was in 1763, when the Common Council raised a subscription for a Lunatic Hospital, and this was opened in 1764, with accommodation for 19 patients. But in the following year the Common Council noted this house to be too small and made plans for a new one to be opened in the Warden's Close. This was an area of open fields and copses on the west side of the city outside the wall.

The new Hospital was opened in 1767; it could accommodate 30 patients and was designated 'The Pauper Hospital for Lunaticks for Newcastle, Northumberland and Durham'. Printed Rules were published in 1766.[5] There are no other official records of the early years of the new Lunatic Hospital, but a lay account in 1795 describes it as 'an elegant extensive brick building with a neat pediment in the centre and spacious gardens', and also records that patients were treated humanely.[6]

The ensuing years, however, became increasingly difficult for the Hospital. The population of Newcastle upon Tyne in 1770 was 21 000, in 1800 28 000 and 1830 54 000. Around this time there was rising national concern for the idiot and lunatic paupers in poor-houses, and in 1808 the County Asylums Act was passed to remedy conditions by authorising the building of county asylums. Appalling conditions in already existing hospitals and asylums were also causing public concern and were exposed in 1815-16 by the Reports of Select Committees of the House of Commons. Perhaps prompted by these investigations, an enquiry was held in 1817 into the conditions of the Newcastle Lunatick Hospital. The Report pointed out that the Hospital was not only for the cure of the insane but was also an asylum for the incurable and a place of relief for the overcrowded poor-houses in the area. It is here that the word 'asylum' is first used in connection with the Hospital. The report gave statistical details of admissions since the first hospital was opened in 1764. It showed a dramatic increase in admissions in the period 1806 to 1817: 402 compared with 172 in the decade 1764 to 1774. A table classified the sexes and attempted to record the outcome of admissions, and it compared the Newcastle results favourably with those of The Retreat, Bethlem and St Luke's, London.

No definite action was taken at that time, but in 1824 a further Committee was appointed to report on the conditions of the Asylum. It revealed that the public subscription had failed and that the Asylum, as it was now referred to, was being run on a private basis. It was grossly overcrowded and ill-ventilated. Chains were in use, there were iron bars on the windows, and the cells resembled dungeons. There was no differentiation between mental diseases, no separation of the sexes, and restraint and coercion were to be seen everywhere. The Report led to a period of hectic reform, and the Council appointed Dr Noel Smith as Physician-in-Charge.

Extensive alterations to the building were made by John Dobson (1787-1865), the celebrated Newcastle architect of the classical style, to provide accommodation for 80 patients in three social classes, one of which was private patients. The new Asylum became known as the Bath Lane Asylum, the street in which it now stood being named after the public baths. It continued in use until 1856, when the patients were moved to the new Durham County Asylum (now Winterton Hospital). This, however, became overcrowded, and in 1864 it was decided to build a new asylum for Newcastle Borough; in the meantime the Newcastle patients were accommodated in the old Bensham Asylum, previously a rather notorious Licensed House. The new Borough Asylum was opened in 1869, and is now St Nicholas Hospital, Gosforth. The Bath Lane building became a warehouse; it was demolished about the middle of this century. Some of the stone wash-basins are kept as a memento in front of the main entrance of St Nicholas Hospital.

Asylums serving the area were also built at Morpeth (1859, later at St George's Hospital) and Stannington (1914, later St Mary's Hospital). These served Northumberland and Gateshead respectively. Mental Handicap Hospitals were built at Morpeth (Northgate Hospital) and at Prudhoe (Prudhoe Hospital).

The Physician-in-Charge of the first two lunatic hospitals was Dr John Hall (1733-1793), a prominent Tyneside physician. He was a man of some enterprise. It was he who founded the public baths in 1781, after which Bath Lane was named. He was the son of a barber-surgeon, was educated at the

Royal Grammar School in Newcastle, studied medicine in Edinburgh, and in 1755 wrote a thesis on Fevers.[7] He was Physician to the General Infirmary, and was President of the Newcastle Philosophical and Medical Society in 1786-87.

When the second lunatic hospital was being built, Hall wanted to provide an extra storey to house private patients. When this was refused by the Common Council he entered into discussion with some of his colleagues about opening a private house elsewhere. For some reason he backed out of the plan; instead he secretly purchased a property which he named St Luke's House and which he opened in October 1766 as a private madhouse. His action incurred the displeasure of his colleagues, and he felt it necessary to publish a book giving his account of the affair.[8]

St Luke's House prospered, and when Hall died in 1793 it was purchased by Dr R Steavenson, another prominent Newcastle Physician. He enlarged the premises and renamed them 'Bellegrove Retreat', a name probably inspired by the York Retreat which was then being projected. The house now had 24 apartments, a separate building for disturbed patients, and pleasant gardens for exercise, recreation and convalescence.[9] It remained in use until 1857, when it was closed, probably the numbers of patients were falling off. In 1852 there were only 10 patients compared with 27 private patients in the Bath Lane Asylum. The house, much altered, still exists as a delightful 17th century residence called White Knights. For many years this was the home of Professor FC Pybus and housed his library; it now belongs to the University of Newcastle.

Private Asylums of Gateshead

Of some interest is the development of Private Asylums in Gateshead.[10] Why it should have been so popular for these ventures is not entirely clear. The population in the 1851 census was about 26 000 and the three institutions that developed there gave a service to paupers in the North East and North West of England. Certainly, there was not enough local population to sustain them. The 1845 Lunacy Act had amongst its main provision proper licensing of Institutions and the formation of the Commissioners of Lunacy. It was the purpose of this Commission to visit all institutions whether public, private or work-house with special provision. Official policy towards these asylums was ambivalent. The profit motive was distrusted and so they were publicly discouraged. However, they gave a service for which there had been no public provision.

The oldest of the private asylums was at Bensham which opened in 1799, as a Licensed House. It eventually closed in 1868 but in the latter part of its life it was known as the Newcastle Borough Asylum because it gave a service to Newcastle prior to the opening of St Nicholas Hospital in 1869. The largest of the four Gateshead asylums was Dunston Lodge, which in 1851 had 157 inmates; this was opened in 1851 but closed in 1900.[11,12] The numbers of patients had fallen, mainly because of the public provision elsewhere. The licence was transferred to a new Asylum at Middleton St George in Cleveland, which lasted well into the 20th century. There was also a Private Asylum at Sheriff Hill (1817-1860) and at Wrekenton (1826-1855).

The Commissioners' Reports for these Institutions were full of criticisms. At Wrekenton there was a cholera epidemic in which 18 of 20 inmates died. The proprietor at Dunston was dismissed for cruelty in 1851. Bensham was constantly criticised for overcrowding.

Disturbed patients had to be physically restrained. Those that were ambulant and amenable were employed and there is a description of patients going out to work in the fields from the Asylum at Sheriff Hill which was, for a time, known as Kent's Asylum after the name of the proprietor. Dunston Lodge is now the site of a council storage depot in Dunston Road.

The Kielder experiment

This therapeutic endeavour in psychiatry should be recorded. In 1980, the Northumbrian Water Authority flooded the new Kielder reservoir, north of Falstone up to the 600 foot contour. Now submerged is the site of a collection of huts which belonged to the Forestry Commission called 'Kielder Camp'. The map reference is NY 648907. It had been used before the Second World War as a Ministry of Labour Training Camp for unemployed men. In 1941, the disused buildings were taken over by the Royal Navy, enlarged and named *HMS Standard.*[13]

As the war progressed, there were increasing concerns for the number of personnel who were subject to psychological and behavioural disabilities, not severe enough to warrant discharge but nevertheless preventing them from giving full and effective service. The vast majority had, in present day nosology, personality disorders and psychopathic disorders and only a few actually had formal mental illness. The site was chosen because of its remoteness; going absent without leave presented real difficulties. There was emphasis on physical work and recreation. It closed in 1945 and during that period there were 842 admissions; 680 men were eventually re-drafted.[14]

It is of interest because it is one of the first experiments of its kind with a large problem group. It featured in the recommendations on Psychopathic Disorders to the Mental Health Commission, which led to the 1959 Mental Health Act. There were recommendations that patients with severe personality disorders should be treated in special units. In fact this did not occur.

Place names and literary associations

There is very little which is permanent left behind from the early history of psychiatry on Tyneside. Perhaps most important is the preservation of the Rules of the Hospital for Lunaticks, printed in 1766, (figure 1) and giving instructions as to the duties of the Manager, who was called the Keeper, the nursers and servants and the relationships of the Keeper with the Committee and the Physician. These rules provide a real record of administration of the early asylums and the Newcastle rules were adopted by other institutions in the country.[15]

R U L E S

OF THE

HOSPITAL FOR LUNATICKS,

For the COUNTIES of

NORTHUMBERLAND, NEWCASTLE UPON TYNE, and DURHAM.

I.

THAT this SOCIETY conſiſt of a Preſident, three Vice-preſidents, Treaſurer, and Governors.

II. THAT all who ſubſcribe One Guinea, or more, be Governors during ſuch Subſcription: And that a Subſcriber of Twenty Pounds, or more, be intitled to all the Privileges of other Governors.

III. THAT a General Court of Governors be held at four ſtated Times in the Year; viz. May-day, Thurſday in the Aſſize Week, Martinmas-day, and Candlemas-day; but in caſe May-day, Martinmas-day, or Candlemas-day, ſhall fall on a Sunday, then the ſame to be held on the Monday following.

Figure 1. First page of the Rules of the Hospital for Lunaticks 1766

There are some place names. Hall's Public Baths, built in 1781 on the same road as the Lunatic Hospital, has already been mentioned. Bath Lane has remained a prominent road in Newcastle, right down to the present day. The Private Hospital, which became known as Bellegrove Retreat, was situated on a strip of land one-and-a-half miles north-west of the city centre, called Spital Tongues. The name Bellegrove has remained applied to a Place, a Terrace and an Hotel in the vicinity of the house itself, which is now called White Knights. Nothing whatsoever remains behind in Gateshead.

There are literary associations. John Boswell (1743-1798) was the younger brother of James Boswell (1740-1795), the famous diarist and biographer. John suffered from periodic attacks of insanity and was several times a patient under Hall's care in St Luke's House. When Boswell visited his brother, he sometimes stayed with Hall at his private residence in Pilgrim Street and he mentions the walk out over the fields to St Luke's House. In his diaries, Boswell describes Hall as 'a sensible, pretty kind man and of a humane appearance', and he subsequently did some legal work for Hall over the reclaiming petition for the freight of a ship.[16] There is a reference to a discussion with Hall about Battie's *Treatise on Madness*, a book then in vogue.[17]

The Martin family originated from Hexham. Their most famous member was John (1789-1854), the painter who produced grandiose romantic paintings, often of biblical subjects, such as The Fall of Babylon and Belshazzar's Feast. He had a brother Jonathan (1782-1838) who was schizophrenic and was preoccupied throughout his life with ideas and delusions of a paranoid, religious nature. He was for a time resident in the Sheriff Hill Private Asylum in Gateshead, having been pronounced insane after a proposed attempt to shoot the Bishop of Oxford. He made two attempts at escaping and was successful on the second in 1821. He had then spent his time working as an itinerant tanner in North Yorkshire and in 1829, under the influence of delusions, set fire to the choir of York Minster. At his trial, which aroused enormous interest, he was found insane and sent to Bethlem in London. A signed portrait by RW Brown remains, (figure 2) showing him whilst in prison awaiting trial, which can be seen at the City of York Art Gallery. Jonathan Martin was something of an artist himself and his work was typical of schizophrenic art: one of his subjects was a bishop with seven heads, rushing to the jaws of a crocodile. He also wrote a first hand description of the Sheriff Hill Private Asylum.[18]

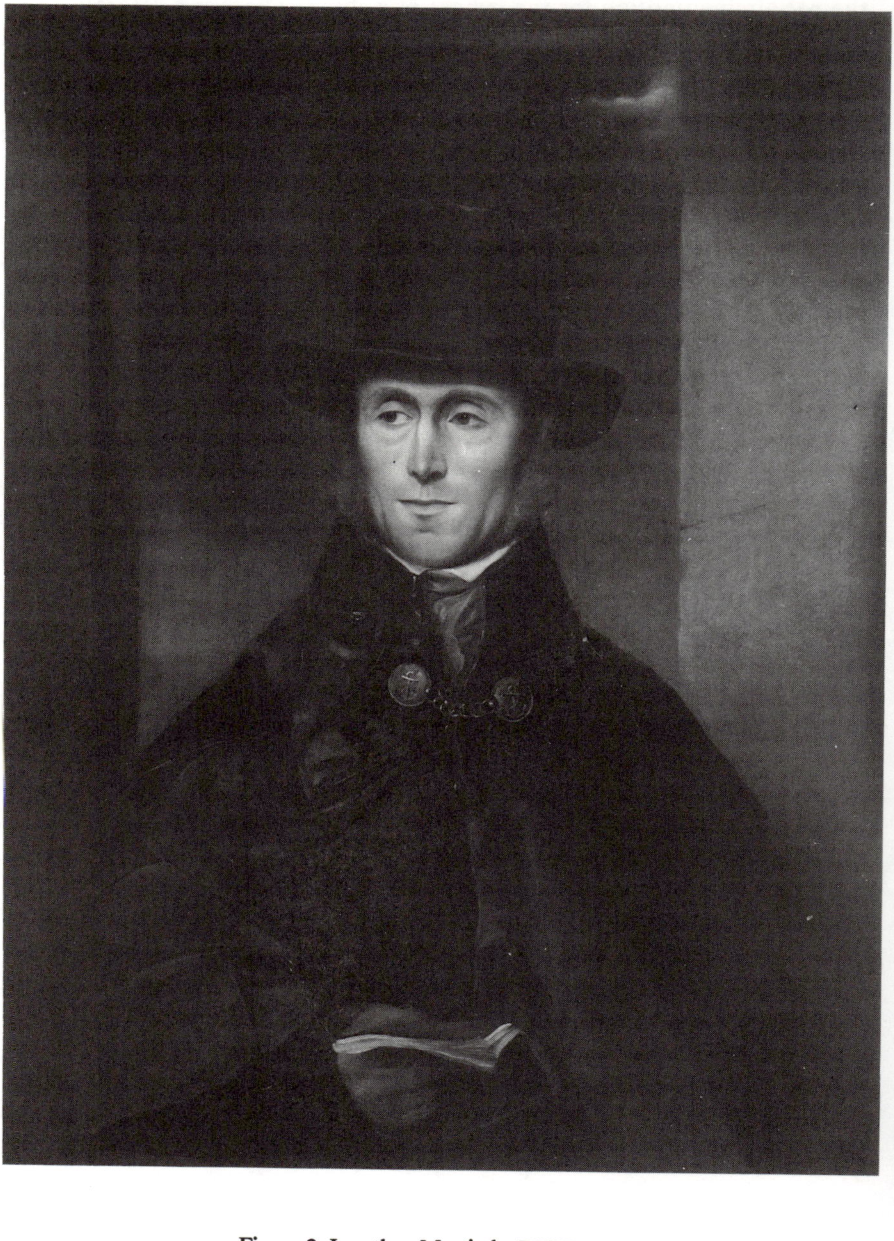

Figure 2. Jonathan Martin by RW Brown:
by permission of the City of York Art Gallery.

References

1. Hunter RA, MacAlpine I. *Three Hundred Years of Psychiatry 1536-1860*. Oxford: OUP, 1963.
2. Jones K. *Lunacy, Law and Conscience*. London: Routledge and Kegan Paul, 1955; 37-40.
3. Le Gassicke J. Early History of Psychiatry in Newcastle upon Tyne. *Brit J Psychiat* 1972; *120*: 419-22.
4. Lunatic Hospital Records. City Archives, Newcastle upon Tyne. 1686.
5. *Rules of the Hospital for Lunaticks for the Counties of Northumberland, Newcastle upon Tyne and Durham 1766*. Central Library, Newcastle upon Tyne. Local Tracts, Miscellaneous I.
6. Harvey J. *A sentimental tour through Newcastle*. Newcastle: Akenhead, 1794.
7. Hall J. *De febra acuta puerperis superveniente*. Edinburgh: Hamilton and Balfour, 1755.
8. Hall J. *A narrative of the proceedings relative to the establishment of St Luke's House, Newcastle*. Newcastle upon Tyne: J White and T Saint, 1767.
9. Mackenzie E. *A descriptive and historical account of the town and county of Newcastle upon Tyne including the Borough of Gateshead*. Newcastle: Mackenzie and Dent, 1827; 527.
10. Manders FWD. *A History of Gateshead*. Gateshead Corporation, 1973.
11. Forest M. *The History of Dunston Lodge Lunatic Asylum*. Gateshead Public Library, 1986.
12. Herring G. *A Day in a Private Lunatic Asylum*. London: Walter Scott, 1884.
13. Le Gassicke J. A Submerged Site of Therapeutic Endeavour. *Bull Roy Coll Psychiat* 1982; *6*: 8.
14. Prewer RR. The Kielder Experiment. *J Mental Science* 1945; *91*: 481-94.
15. Roberts N. *Cheadle Royal Hospital*. Altrincham: J Sherrat & Son, 1967; 12.
16. Boswell J. *Private Papers of James Boswell from Malahide Castle: In the Isham Collection*. Edit Scott G and Pottle FA. Privately printed 1928-34, 10, 66.
17. Battie J. *A Treatise on Madness*. London: J Whiston and B White, 1758.
18. Balston T. *The Life of Jonathan Martin*. London: MacMillan, 1945.

Chapter 20

THE PORT OF TYNE SANITARY AUTHORITY: FLOATING HOSPITALS, BERI-BERI AND BUBONIC PLAGUE

JR Guy

> Port Sanitary Regulations in the United Kingdom had as their principal object the safeguarding of the health of the inhabitants of the ports themselves.

That was the view of Dr Thomas Clark, chairman of the Liverpool Port Sanitary Committee in 1896. Few would have quarrelled with this interpretation. He was reiterating the prevailing medical orthodoxy, as it had been summarized by one of the medical inspectors of the Local Government Board, Dr Francis Blaxall, in 1885. The regulations applied by the Port Sanitary Districts, acting in concert with the Customs authorities, were to provide the United Kingdom with its 'first line of defence against the introduction and spread of dangerous infectious disease, and the preservation of the health of crews and passengers by securing that vessels should be kept in a wholesome condition'.[1]

Soon after its constitution by act of parliament in 1871 the Local Government Board had established certain of the Customs ports as Port Sanitary Districts, and began the appointing of the pre-existing local sanitary authorities, urban or rural as the case might be, as the Port Sanitary Authorities. The new authorities were required to appoint a Medical Officer of Health and an Inspector of Nuisances, and make due hospital provision for cases of infectious disease entering their jurisdiction.

Dr Clark was echoing Blaxall's words:[2]

> It might indeed be said that not only the health of the port was safeguarded, but the health of the whole community, since seaborne diseases might in the absence of suitable regulations and preventive measures be disseminated far and wide throughout the country.

Although the health and welfare of the seafarers was never ignored by the Port Sanitary Authorities, their concern, certainly before the end of the 19th century, was primarily with preventive medicine. The lesson from the history of infectious diseases which had gained access through the ports and then spread rapidly inland, with consequent suffering and death, was there for anyone to learn. No one had forgotten that the cholera epidemics of 1831-2, 1848-9, 1853-4 and 1865-66 had all gained their first foothold in port towns (in 1831 Sunderland and in 1853 through the Tyne itself). The Port Sanitary Authorities had been brought into existence to prevent history repeating itself.

The River Tyne Port Sanitary Authority, after a provisional existence of some years, had been permanently constituted under the Local Government Board's Provisional Orders Confirmation (No 7) Act of 1882. However, as Dr Henry Armstrong noted in his history of the early days of the Authority, what he called 'the sanitary charge of the Tyne' dated in fact from 1871, when a joint committee of the local sanitary authorities had been formed, for the purpose of inspecting vessels entering the river from ports where the presence of cholera was suspected.[3]

The 1871 committee consisted of representatives from the corporations of Newcastle, Gateshead, Tynemouth, South Shields, Jarrow and the smaller communities along the north and south banks of the river. From the outset it adopted what were the classic means of preventing the importation of infectious disease into their heavily populated districts: inspection, medical supervision, and the hospital isolation of reported or suspect cases. The year 1870 had seen the beginning of what has been called 'a most intense cholera prevalence in Europe', particularly in Russia and Prussian Poland, with which countries the Tyne Ports carried on a considerable trade.[4]

Both the extension of railway networks and the shortening of journeys consequent upon the advent and the continuing improvement of the steamship facilitated trade and travel. Because passengers might now arrive at their destinations before symptoms of disease became apparent, these improvements were also perceived as intensifying the threat of infectious diseases being imported. The formal opening of the Suez Canal in 1869, greatly reducing the passenger-time from cholera's heartland in India to European ports, had only served to heighten the anxiety.

The Tyne Ports committee of 1871 initially placed the sanitary policing of the river in the hands of a medical officer and two inspectors who were also medically qualified. It was their duty to visit ships entering the river which were suspected of having cholera on board. In addition a former steam ferry boat, the *Tyne*, was acquired, having been donated by the river commissioners, and a wooden pavilion, 43 x 23 feet, with accommodation for a 14-bed ward, water closets and a nurses' room fitted up as a surgery, was erected upon the hull.

The lower deck was divided up to provide a coal store to supply the ward and surgery stoves, a blanket store, a pantry and kitchen, nurses' bedrooms, a room for the ship-keeper and his wife, and a mess. Alongside was moored a second hulk, reached by a gangplank, upon which a laundry and disinfecting plant were erected. The hospital, designed by Newcastle's Borough Surveyor, was staffed by a matron and a steward, the medical superintendent being the assistant port medical officer, Dr Byrom Bramwell. The hospital was described and illustrated in *The Lancet* of 6 January 1872, whose verdict was that it was 'an excellent undertaking'.[5]

The hospital was intended to be a temporary expedient, to facilitate the isolation and treatment of any cholera cases brought into the river by shipping from 'foul' ports. The spread of cholera in 1872 into Asia Minor and Arabia, where it attacked the Mecca pilgrims, resulted in the ports committee resolving upon the hospital's permanent maintenance. In 1871-72 the expense of equipping it and paying for the medical inspection of vessels entering the river had amounted to £1717, a sum met by levying a rate of $^{1}/_{4}$d in the £ on the riparian authorities. It was felt to be money well spent.[6]

The Tyne committee in 1871 may well have been among the first port authorities to provide what was in many ways a virtually purpose-built floating hospital. Another east coast port, Lowestoft, had a similar arrangement, with a two-ward pavilion housing six beds erected upon the hulk of a 45-ton wherry. The Lowestoft hospital was not, however, commissioned until 1872.[7]

The idea of floating hospitals was not new. Naval ports, both in Britain and her colonies, where there was no hospital facility on shore, frequently made use of superannuated ships-of-the-line; the old *Blenheim* (90), serving as a floating hospital in 1743, had even had a separate fever ward.[8]

Medical opinion was, however, divided over the wisdom of using hulks as floating hospitals. Dr F Oppert, in his *Hospitals, Infirmaries and Dispensaries*, had said in 1867 that 'ships should not be used ... in time of peace'. He does not seem to have reflected the majority view.[9]

Their utility had, nonetheless, been demonstrated, especially for the isolation of infectious cases. Cardiff's reforming Medical Officer, Dr Henry Paine, in 1858 had called for the establishment of a seamen's receiving house in the increasingly busy south Wales port, to prevent the spread of disease into the town itself. In 1866, when the frigate *HMS Hamadryad* was moored there to serve as a seamen's hospital, Paine made use of her to isolate and treat infectious diseases.[10] Even earlier *HMS Grampus* had been moored at Greenwich and opened as a hospital for sick seamen in October 1821. The location had been chosen as the most convenient for the receiving of the sick from ships before they passed upstream and into the port of London.[11]

There was, then, no lack of precedent for the Tyne committee's initiative. In addition, as an anonymous correspondent of *The Lancet* in September 1873 was to point out, because such isolation hulks were required only for occasional occupation by the sick, they could be run economically on a 'care-and-maintenance' basis. Perhaps with the Tyne and Lowestoft hospitals in mind, the same correspondent nonetheless expressed reservations about the use of old government vessels. These, he felt, were unwieldy, could be unhygienic and were more costly to maintain than purpose-built floating hospitals.[12]

The cholera pandemic which had brought about the Tyne committee's initiative waned as the decade advanced, so that the immediate danger receded. There were two resultant changes in the sanitary supervision of the Ports of Tyne, both underpinned by the passing in 1875 of the Public Health Act. The two medically-qualified inspecting officers were replaced in 1879 by a lay Inspector of Nuisances, and the single hospital ward was divided. Both changes are indicative of a shift in the emphasis of the sanitary administration. Although a continuing threat from cholera was not discounted, under the provisions of the 1875 Act the removal to hospital of every patient suffering from infectious disease on shipboard became compulsory. The disease 'catchment' was therefore considerably widened. A single-ward hospital, where cross-infection would be possible if not inevitable, was no longer adequate, and the *Tyne* was adapted accordingly.

Initially the single ward was divided into two, and then, in 1883, with cases of several different diseases being nursed at the same time, and with a threat of the recrudescence of cholera in the Mediterranean, the Authority chartered and then subsequently purchased the Dutch galliot *Alliance* to provide extra accommodation. (A galliot of the time was usually strongly-built, ketch-rigged, and of approximately 150 tons, and therefore suitable for the purpose.) On her deck a block of two wards comprising ten beds with the necessary offices was built and equipped.[13]

The hospital now consisted of three converted vessels moored together in front of the large open stretch of water known as Jarrow Slake, about 6½ miles below Newcastle. They were protected from the danger of collision from traffic on the river itself by an enclosure of piling. The Slake, though a large expanse of water, was too shallow to be used for shipping purposes, and the site was consequently left open. The hospital thus met the criteria laid down by one of the medical officers of the Local Government Board (and later its Chief Medical Officer), Dr Richard Thorne:[14]

> If [floating hospitals] can be placed where communication with them, both for the reception of patients and for administration purposes, is not likely to be interfered with by weather, the more complete isolation which is secured by means of their use is an element well worthy of consideration.

The Jarrow Slake certainly provided complete isolation. Shallow and relatively sheltered – it was partly occupied by the Tyne Improvement Commissioners' Timber Ponds – nonetheless at high or low tide the hospital was accessible only by boat. In 1883 the Authority purchased the steam launch *Midge*, with a specially equipped forecabin, heated and provided with an ambulance hammock, so that patients could be removed directly from ship to hospital. *Midge*, replacing a steam-launch acquired in 1882 (but found unsuitable) and normally moored at the Authority's South Shields station, Corporation Quay, also served to transport the inspectors from ship to ship.[15] In 1893 a second launch, *Spark*, was acquired to supplement her. *Midge* was eventually sold (for £56 10 0d) in 1899 and in turn replaced by the *JF Spence*, purchased through a Local Government Board loan.

The replacement of the medical inspecting officers by a lay Inspector of Nuisances may be thought to have undermined the effectiveness of the sanitary administration of the ports. In fact this was not the case. Rather it was a more rational use of resources, and entirely in line with the Local Government Board's philosophy. The inspector appointed in 1879 was an experienced merchant seaman, who had sailed as a chief mate; at all times he acted under the instruction, and if necessary under the superintendence, of one of the port's medical officers. However, even after 1882, when the Port of Tyne Sanitary Authority was officially constituted by the Local

Government Board, and an assistant inspector engaged, it was not possible to inspect personally every vessel entering the river; by the 1880s the annual average number of arrivals in the port was no fewer than 14 848, of both coasters and deep-sea traders.

Dr Armstrong recorded in great detail how the system of inspection worked on the river during his period as Medical Officer of Health in this decade. Under the provisions of the Quarantine Act all cases of disease occurring on vessels arriving at the port from overseas were to be reported to HM Customs. Normally that arrangement worked well. Very few Masters deliberately witheld information, since they could be prosecuted and heavily fined for so doing; more often than not, misrepresentation was the result of misdiagnosis on the part of the captain. The Port Sanitary Authority did not rely wholly upon the Customs' reports. It merely used them as indicators, and previously unreported or undetected cases of infectious disease on ships which had signalled 'all well' were often picked up by the Inspectors of Nuisances.

The Port Authority concentrated its attention upon vessels deemed to be in a 'high risk' category. Dr Armstrong described the procedure thus:[16]

> The medical and daily press, the *Shipping Gazette*, etc. are regularly examined for the purpose of learning of disease abroad. A list of vessels bound to the Tyne from ports so infected (called the "Homeward Bound Register") is systematically kept by the chief inspector, who enters in it the name of the ship, the dates of passing different ports on her voyage, the time of her expected arrival, etc. Ships on this register are visited by our officers without delay on entering the port. The inspectors on boarding any vessel are in the practice of interrogating the master as to reports of disease at the places the ship has come from. Free intercommunication is maintained with other port sanitary authorities as to vessels likely to arrive, which should be kept under observation on account of recently having had infectious disease on board.

Armstrong provided a number of examples of how the system worked in practice:[17]

> The information gained in 1881 as to the prevalence of small-pox at Bilbao led to the visiting at each arrival of every vessel trading regularly from that port to the Tyne with iron ore. As vessels came here every few weeks, and as the number of vessels was considerable, the duty represents a large amount of work.

The system relied upon informed judgement as to which vessels were to be placed in a 'high risk' category, and therefore given priority when it came to inspection. It relied also upon co-operation with other Authorities and HM Customs, to provide the earliest possible information, and upon a skilled, rigorous but tactful interrogation of shipmasters. At least for this last, an inspector who was or had been himself a ship's officer rather than a medical man was almost certainly an advantage.

When a case of infectious disease was reported or detected, the sufferer was removed to the floating hospital, and the required disinfecting procedures carried out aboard the vessel before she was permitted to disembark her passengers. The number of such cases was not large, between 1881 and 1887 never rising above thirteen in any one year. Smallpox, enteric fever and what Dr Armstrong referred to as 'continued fever' were the most common causes of admission, followed by scarlet fever.

The Port Medical Officer, who was also the Medical Officer of Health for Newcastle, sometimes found himself involved in a conflict of interest. In his former capacity he administered a hospital, equipped and maintained at public expense, but whose wards were rarely occupied by more than one or two patients at a time and who were usually suffering from infectious diseases common enough in the riparian districts themselves. (The exception was 'African Coast Fever' – probably Blackwater Fever – 1 case in 7 years.) As Newcastle's MOH he could be placed under pressure from colleagues in the riparian districts to admit their cases, as he evidently had beds available in the port hospital. Such requests were always refused. It cannot have been easy to explain that the empty beds might be needed at very short notice, or for the precautionary admission of suspect but not fully developed cases. The admission of cases for observation resulted in German measles, tonsillitis and bronchitis appearing in the hospital's statistics. Patients thus diagnosed were speedily discharged, but, as Armstrong said, 'It is safer to act on this principle than to leave the cases to develop and become dangerous in a crowded forecastle'.[18]

The support of the Local Government Board for floating hospitals, even to the point of the publication of model plans in 1886, and its willingness to advance loans for the provision of new hospitals gave impetus to the Port of Tyne Authority's resolution to replace its three hulks with a purpose-built facility. In his Annual Report for 1884 the medical officer had reported that the hospital was becoming defective through old age, and was deemed incapable of repair. It leaked. Accordingly WG Laws, Newcastle's Civil Engineer, designed a 30-bed hospital in three ward blocks, mounted on a platform 140ft long and 80ft wide, to be floated on ten cylindrical pontoons in the Jarrow Slake. Laws' hospital was to provide the Authority with one of the best facilities available in the United Kingdom.[19]

George Laws had been first approached in 1884, and asked to advise on the replacement of the old hospital. Originally the intention was to acquire another hulk, and build upon it as before. Several vessels had been inspected, and the Admiralty had offered to sell a gunboat, then laid up in ordinary, for £2450. However she lay at Portsmouth, and the cost of bringing her to the Tyne and effecting the necessary repair and conversion work was deemed too high. In 1885 Laws therefore prepared plans for the pontoon hospital, the contract for which was awarded to Wood & Skinner of Bill Quay. The Wood Skinner Yard specialised in the building of cargo steamers for coastal and European trade, the so-called 'short sea trade'. They produced economically priced vessels of anything between 100-2000 gross register tons, and sold many of them to Scandinavian owners.[20]

Wood Skinner was convinced that they could build the whole hospital on the slipways of their No 3 yard, launch it, and then tow it the four miles downstream to the mooring. It was a bold and risky undertaking, but ultimately a successful one. The hospital took to the river on 2 August 1885 without the breaking of a single pane of glass in the windows. Within four hours the pontoon was safely at the mooring which it was to occupy for more than forty years. The initial £5000 cost was met by a loan from the Local Government Board, repayable at $3\frac{1}{2}\%$ interest over 20 years, though additional funding was necessary in 1891 and in 1894, the latter loan to cover the cost of a new disinfecting apparatus. By 1897 the original loans had been paid off, and all loan debt was liquidated by 1911.[21]

Laws gave a full description of the new hospital to the local branch of the Association of Municipal and Sanitary Engineers at its Newcastle meeting in 1887.[22] The hospital consisted of ten cylindrical iron pontoons, up to 70ft long and 6ft in diameter, each weighing $53\frac{1}{2}$ tons, supporting an iron framework upon which was carried a deck of creosoted timber (figure 1). The deck provided space for three pavilions, each containing two wards divided by a nursing station and a bathroom, some smaller structures and a mortuary. The hospital had a floating weight of 535 tons.

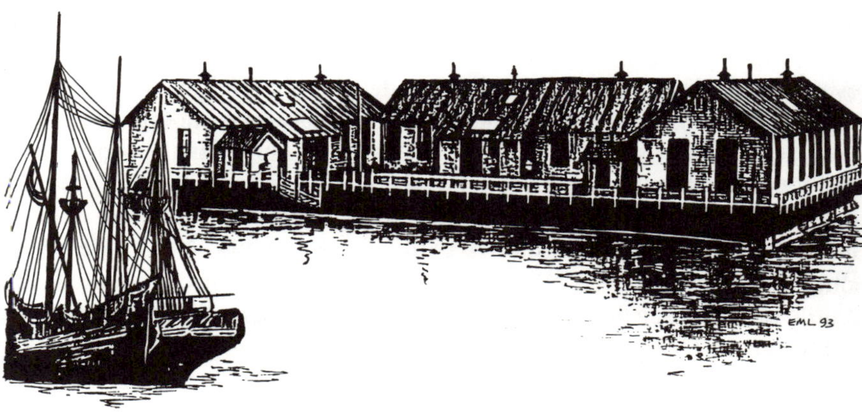

Figure 1. The Floating Hospital: drawn from a photograph by E Lazenby.

Originally a fourth block was planned, to house the caretaker, kitchen, storerooms and dispensary, but there is no record of this having been built. Plans for the work were described as 'in progress' soon after the launch, but later seem to have been abandoned. The old three-hulk hospital was retained for a while; *Tyne* was disinfected in 1890 and sold in 1891 to be broken up, and the Disinfecting Hulk likewise disposed of. The *Alliance* remained in service, no longer as the cholera unit, but as the new administrative block. She was, however, accident prone. In 1888, during a gale in May, her mooring chain carried away. In July she developed a list and then at high tide on the 25th suddenly sank; fortunately there was no one on board and the Slake being shallow, the water only reached the pavilion. She had to be raised and beached for repair. Then, in the Northumberland Dock in 1890 undergoing further work, she became displaced, collided with the dockside, started filling with water again and had to be pumped out by the Tyne Commissioners' Tug.

The Tyne Floating Hospital was not the only one designed by George Laws. The River Tees Authority, which possessed a six-bed hospital accommodated on the hulk of an old sailing brig, sought Laws' advice in 1892 over its replacement, and the new floating hospital, designed by himself and TW Stainthorpe, Surveyor to the Eston Local Board, was in many respects similar to that which had proved its worth on the Tyne.[23]

The Annual Reports of the Port Medical Officer, Henry Armstrong (until his forced resignation in 1895), and then Edmund Harker MD, contain detailed accounts of the working of the Tyne hospital, the number of patients treated and the range of disease. At the outbreak of war in 1914 Harker anticipated an increase in shipborne disease, and to this end the river staff had been increased and a new steam launch, the *George C Coates* acquired. Built by Hepple & Co of South Shields, like her predecessors she had an ambulance saloon aft, and was provided with electric light.

Harker's precautions were justified, for there was indeed a marked increase in the number of patients admitted to the hospital during the war years, many from serving units of the Royal Navy. In 1917, 104 patients were treated on board, only eight of whom were from the mercantile marine. The spread of common complaints was inevitable among the concentrations of men aboard units of the Grand Fleet, many living in close proximity with others for the first time. In his Annual Report for 1917 the MOH tabulated scabies, rubella, diphtheria, measles, chickenpox and septic throat among admissions from the Royal Navy. (One patient from *HMS Satellite*, a very elderly corvette used as a drill-ship for the Naval Reserve, was admitted with scabies on 28 May but recorded as having 'escaped' from the hospital on 3 June!)

The 1917 figures were inflated by the agreement reached in February by the Port Sanitary Authority to admit cases of scabies to the hospital from the Navy. No fewer than 79 were treated during the year, something of a comment upon the inadequate standards of hygiene on board the ships, *Sarcoptes scabiei* flourishing when men are living in cramped conditions and where ablution and laundry facilities are overstretched. However, all cases may not have been genuine. Scabies could be simulated by pricking the skin of the interdigital spaces with a needle and then vigorously rubbing the pricks with a concentrated solution of brine. Perhaps it is not surprising that one patient found it necessary to 'escape'![24]

In his historical retrospect Henry Armstrong demonstrated that example was the best way of illustrating the working of the Port of Tyne Sanitary Authority. This chapter therefore concludes with two cases which reveal the careful, integrated approach of its officials in response to the threat of imported disease.

Case I

On 12 August 1910 the Brazilian Navy protected cruiser *Barrozo*, with a crew of 434, arrived in the Tyne. She was an elderly ship, having been laid down in 1895. Built to specifications popular at the time, with armoured deck but largely unprotected sides, she was by 1910 obsolescent if not obsolete (figure 2).[25] She was also coming home, having been designed and built by Swan Hunter at their Elswick yards. She had been at sea for more than a month, sailing from Rio de Janeiro on 3 July, and calling at Pernambuco, St Vincent, Las Palmas and Plymouth. Here two seamen complained of illness, and on the voyage to the Tyne the ship's surgeon diagnosed their complaint as beri-beri. On arrival Dr Edmund Harker was notified, went aboard and examined the patients, and then admitted them to the Floating Hospital.

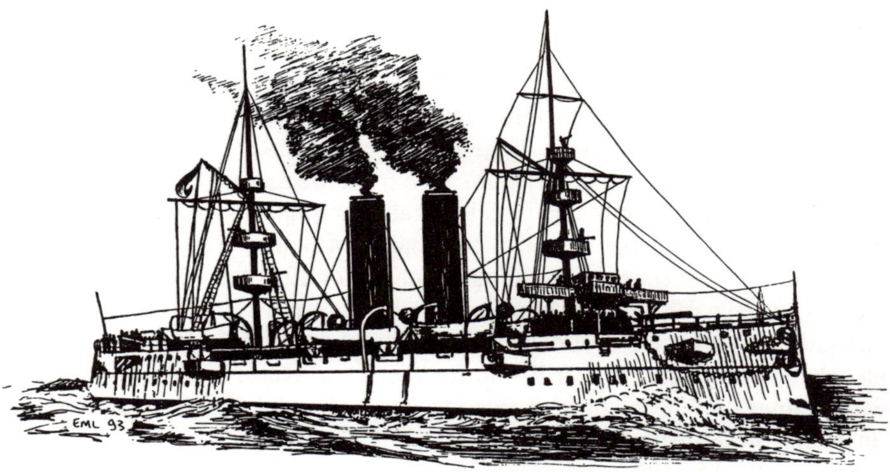

Figure 2. *Barrozo*. The Brazilian Navy Cruiser (length 330ft, 20 guns): redrawn from *Jane's Fighting Ships* 1914 edition by E Lazenby.

In 1910 there was still considerable debate over the cause and nature of beri-beri. In 1903 Cecil Bullmore, MOH for the Port of Falmouth and Truro, had published an analysis of cases of beri-beri diagnosed on board ships entering his jurisdiction between 1896 and 1901, but although he had investigated possible links between the disease and diet, he had reached no definite conclusions. As many of the vessels examined had come from Scandinavian ports, there was insufficient evidence to connect beri-beri with rice. Nonetheless he was not altogether happy about the diet usually provided.[26]

By the time of the *Barrozo*'s arrival in the Tyne seven years later, a link between beri-beri and dietary deficiency was generally accepted, though there were still those who believed that it was the result of an organism causing acute infection. Even Sir William Osler, in the thoroughly revised 8th edition of his classic *Principles and Practice of Medicine*, issued two years later in 1912, remained cautious.[27] There was also little doubt that attacks of beri-beri could be precipitated by unhygienic conditions, such as those met with all too often in the overcrowded forecastles of both sailing and steamships.

The number of Harker's patients from the *Barrozo* grew in early September, until 36 had been admitted to the floating hospital. All suffered from peripheral neuritis and dropsy, the former so severe in some cases as to amount to almost complete paraplegia. Most suffered some cardiac distress after exertion; the one and only fatality occurred after a meal when a seaman complained of sudden chest pain, and succumbed to a cardiac arrest.

Harker had closely examined the cruiser, and concluded that the seamen's berths were overcrowded and woefully inadequate, some men having to sling their hammocks on the upper decks. The only ventilation came via open hatchways. The diet was also inadequate.

Removal to the floating hospital proved to be, in all but the one fatal case, beneficial. Here the overcrowded forecastle was exchanged for 'a lofty, airy, sunlit hospital ward' in Harker's words. Rice was excluded from the diet, and emphasis placed instead on fresh vegetables, fruit and milk. Rest, gentle exercise and massage replaced the warship's sick-bay or normal routine.

However the *Barrozo* outbreak faced Harker and the Port Authority with an important question. Beri-beri carried with it little risk of communication from the sick to the healthy. Should cases therefore be treated in the floating hospital, taking up beds reserved for the admission of infectious diseases, or should the beds stay empty and the sufferers be nursed on shore in the general or voluntary hospitals? By admitting beri-beri cases to the floating hospital in 1910 Harker modified the absolutist stance of his predecessor, concluding that it was unreasonable to tax the resources of the general hospital wards by sending his patients to them. Harker's more flexible approach made subsequent, wartime, decisions easier, for example that in 1917 over scabies.[28]

Case II

Two years later Harker was confronted with the kind of case for which the hospital had been designed and built. On 2 July 1912 the *SS Bellailsa* sailed from Rosario with a cargo of maize, bound for Hamburg. *Bellailsa* was a 16-year old, 3797grt schooner-rigged, single-screw steamer, built by D & W Henderson & Co and sailing under the British flag for Bell Bros and Co's Bellailsa Steamship Company. Her master was a 56-year old Norwegian, Ole Olsen Aagaard, who had been with Bell Bros since 1885, and had commanded the *Bellailsa* since her launch. A senior and experienced captain with the company, Aagaard had with him on board four apprentices.[29]

Whilst discharging her cargo at Hamburg in late August, one apprentice, Robert Hirst Morton, fell ill. A doctor was called on board, but on 4 September Morton died. His body was taken on shore for post-mortem examination. On 8 September *Bellailsa* sailed for the Tyne, but a second apprentice, John Rewcastle McWhirter, was now taken ill. Immediately Aagaard put back to Cuxhaven, a doctor was called, and McWhirter taken ashore. *Bellailsa* sailed again, and arrived in the Tyne on the 10th, berthing at the Mercantile Dry Dock in Jarrow. Now a third apprentice, John William Raeburn, was ill, and Aagaard informed the Customs, who immediately telephoned the Port Sanitary Authority.

Harker and his inspector went aboard, interviewed the captain, and examined both the patient and the post-mortem certificate from Hamburg of Robert Morton, which stated that he had died of 'abdominal typhoid'. Harker, as a result, made a provisional diagnosis of enteric fever in the case of Raeburn, who was immediately removed to the floating hospital. The normal procedures were then adopted by his inspector. The *Bellailsa* was fumigated, and her water tanks discharged and cleansed.

By 11 September Harker was sure that Raeburn was suffering from bubonic plague and not enteric fever, despite the fact that a microscopical examination of a blood-sample for *Bacillus pestis* had proved negative in this respect, but examined bacteriologically had given a positive Vidal reaction when tested for enteric. Exactly the same results had been obtained at the post-mortem examination of Morton in Hamburg.

Harker stuck to his guns. Culture tubes were inoculated from the sample and incubated, and a guinea-pig also inoculated. The latter sickened and died, the cause of death after post-mortem examination being demonstrated as plague, and within 48 hours the inoculated tubes were also showing all the characteristics of plague. It was too late to save Raeburn. His disease, complicated by double pneumonia, proved fatal on 16 September. Harker's post-mortem conducted on the floating hospital gave conclusive proof.

On 20 September the Hamburg Port Doctor, Saunemann, communicated the results of the bacteriological investigations in the cases of Morton and McWhirter (who himself died on the 29th). Despite the post-mortem diagnosis in the case of the former, both were shown to have suffered from plague. Five days later Harker heard from the Local Government Board. Their parallel bacteriological investigations, undertaken on a sample he had sent them, confirmed his own diagnosis.

The *Bellailsa* was now thoroughly fumigated for rats, twelve corpses collected, and all bacteriologically examined, some being sent to the Local Government Board for the purpose. One was found to be plague-infected. Of the four apprentices on board, three had fallen victim to a virulent strain of *B. pestis* and all three had died. The questions remained: how did it come about, and why had the fourth remained in good health? Harker continued his investigation, and the outcome provides a classic example of epidemiological research.

All four apprentices were berthed in the after part of the *Bellailsa* by themselves. The three who died lived together in a spacious berth on the port side. The fourth, Rogerson, occupied a berth on his own on the starboard side. The plague-infected rat had been found below the apprentices' berths. Although living apart from the others, Rogerson had been theoretically just as much at risk. Harker persevered. The three who succumbed had purchased in Rosario a tame rabbit, and had kept it in a hutch in close proximity to the lazarette which was home to the infected rat. In Hamburg a workman offered to purchase the rabbit as a pet for his children, but it died before the transaction could be completed. The second officer threw it overboard, noting that there was vermin on its fur.

Harker's case was complete. The three boys had frequently played with their pet in the berth. The day after the rabbit, whose hutch and food-supply were easily accessible to rats and their fleas, had died, Morton was taken ill. Four days later McWhirter followed, and two days after that, Raeburn. Rogerson survived unscathed: he had a berth to himself; he did not like rabbits; he had not played with his fellows' pet.[30]

As a result of the procedure carefully adopted in both Hamburg and on the Tyne, the plague did not spread. Aagaard, an experienced and conscientious captain, concerned for the health and welfare of his apprentices and crew, had called in a doctor as soon as illness was reported, in one case even putting back to port – and thus, perhaps, saving his men from a wider visitation. Both in Germany and England the patients were isolated, and bacteriological and post-mortem examinations carried out, the medical officers involved keeping each other informed. The ship involved was thoroughly cleansed and fumigated. The names and addresses of the paid-off crew were sent to their local medical officers of health, and the men monitored for any suspicious symptoms.

The 1912 plague case very clearly demonstrated the worth of the Port Sanitary Authority system and the value of the Tyne's floating hospital, but not everything was sweetness and light. There were occasionally tensions between the Authority and its medical officers, as the bitterness engendered by the forced resignation of Dr Henry Armstrong illustrates. In May 1895 Armstrong was absent, as a member of a deputation to the Local Government Board. During his absence the *SS Regulus* arrived in the Tyne, with smallpox on board. She was visited, patients removed to the hospital, and the forecastle and contents disinfected. However some infected bedclothes were concealed from the inspector, taken ashore, and three cases of the disease in Jarrow were alleged to have been the result.

The Port Sanitary Authority met without their MOH, and passed a vote of censure on him. Though the Authority subsequently decided to take no further action, when the Local Government Board had informed them that there was nothing in Armstrong's conduct which required either further investigation or censure, they did not rescind the censure motion. He resigned. Armstrong himself was convinced that, having made some comments upon the poor sanitary state of some of the vessels trading from the port, he had fallen foul of certain shipowning members of the authority, who had taken his remarks personally and were determined to force him out of office. He concluded:[31]

> Any outspoken public officer who tries to do his duty must occasionally tread on the toes of men who, having the power to injure him, find the temptation irresistible. He is not the first, and does not expect to be the last, who has so suffered.

The work, despite such clashes, was not interrupted. As he prepared his Annual Report for 1914, writing on board HM Hospital Ship *Plassy*, where he was serving with the Naval Reserve, Edmund Harker commented thus:[32]

> In our work as a Port Sanitary Authority we wage a continual war against unseen foes in the form of foreign infectious diseases, which are transported from country to country by the peaceful Mercantile Marine and which become a menace to the Public Health when they gain a foothold in our midst....

It was the task of the Authorities, their inspectors, medical officers, and their hospital staffs to see that no such foothold was obtained. The Tyne Authority, in common with all the others, was almost completely successful. It occasionally lost a skirmish with its unseen foes. It never lost a battle.

The war, however, goes on.

References

Note: The published Annual Reports of the Port Medical Officers of Health, with associated manuscripts and papers, are deposited with the Tyne & Wear Archives Department, Blandford House, Newcastle upon Tyne. Information otherwise unattributed has been drawn from these Reports and papers (TWAD 604R1195, 1208, 1236-1238 for the Reports, TWAD 604R1180, 1188-1191, 1248 for Statements of Receipts and Expenditure).

1. Blaxall FH. *Report on the Sanitary Survey of Port and Principal Riparian Sanitary Districts 1885-1886. Supplement to the Fifteenth Annual Report of the Local Government Board*. London: HMSO, 1886, 129.
2. Conference Report in *The Sanitary Record* 18 Sept 1896:244-247 for Dr Clark's remarks and a re-statement of the prevailing view.
3. Armstrong HE. Port sanitary administration on the Tyne: A seven years' retrospect, 1881-1887. *Pub Health* 1888-89:33-43.

4. Clemow FG. *The Geography of Disease*. Cambridge: U Press, 1903:98.

5. Ports of Tyne floating cholera hospital. *The Lancet* 1872; *i*:15-16.

6. Clemow FG, *op cit* note 4:98; Armstrong HE, *op cit* note 3:34.

7. Clubbe WH. Floating hospitals for cholera patients. *The Lancet* 1872; *ii*: 468.

8. Lavery B. Support Craft. In: Gardiner R, ed. *The Line of Battle. The Sailing Warship 1650-1840*. London: Conway Maritime Press, 1992:112. The subject of floating hospitals is explored in Guy JR, Ahoy! Patient coming aboard. Floating hospitals for infectious diseases. *Bull Med Sci Hist Soc* 1991; *10*:11-22.

9. Oppert F. *Hospitals, Infirmaries and Dispensaries*. London: J Churchill & Sons, 1867:154.

10. Mayberry JF. The Hamadryad Hospital Ship for Seamen 1866- 1905. *Brit Med J* 1980; *ii*:1690-1692. See also the same author's *I Saw Three Ships. The Story of HMS Hamadryad, Cardiff's Hospital Ship 1866-1905 and Gospel and Educational Ships HMS Thisbe and HMS Havannah*. Lancs, St Michael's: nd; *The Lancet* 1869; *i*:333.

11. Goldsmith E, McBride AG. Dreadnought Seamen's Hospital. *Brit Med J* 1976; *ii*:1511-1513.

12. *The Lancet* 1873; *ii*:428.

13. Tyne & Wear Archives Department (hereafter TWAD) 604R1236. *Annual Report* for 1883:3-4.

14. Thorne RT. *Report to the Local Government Board on the use and influence of hospitals for infectious diseases*. London: HMSO, 1882:394-410.

15. The plans for *Midge* can be seen in the Dept of Maritime History, Newcastle Museum of Science and Engineering.

16. Armstrong HE, *op cit* note 3:38.

17. *ibid*: 39-40.

18. *ibid*: 39.

19. Laws WG. The floating hospital of the River Tyne Port Sanitary Authority. *Proc Munic & Sanit Eng*. 1887-88; *14*:7-18, and TWAD 604R1236 *Annual Report* for 1886, with appended plans and elevations.

20. The *SS Transit* (1334 grt), built for Wilhelm Wilhelmsen in 1889, with her straight stem, well deck, long raised quarter deck and counter stern, was a typical product of the yard. Turnbull L. *Discovering your Neighbourhood: an Introduction to Local Studies*. Gateshead Metrop Bor Counc Dept of Educ. nd, unpag.

21. TWAD 604R1180 & 1191 (Annual statements of receipts and expenditure by the Port Sanitary Authority).

22. See n19. See also TWAD 604R1236, *Annual Report* for 1888:13. 'The pontoon hospital floats steadily in the roughest weather. There is sufficient depth of water round her at low water neap tides.' There is a fine scale model of the hospital in the Dept of Maritime History, Newcastle Museum of Science and Engineering.

23. Stainthorpe TW. The floating hospital belonging to the River Tees Port Sanitary Authority. *Proc Incorp Ass Munic & County Eng* 1894-95; *21*:55-68.

24. War Office. *Memoranda on Medical Diseases in Tropical & Sub- Tropical Areas*, 1941. London: HMSO, 1941:23.

25. Humble R. *Before the Dreadnought. The Royal Navy from Nelson to Fisher*. London: Macdonald and Jane's, 1976:164-5. I am grateful to the Maritime Information Centre at the National Maritime Museum for providing me with details of the *Barrozo*.

26. Bullmore C. Notes on beri-beri at Falmouth. *Pub Health* Jan 1903:198-211.

27. Osler W. *Principles and Practice of Medicine*. New York & London: D Appleton & Co (8th ed), 1912:414-5.

28. The outbreak of beri-beri on the *Barrozo* was fully reported by Edmund Harker in his *Annual Report* for 1909 (pub 1910):30-32. TWAD 604R1195.

29. I am grateful to the Maritime Information Centre at the National Maritime Museum for providing me with details of the *Bellailsa* and a copy of the British Master's Certificate of Competency (No 010168) of Captain Ole Olsen Aagaard, which records his career.

30. Edmund Harker gives full details of this outbreak of plague in his *Annual Report* for 1912 (pub 1913):24-26. TWAD 604R1195.

31. TWAD 604R1237 *Annual Report* for 1895 (pub 1896):17-18.

32. TWAD 604R1195 *Annual Report* for 1914 (pub 1915):6.

Chapter 21

DENTAL EDUCATION AND PROVISION OF SERVICES IN THE NORTH EAST OF ENGLAND

GEM Hallett

Dental disease is as old as mankind, capable of causing great pain and discomfort and, in ancient times, occasionally death. Yet dentistry was not to develop into an organized discipline in Great Britain until the mid-19th century. The first landmark was the formation of the General Medical Council in 1858, representing all the Licensing Bodies and Universities, with additional members nominated by the Privy Council, but it was not until 1898 that the first practising dentist was appointed to this body, namely Charles Tomes. In mid-century there was no restriction upon the type or qualifications of any person engaging in the practice of dentistry so, in an effort to impose such control in the public interest and to encourage ethical professional standards, the Dentists' Act of 1878 created a register of those approved as 'specially qualified to practise dentistry', together with their approved titles. All legally qualified medical practitioners were also entitled to practise dentistry. By 1902, out of 4641 enrolled on the Dentists' Register, 43.3% were in possession of a dental qualification granted by the Royal Colleges of Surgeons of England, Edinburgh, Glasgow or Ireland, whilst 55.8% were admitted solely on their being able to demonstrate that they were over 21 years of age and in *bona fide* dental practice.

The 1878 act had certain weaknesses and in 1921 a new Act was passed to confine the practice of dentistry to those who had followed a GMC-approved course and who had qualified for a recognised diploma or degree. But, as in 1878, all those who were then in dental practice and over 21 years of age were admitted to the Dentists' Register. Once more a large influx of the latter group were admitted so that by 1924, although the number of qualified dentists had risen to 5032, 'dentists 1921' (as they came to be known) had risen from 2587 in 1902 to 7301. Control of the dental profession now reposed in a Dental Board which was under the aegis of the General Medical Council, but with cross-representation between the two bodies. A further Act of Parliament in 1956 defined the profession of dentistry and its regulation, this time by a totally independent General Dental Council replacing the old Dental Board. Six members of the GMC however still sat as members of the GDC, but for matters of education only.

The establishment of the Newcastle Dental Hospital

If dentistry hardly existed as a cohesive profession in London in the mid-19th century, the provinces were even less organized. There had been some resident and highly-regarded full-time practitioners in Newcastle since the beginning of the century, but others merely combined cupping with extractions, or were primarily pharmacists (such as James Eno), but extended their services to dentistry, which in some instances became their principal occupation. There was also a small coterie of medically-qualified men styling themselves 'surgeons practising dental surgery' who wielded considerable political influence. Otherwise there was little professional unity, with the result that, when in 1894 all six licentiates in dental surgery practising in the city were called together by Robert Lacy Markham, it was remarked how little personal contact each had with his colleagues; until 1890 they had largely practised as single individuals, privately and for their own financial interests. However the honorary dental surgeons attached to various medical charities in the city had treated dental patients, albeit predominantly by extractions.

In 1894, the annual meeting of the British Dental Association had met for the first time in Newcastle, undoubtedly providing a spur for many of the northern practitioners to meet each other and exchange ideas. This, together with the simultaneous release by the BDA of their sponsored 'Fourth Report on School Children's Teeth', most probably underlay Markham's proposition in the December that Newcastle should become an academic and collegiate centre for northern dentistry. There was an urgent need for the establishment of a dental hospital, both for the treatment of the necessitous poor, and as a centre which would be recognised by the Royal Colleges as providing suitable clinical training for dental students. An organising committee was formed, and advice sought from the staff of the existing Edinburgh Dental Hospital; following these investigations a Committee of Management met officially for the first time on 23 May 1895. Premises were leased on the corner of Clayton and Nelson Streets, and on 22 April 1895 there was a formal (and widely reported) opening of the new dental hospital by the Mayor of Newcastle. This marked the real start for dentistry as a formal profession in the North of England. In London, the Odontological Society for the scientific study of aspects of dentistry had been formed in 1857, but it had very few provincial members. So, in Newcastle in 1894, the North of England Odontological Society was formed with the same objectives; it remains an active body to this day.

Earlier, in 1881, a notice had appeared in the *Sunderland Daily Post*, proposing that a dental hospital should be built for the town (population then 130 000) and that a local dentist, Mr GF Tate LDS RCS (1880), who also practised in Blackett Street, Newcastle, should have an honorary appointment to it. This scheme provoked much acrimonious comment in the lay and professional press regarding Tate's personal standing, with the result that it all came to naught. Tate left Newcastle for Cairo, and thence to Smyrna, disappearing from the Dentists' Register in 1900. It is interesting to speculate upon the possible development of dentistry in the North of England had the suggested dental hospital been actively supported and achieved by the Sunderland civic authority and the regional dentists at that time.

During the twelve years the Nelson Street hospital was functioning there was such a demand for treatment that it became quite clear that more commodious premises were urgently needed. Various abortive alternatives were explored, until finally the Committee of Management negotiated a lease on the top floor of Handyside's Building (now demolished). The move took place in 1907 and occupation lasted until 1931. In the meantime the Newcastle Dental Hospital had become the centre for dental education in the North of England, with a close association with the College of Medicine, and its training was recognised by all four Royal Colleges of Surgeons for their Licence in Dental Surgery. In 1916 the University of Durham instituted its own Licence in Dental Surgery and thereby became a Dental Authority recognised by the GMC. (After 1963, when the then Federated Colleges of Durham and Newcastle divided to form separate universities, Newcastle became a Dental Authority in place of Durham and granted Bachelor and Doctoral degrees in Dental Surgery. The former Licence in Dental Surgery (Dunelm) was abandoned).

The First World War years

This was a period of upheaval for all training establishments and, there being no national military service at this time, many recruits and volunteers had to be rejected on account of their dental inadequacy. At the outbreak of war no dental surgeons were included in the army medical services. Dentists and dental students were not excused from military service, with the result that at Newcastle both staff and student numbers were seriously depleted; indeed, four students lost their lives overseas through enemy action. At the hospital the staff, who were all part-time, agreed early in 1915 that the hospital should be opened in the afternoon and evenings for the dental treatment of HM Forces, and in particular for the Tyneside Scottish Battalion of the Northumberland Fusiliers. A great deal of treatment was effected, mainly tooth extractions and the supply of dentures. Later, this arrangement gave way to the formation of a 'Panel of Dental Surgeons' for the district to undertake military dental work. The operative procedures were thus transferred to the individual dentists' surgeries and controlled by an executive committee which had been set up, the Newcastle Dental Hospital becoming the 'Distributive Centre'; an Indenture was published (approved by the BDA) and was signed by 46 dentists. This arrangement worked for nearly a year, but by the end of 1916 the Army had decided to assume independent responsibility for the dental treatment of troops. The details of how this service operated are difficult to elucidate. Although the Navy had serving dental officers with the rank of t/surgeon lieutenant(D) RNVR in November 1918, and an established Royal Naval Dental Service by January 1920, it was not until January 1921 that the Army Dental Corps was authorised by Royal Warrant (becoming the Royal Army Dental Corps in December 1946).

Another public service was the provision of dental examinations and treatment for children in approved homes. Arrangements had been made in 1910 for them to be examined by various members of the dental hospital staff, but in 1913 this service was discontinued and letters written to the Boards of

Guardians suggested that they should appoint a private practitioner to do this work. It may be noted that the children from these homes displayed a remarkable relative immunity to dental caries which attracted national interest and which tended to be attributed to the simple institutional dietary regime. By the end of the war there was an acute national dearth of dental surgeons and the Services began to return some of the former dental students who had been combatants, to enable them to resume their dental studies. At Newcastle the number of students had fallen until, in 1917, only three students remained in the Hospital. By 1920 grants had been made by the Board of Education to 27 students, and by the following year 34 students were in receipt of bursaries.

The establishment of school dental services

Throughout the 19th century and for the first quarter of the 20th, very little attention had been given in the UK to the dental needs of children, although at one of the earliest meetings of the Odontological Society in London in 1857, Samuel Maclean had drawn attention to the very bad state of many young people in the first decade of life and had recommended the early extraction of all four permanent molars when 'attacked with caries at an early period of life'. The BDA had sponsored a series of investigations into the condition of children's teeth and had published seven reports between 1891 and 1898 (the 1894 one in Newcastle); recommendations regarding dental inspection and treatment had also been made to Boards of Guardians or Management of schools. In 1895 William McPherson Fisher of Dundee, at an annual meeting of the BDA held in Cambridge, stressed the urgent need for compulsory attention to the teeth of schoolchildren. This paper was one of the most influential in the annals of dentistry for children, but it was not until 1926 that there were appointments of Dental Staff to the Ministry of Health and to the Board of Education.

In Northumberland in 1931 the school dental service consisted of one full-time and one part-time dental officer for 40 000 school children. They worked entirely from a 'mobile dental van'. At this time Mr AE Robinson was appointed as whole-time senior dental officer; the measure of his zeal and the efficient development of the dental services during his direction is the fact that when he retired, in 1972, the school dental service was staffed by 31 dental officers, and there were 17 mobile surgeries and a laboratory with 5 technicians. He was also appointed in 1942 as part-time lecturer in Community Dentistry at the University, a post which he held for 30 years. His successor as chief dental officer for Northumberland, Mr Colin Carmichael, also held this part-time lectureship until his retirement in 1990, by which time he was (following changes in the pattern of National Health Service and Local Authority Community Health Service Administration) first, Area Dental Officer to the Newcastle AHA(T) and subsequently, District Dental Officer to the Newcastle Health Authority. During this period of change the Northumberland Community Dental Service shrank to some 10 officers as other Districts were created and took over much of Northumberland County Council's former Health responsibilities.

The third Dental Hospital building

The Handyside's buildings in Percy Street functioned as the Dental Hospital for nearly a quarter of a century (always staffed by part-time practitioners), but the ever present ambition of the successive deans, JT Jameson and J Coltman, had been to see a dental hospital and school within the precincts of the Royal Victoria Infirmary. It was Coltman who succeeded in attracting the interest of a local industrialist/ship builder, Sir Arthur Sutherland, who in 1931 gave £12 000 to the furtherance of these objectives. Together with supplementary funds from the Dental Board of the United Kingdom, this enabled a new school building to be erected on Queen Victoria Road. It was grafted on to a 'temporary building' which had been erected during the 1914 - 18 war for the rehabilitation of war wounded, and was converted into the new Dental Hospital and equipped with all that was then considered clinically necessary. Only minimal provision was made at this time for research into dental disease and associated afflictions, but these two buildings became the third home for dental education in the North of England, the only establishment of its kind between Edinburgh and Leeds. The new premises were opened on 28 Jan 1932 by the Marquis of Londonderry, Chancellor of the University of Durham.

Members of the Dental Board in London were ever anxious to promote dentistry as an academic discipline. Liverpool had had the first full-time Chair of Dental Surgery (established in 1920), followed soon afterwards by Leeds, Manchester, Birmingham and Edinburgh, with most of these (though not Liverpool) being supported 50% financially by the Dental Board. By 1932 Coltman was approaching retirement, and it was felt to be an urgent matter to appoint a full-time Professor of Dental Surgery at Newcastle. A chair was established to which Dr Robert Bradlaw from London was appointed in 1936, and his arrival produced a dynamic surge forward in dental education. This was well demonstrated when the annual meeting of the BDA took place in Newcastle in 1939, attended by many distinguished dentists from both home and abroad, and again forming a focus for national and northern regional practitioners to meet.

With the outbreak of the second World War history repeated itself: public dental services and practitioners' services inevitably diminished as students, younger staff and practitioners left for the now established Dental Services of the Army, Navy and Air Force. By 1945 Robert Bradlaw, who was well aware of the great demand there would be for dentistry on a national scale in the near future, was pressing the authorities for much larger accommodation and increased staff. The only way to accomplish this was to leave the RVI site, move to the former Medical College in Northumberland Road (by now empty) and convert it into a dental school and hospital. Once more Sir Arthur Sutherland provided substantial funds (£50 000) towards the cost of the necessary extensive alterations and thus Dental School and Hospital number 4 was opened on the 28 May 1948 by the Rt Hon Aneurin Bevan MP, the Minister of Health. By this time the staff had been augmented to 3 full time professors, 2 readers and 3 lecturers, and there were five separate departments, including for the first time one of Children's Dentistry (later named the Department of Child Dental Health). Preventive measures now began to assume a much more dominant role in dental education than heretofore and the first chair in children's dentistry in the UK was created in Newcastle in 1951.

The introduction of the National Health Service

The School and Hospital remained in Northumberland Road for 30 years. During this time the impact of the National Health Service was enormous and dentistry was wrenched almost forcibly out of its traditional pattern of education and delivery of service to the public. Suitably qualified practitioners were graded as consultants; oral surgery and orthodontics became the first two recognised dental specialties, and a proper training scheme was formulated. It was clear that Cumberland, Co Durham, and Northumberland would need specialist dental services, so an advisory dental committee to the Regional Hospital Board was set up with two specialist advisers, which led in the 1950s to the establishment of dental centres at Sunderland General Hospital and at Carlisle. At first one oral surgeon and one orthodontist were appointed, having the onerous task of dividing their services between these widely separated centres. In the early 1960s these appointments were doubled and a dental centre was set up in Middlesborough General Hospital, officially opened in October 1963. More recently these centres have enlarged further and in concert with the Regional Post-graduate Institute for Medicine and Dentistry in Newcastle have formed an integral part of the delivery of post-graduate dental education in the North of England.

The North of England Regional Hospital Board was the Authority dealing with an enormous geographic area: its northern boundary was the Scottish border; on the east coast it stretched south to Staithes and crossed England to Barrow-in-Furness in the west. The population in the 1950s was about 3 200 000, largely concentrated on Tyneside, Teesside, Sunderland, Durham and Carlisle. The logistics, which were formidable, led over the years to several re-organisations of the administrative systems, during which a considerable number of new hospitals were commissioned. But this time, as each was planned, first-class dental accommodation was included, together with permanent or visiting clinical dental and supporting staff. By 1992 the number of full time dental consultants for the northern region, outwith the Newcastle Teaching School and Hospital, had risen to 12 (8 oral surgeons and 4 orthodontists).

In the decades following 1948 there were a series of cathartic upheavals in the field of general practice. The long-established pattern of a single-handed practitioner with one or two dental technicians working on the premises could no longer sustain the demands of a busy NHS practice. The dentist's remuneration was derived on a quite different basis from that of medical practices and was assessed from time to time by reviews of fees for items of treatment. The rapid development of technical methods and the advances in clinical knowledge emanating from the teaching and research centres meant that the necessary range of expertise could no longer be provided by one practitioner. Technical work was increasingly sent out to laboratories where technicians to the profession set up entrepreneurial establishments, independent of the dentist and making their own charges.

This produced an irreversible change in pattern of the delivery of dentistry to the patient. It also made it more expensive. Except for certain priority groups, all NHS patients now have to contribute substantially towards the cost of their dental treatment; the one-time cornerstone of free treatment for all is unlikely to be restored. However the importance of dental health has, since the last war, been progressively recognised by the public. In the North of England the era when young people, especially young women, were encouraged to have all their relatively sound teeth extracted and replaced by dentures before getting married, so as to forestall future dental expense, is now mercifully consigned to history. Dentistry, costly though undoubtedly it often is, is now widely accepted as one of the ineluctable health measures for children, adults and the ever increasing number of elderly and aged persons in our modern society.

The Dental School and Hospital since 1960

Towards the end of the 1950s, the School and Hospital in Northumberland Road had become alarmingly restricted, both in internal space and surroundings (especially in the matter of car parking). For two years Professor Bradlaw and the senior staff studied with an appointed architect the possibility of extending the existing building by completing the fourth side of the square, but in 1960 Bradlaw accepted the headship of the Dental Post-Graduate Institute in London and soon afterwards also became President of the General Dental Council. At the time of his departure there were 333 dental students and the school had an intake of 75 each year, although it had the equipment and clinical accommodation for a yearly entry of only 50–55. Professor Maurice Hallett, who had held the Chair of Children's Dentistry since 1952, was appointed Dean in succession to Bradlaw, and together with senior colleagues studied the problem afresh. There was only one solution – to build a completely new Dental School and Hospital to accommodate an annual intake of 75 students, to return to the RVI site, and to build there in such a way that the projected new Medical School and Ward Block would be contiguous.

This is not the place to describe the tortuous planning problems of the next fifteen years. Suffice it to say that the urgency of the situation was recognised by the University, the Regional Hospital Board and the Board of

Governors of the RVI. The University Grants Committee and the Department of Health and Social Security concurred, and the Dental School and Hospital were accepted as being in Phase I of the development of the 8.5 acre site north of the RVI. Eventually building operations started in 1974 and the new Dental School and Hospital, with an overall area of nearly 100 000 sq ft and costing over £5m (the fifth in its long history since 1895 and the first to be custom planned), was opened on 15 Sept 1978 by the Chancellor of the University, the Duke of Northumberland. By this time Hallett, who had been Dean since 1960, had retired, to be succeeded by Professor Roy Storer, who had held the Chair of Dental Prosthetics since 1968. He held the deanship until his retirement in September 1992 and saw through the important period when the Dental School and Hospital were joined by the new Medical School, opened by the Queen Mother on 6 Nov 1984, and the later completion of the new Ward Block and the full development of the site. Storer's successor as Dean of Dentistry has been John Murray, formerly Professor of Child Dental Health, who had succeeded Hallett in 1977. Although the School had been planned for an agreed yearly intake of 75 students there was a change in government policy in the early 1980s, when it was thought that the total national intake of dental students should be reduced, with the closure of some schools and the amalgamation of others. Newcastle's intake was reduced to 70, but it nevertheless remains one of the largest dental schools and hospitals in the country and a vigorous centre for academic advancement and research.

Supporting services

Clinical dentistry has always required support services. The earliest of these were the dental mechanics, from whose ranks before 1921 many practising dentists evolved. After the war, the term 'mechanic' was rejected in favour of 'technician'. There has long been a wish on a part of the technician body to include the clinical provision of dentures within their legal remit; in Canada they already do this as 'denturists', but such practice is not currently permitted in the UK.

Dentists have always also needed chairside assistance for efficient treatment of patients. There is now a training school for dental surgery assistants at Newcastle; they form an essential part of the team. Since the creation of the GDC, dental hygienists have also been recognised as essential members of the same team and formal training centres have been created in all dental hospitals.

In the early 1950s there was much interest in the vocation of a 2-year trained person who could carry out what were termed certain simple fillings and extractions. Such a system had been set up first in Malaya and then in New Zealand, where they were known as 'dental nurses', and the training school was at Wellington. In this country a school for a 2-year training course was opened at New Cross Hospital, London, by Enoch Powell on 9 Dec 1960; the enterprise was monitored and funded by the DHSS and the new profession governed by the GDC. Those qualified were first called 'dental auxiliaries' and later 'dental therapists'. Many local authorities, including some in the north of England, furbished their existing dental centres expensively with new equipment, hoping that economies could be made by employing personnel less costly than fully trained dentists. In the event, the scheme did not have the success for which the government had hoped because manpower in the Community services improved, caries in children lessened (as a result of fluoridation), and more dental practitioners were prepared to treat them. The New Cross School closed on the recommendation of the Dental Strategy Review Group in 1981, although the London Dental Hospital continues to train a small number of young women for this work.

The future of the dental services

The future of general dental practice in 1993 and beyond is fraught with considerable anxiety. No system of remuneration has, so far, been found which satisfies for long the government (as pay master) and the practitioners of NHS dentistry equally. Many dentists are today changing from whole-time NHS to part-time, or even whole-time private practice. A distressing number have already been declared bankrupt. Yet since the implementation of the National Health Service Act of 1946 in May 1948, by which dentistry probably received its greatest impetus by becoming an integral part of the NHS, the political shibboleth of 'free health treatment for all' has been found to be not economically sustainable. A recent Parliamentary Committee under the chairmanship of a distinguished civil servant, Sir Kenneth Bloomfield, has carried out an intensive survey of the many problems of finance and administration in National Health dentistry. The result, reported in January 1993, is an extensive document of observation and suggestions but without definite recommendations. It has been cautiously received by the profession, and a great deal of debate will follow. It would be most unwise to attempt any prediction of what changes it may lead to, but it is devoutly to be hoped that, as a result, a formula may be achieved to which the dental profession can accede and thus consolidate the great advances in the provision of dental care made in the UK, to which the North of England with its academic centre in Newcastle upon Tyne has contributed so much over the last century.

Acknowledgments

I am indebted to Dr AS Hargreaves for her great help in the preparation of my manuscript and also for many valuable editorial suggestions. Also, I must thank Mrs Vera Dyer, my former secretary, for so diligently extracting many important items of interest from the early annals of the Dental Hospital and School. I am grateful to Mrs Muriel Cohen, former librarian of the British Dental Association, who discovered the interesting and enigmatic item regarding Mr GF Tate in 1880.

Chapter 22

GEORGE REDMAYNE MURRAY 1865 – 1939

The first use of thyroid extract for the treatment of myxoedema

C N Armstrong

George Murray was born in Newcastle upon Tyne in 1865, son of a physician, William Murray. He was educated at Eton where he rowed in the Eton crew, then at Trinity College, Cambridge, and he had his clinical training at University College Hospital, London, where he won a gold medal. He graduated MB (Cantab) in 1889 and MD in 1896. After graduating at Cambridge he spent two years in Paris and Berlin. He then returned to Newcastle upon Tyne in 1890 where he was appointed Pathologist to the Hospital for Sick Children and Lecturer in Bacteriology and Comparative Anatomy at the University of Durham.

At the monthly meeting of the Northumberland and Durham Medical Society on Thursday 12 February 1891, held in the library of the Royal Infirmary, Newcastle upon Tyne, with Dr Drummond in the chair and 54 members present (no cars! they had to come on foot, by horse or in a carriage), George Murray was present and showed a case of myxoedema. The minutes give a detailed record of the case, of Murray's opinion that myxoedema was due to loss of an active internal secretion of the thyroid gland, and of his proposal to treat the patient with an extract of the thyroid (Appendix 1).

Sir Walter Langdon-Brown in his Inaugural Presidential Address to the Section of Endocrinology, Royal Society of Medicine in 1946 entitled 'The Birth of Modern Endocrinology' said the birth took place in Newcastle upon Tyne. He had been a personal friend of George Murray and he had from Murray's own lips what took place at the meeting in 1891.

> Modern endocrinology dates from 1891. A Committee had been appointed to investigate the cause of myxoedema, which was recognised to be associated with the failure of function of the thyroid gland. But the tendency was to regard the disease as due to a failure of excretion, which, indeed, the bloated aspect of the myxoedematous patient might well suggest. ... Victor Horsley was the secretary of this Committee and G.R.Murray, who had worked with him at University College Hospital, suggested that the condition was due not to a failure of excretion but to the loss of an active internal secretion. To emphasize his faith in his hypothesis, he showed a case of myxoedema at a meeting of the Newcastle and Northumberland Medical Society and said that he proposed to treat it by an extract of thyroid gland.
>
> I had the story of what followed from Murray's own lips. A senior member of the Society said that it would be just as sensible to treat a case of locomotor ataxy with an emulsion of spinal cord. Undeterred Murray made arrangements with a slaughterhouse to be allowed to

dissect out sheep's thyroids under antiseptic precautions. The Medical School at Newcastle refused him any facilities, but Armstrong College came to his assistance and gave him a room in which to prepare his extracts. A year later he triumphantly showed the case of myxoedema which had been cured by his extracts before the same Society.[1]

At the meeting of the Northumberland Durham Medical Society on 8 October 1891, with Dr Gowan in the chair and 46 members present, Murray showed his case again after six months treatment with injection of thyroid extract, cured (Appendix 2).

Murray reported the case at the Annual Meeting of the British Medical Association at Bournemouth, in July 1891, and published his 'Note on the treatment of myxoedema by hypodermic injections of an extract of the thyroid gland of a sheep' in the BMJ on 10 October.[2] In Aug 1892 he published further results in a paper entitled 'Remarks on the treatment of myxoedema with thyroid juice, with notes of four cases'[3] and later, in 1900, his book *Diseases of the thyroid gland*.[4]

In 1893 Murray was appointed Heath Professor in Comparative Pathology at the University of Durham and, in 1898, Honorary Physician to the Royal Infirmary. In the same year he became a Fellow of the Royal College of Physicians of London; he delivered the Goulstonian Lecture in 1899 and the Bradshaw Lecture in 1905 on 'Exophthalmic goitre and its treatment'. In 1908 he was offered, and accepted, the Chair of Medicine at the University of Manchester, and was also appointed Physician to the Royal Infirmary, Manchester. He continued his interest in thyroid diseases. During the 1914-18 War he served in the Royal Army Medical Corps, and for a short time afterwards, with the grade of Colonel, he served in Italy. He became a member of the Medical Research Committee. He retired in 1925, and died in 1939.

Appendix 1[5]

Northumberland and Durham Medical Society Session 1890-91

February Meeting

THE FIFTH MONTHLY MEETING of this Society was held in the Library of the Royal Infirmary, Newcastle upon Tyne, on the evening of Thursday, 12th February, 1891 — Dr Drummond (President) in the chair. Fifty four members present.

Myxoedema

Dr GEORGE MURRAY: I have brought this patient before you this evening as a good typical case of myxoedema, and also because I wish to have your opinion upon a mode of treatment which I believe to be new, and which I propose to try in this case.

This patient is a woman of 46, she has had a family of nine children, of whom six are living. Four or five years ago, her relations first noticed that her speech and actions were becoming very slow, and she, herself, began to feel that it was a great effort to do her ordinary housework. Her features gradually became enlarged and thickened. The hands and feet also increased in size and altered somewhat in shape. At the present time she presents most of the characteristic symptoms of myxoedema. She complains of langour, great sensitiveness to cold, and a disinclination to see strangers. The features are notably thickened. This change is well seen in the alae nasi and lips. The connective tissue of the eyelids and beneath the eyes is swollen and oedematous in appearance. It, however, does not "pit" on pressure being made, nor would any fluid exude if it were pricked as in the oedema of Bright's disease. The cheeks have the characteristic pink colouration in the centre. The tongue is not unusually large at the present time, though the patient tells me that it was enlarged at an earlier period of her illness. The hands and feet are both enlarged; the former have that peculiar shape which has been described as "spade-like". The skin is dry, and the superficial layers of the epidermis are constantly being shed. The hair is very fine in texture, and a considerable quantity of it has been lost. Her speech, you will notice, is remarkably slow. No thyroid gland can be felt in the neck. The urine contains no albumin.

This peculiar disease, as is now well known, is due to the absence of the thyroid gland. It has followed the removal of this gland for goitre in man, as was pointed out by Prof. Kocher of Berne. Mr Victor Horsley has also succeeded in producing the same disease in monkeys by the removal of the thyroid. The symptoms, then, are due to the absence from the system of some substance which is secreted by the normal thyroid gland. Attempts have been made to supply this deficiency, by grafting portions of the thyroid gland of one of the lower animals under the skin or in the peritoneal cavity of myxoedematous patients. This operation has been followed by great improvement in the patient's condition, though the symptoms have reappeared when the grafted piece of gland atrophied.

In one case, Bettencourt and Serrano, of Lisbon, introduced the half of a sheep's thyroid gland beneath the skin of the infra-mammary region on each side. This was followed by an improvement which commenced the day after the operation. They concluded from this that the improvement was not due to the implanted gland becoming vascularised, and so able to carry out its normal function, but to the absorption of the juice of the grafted thyroid into the circulation.

It has occurred to me that it would be worthwhile to try the hypodermic injection of an emulsion or extract of the thyroid gland of a sheep. This treatment appears to be rational, and, at any rate, would not harm the patient. We may, I think, by this means hope to produce as much improvement in a case of myxoedema as was brought about by the absorption of the juice of the gland which had been introduced beneath the skin, and it has the advantage of being a much simpler proceeding.

Dr. GOWANS said the case that Dr. Murray has just shown to the Society is undoubtedly one of myxoedema. Besides the usual facial and cutaneous symptoms which characterise the peculiar malady, he wished to draw attention to a sub-normal temperature of no less that two degrees in Dr. Murray's patient; also the thyroid gland could not be felt; and an interesting fact in the life history of the patient, that of severe haemorrhages at one period. In his experience, extending over a considerable number of cases, the history of severe bleedings was almost invariably present. In regard to the treatment, Dr. Murray proposed to adopt in his case, it certainly was a novel and original one. He, however, cautioned Dr. Murray against hurriedly coming to a favourable opinion of its effects, as patients suffering from myxoedema frequently had periods of apparent improvement, especially during mild weather. As a surgeon he felt much inclined to adopt the procedure recommended by Horsley, of grafting thyroid tissue. In answer to Dr. Morison's question as to how long he had had cases of myxoedema under observation, he begged to state that he had the pleasure of exhibiting the first case recognised in the North of England, about twelve years ago, to the members of the Society; and that the patient he has had under his observation for eighteen or nineteen years. She is still alive, and in somewhat better condition than when exhibited here.

Appendix 2[6]

A Case of Myxoedema Treated by Hypodermic Injections of the Thyroid Gland of a Sheep

Dr. GEORGE MURRAY: I showed this patient at the February meeting of this Society, and then suggested treating her by means of hypodermic injections of an extract of the thyroid gland of a sheep. As is well known this disease is due to the loss of function of the thyroid gland, so it was hoped that this treatment would in part, at least, compensate for that deficiency and relieve the symptoms of the disease.

The patient, a woman of 46, has been ill for about five years, and last February she was a typical case of myxoedema. There was a considerable amount of solid oedema of the face and hands especially. The upper eyelids were so much enlarged that she found it difficult to look upwards, and all the features were considerably thickened. The hands were large and "spade-like", the skin was dry and scaly, for she had not perspired for four years; the hair was fine and scanty; the speech was slow and drawling; she was slow in thought and action; she complained of languor, disinclination to see strangers, and sensitiveness to cold. The temperature was sub-normal, as it varied between 96.4 and 97.2 deg.F.

The treatment commenced in April, and during the last six months extracts of eight lobes of thyroid glands of sheep have been injected. Those of you who have seen the patient before will notice that a striking improvement has taken place. The subcutaneous solid oedema has greatly diminished and has practically disappeared from the hands; the lips are much smaller; the swelling of the upper eyelids has so much diminished and most of the natural wrinkles have returned; the speech has improved so that scarcely any drawl is now to be noticed; her mental processes seem to take place more rapidly, and the memory has improved, so that she is no longer afraid of going out alone. She menstruated normally in May, June and July. The skin is much less dry, and she perspires when out walking. She is no longer so sensitive to cold, and the temperature, is practically normal. The hair has begun to grow again so that she now has a considerable quantity of new short hair on the head.

The extract is prepared in the following manner: – One lobe of the thyroid gland of a freshly killed sheep is cut into small pieces, and mixed with 1 cubic centimetre of glycerine and 1 cubic centimetre of a 0.5% solution of carbolic acid. This mixture is allowed to stand in a test tube closed with a plug of cotton wool for 18 to 24 hours. All vessels and instruments used in the preparation should either be sterilised by heat or thoroughly cleansed with a 1 in 20 solution of carbolic acid. The mixture is placed in a fine handkerchief which has previously been placed for a few minutes in boiling water, and as much fluid as possible is squeezed through it. By this means 3 cubic centimetres of a turbid pink liquid are obtained. 1.5 cubic centimetres (25 minims) of this may be injected twice during a week, and should be repeated every other week. In this way a patient receives the extract of one lobe each fortnight. The injections are made with an ordinary hypodermic syringe beneath the loose skin of the back between the shoulder blades. The syringe and the surface of the skin are both carefully cleansed with a 1 in 20 solution of carbolic acid.

Dr. REDMOND remembered the condition of the patient when before the Society in February, and thought Dr. Murray was to be congratulated upon the manifest improvement resulting from the original treatment he had been since carrying out; and hoped the Society would, later on, be afforded an opportunity of observing its further progress.

The PRESIDENT endorsed the improvement detailed by Dr. Murray. When the case was first shewn he had warned members not to jump to any conclusions while treating such cases, since the patients varied greatly, being better in summer and worse in winter. He had not been prepared to find such an improvement as he now saw in the patient, and he was inclined to believe that this improvement was due to the treatment.

He understood Dr. Murray to say that he did not expect to cure the case, but merely to stay its progress and improve the general condition of the patient.

Appendix 3

There are further related entries in the *Proceedings*. On 11 Feb 1892 Murray showed another case of myxoedema (a woman of 52 who had a 12 year history and had been in the Hospital for Incurables for 5 years). Injections of thyroid extract, started in Nov 1891, had continued weekly for 16 weeks and she had improved impressively. He also showed his first patient again:

> The third patient is the case I have shewn here twice before. I have brought her here this evening, to shew you the improvement which you saw had taken place in her last October, after six months' treatment, has been fully maintained through the winter, though she has only had eight injections of 25 minims each since October. At one time I left off the injections, as I wished to see how soon the symptoms of myxoedema would return. After five weeks the old symptoms began to reappear, but they soon disappeared again on renewing the injections once a week.[7]

On 22 Dec 1892 he showed a third case, also improving with the same treatment, and 'some photographs of men and women with myxoedema who had been treated by the same method, and who were very greatly improved.' In discussion 'Dr. Allison mentioned a case of myxoedema in which he had obtained much improvement by the patient eating a fried fresh sheep's thyroid every morning at breakfast.'[8]

Finally, at the meeting on 9 Feb 1893 Murray reported, under the title 'Two cases of myxoedema treated by taking thyroid extract by the mouth',

> I am sorry that the first patient I wished to shew you has not arrived. She was the first case of myxoedema which was successfully treated by thyroid extract. I first shewed her here two years ago, and at that time suggested the treatment by injections of thyroid extract, which I soon after carried out. Eight months later (October, 1891), I shewed her here again, and you were able to see what a great improvement had taken place in her condition. At the present time she shews no sign of myxoedema, and is kept in this excellent state of health by taking one drachm of thyroid extract during each week in doses of ten minims in water each morning by the mouth.'

He also showed his second case again who now had 'scarcely a sign of myxoedema', and he mentioned other successfully treated cases. The extract for oral use, consisting of equal parts of thyroid juice and glycerine, was prepared for him by Messrs Brady and Martin, the Newcastle pharmacists. He was able to report that Dr. Robin of Lyons had successfully treated cases of sporadic cretinism (by injections) and that Dr. Vermehren of Copenhagen gave 'the white precipitate, which is obtained by adding alcohol to thyroid extract, in pills'.[9]

References

1. Langdon-Brown W. The birth of modern endocrinology. *Proc Roy Soc Med* 1946, *39*: 570-510.
2. Murray GR. Note on the treatment of myxoedema by hypodermic injections of an extract of the thyroid gland of a sheep. *Brit Med J* 1891, *2*: 796-7. On the next page appeared a short note by E Hurry Fenwick, Surgeon to the London Hospital, reporting success in treating myxoedema by the same technique, but his observations were short-term and he concentrated on the diuretic effect of the injected extract.
3. Murray GR. Remarks on the treatment of myxoedema with thyroid juice, with notes of four cases. *Brit Med J* 1892, *2*: 449-50. The paper had been presented to the Pathology Section at the BMA Annual Meeting in Nottingham, in July, with Victor Horsley, the President, in the chair. There was discussion by several speakers with experience of using injections of thyroid extract. In this paper Murray published photographs of his second case before and after treatment.

   It was actually during this meeting (on 27 July 1892) that HW Mackenzie first tried the effect of treating myxoedema by mouth with fresh thyroid glands (Mackenzie HW. A case of myxoedema treated with great benefit by feeding with fresh thyroid glands. *Brit Med J* 1892, *2*: 940- 41.) His paper was published together with one by Dr. Fox of Plymouth who treated his patients with a combination of oral thyroid extract, and 'half a thyroid, lightly fried and minced, to be taken with currant jelly once a week.' Twice a week, he found, caused thyrotoxic symptoms.
4. Murray GR. *Diseases of the thyroid gland*. London: HK Lewis, 1900.
5. *Proc Northumb Durh Med Soc* Session 1890-91, pp 91-3.
6. Minutes of the Oct 1891 meeting of the Society. *Proc Northumb Durh Med Soc* Session 1891-2, pp 12-14.
7. *ibid* pp 63-65.
8. *ibid* Session 1892-3, pp 100-101.
9. *ibid* Session 1892-3, pp 129-30.

Chapter 23

CARDIOLOGY IN NEWCASTLE – THE FIRST 60 YEARS

H A Dewar

The first name that appears to link Newcastle with cardiology is that of Andrew Wilson MD of Newcastle upon Tyne who, in 1774 when he was physician to the Infirmary, published *An Enquiry into the Moving Powers employed in the Circulation of the Blood.*[1] Next would seem to be Professor Sir David Drummond (1852 – 1932), a physician whom Professor Sir William Hume greatly admired and whose chief interests were in nervous and cardiovascular disease.[2] But it was with Hume himself that cardiology in Newcastle effectively began. Son of George Haliburton Hume, a surgeon on the staff of the Infirmary, he was educated in medicine at Cambridge and the London Hospital. He was appointed to the honorary staff of the Royal Victoria Infirmary in 1908 when he was 28 years of age, soon after the hospital had moved from its old position on Forth Banks to its present site. The date of his appointment makes a convenient starting point for this history.

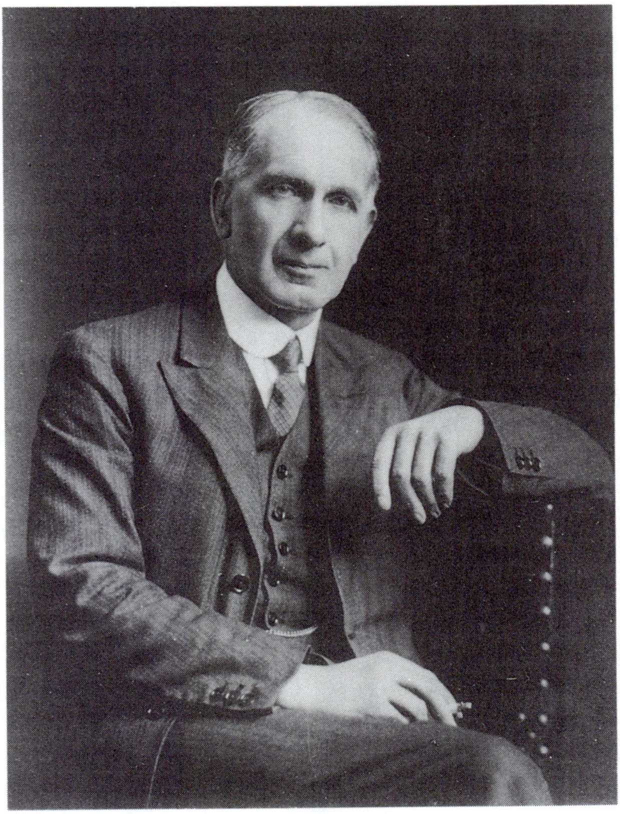

Figure 1. Sir William Hume (1879 – 1960)

In 1908 Newcastle was at the peak of its prosperity. Ships from all over the world docked at its quayside, the swing-bridge opened daily to allow colliers up to load coal at Dunston Staithes and then to pass down again to carry it to London or ports on the Continent. Where now Vickers factory makes a somewhat precarious living manufacturing tanks, Lord Armstrong's Elswick works were turning out every possible kind of armament for the British Army and for the British, Japanese and other navies of the world, and also built the ships that carried them. Huge profits were made, of which the workers received a tiny share, and there was no unemployment. But by modern standards the health of the workforce was deplorable. Industrial injuries were common and uncompensated; tuberculosis and other infective ailments were rampant; and workers' children, if they did not succumb to the complications of measles and whooping cough, would not infrequently become deformed by rickets.

For anyone interested in heart disease, diphtheria and rheumatism in particular invited study. Diphtheria anti-toxin was available and used but there was no prophylaxis and only too often children would present with a choking exudate on tonsils or larynx and a toxic myocarditis whose lethal consequences no amount of anti-toxin could avert. The one remarkable feature was that, if the victim did recover, he or she always did so completely and chronic diphtheritic myocarditis was not an entity. Rheumatism had three classical manifestations – acute rheumatism, commonly called rheumatic fever, with severe but transient arthritis, high fever with night sweats and erythematous rashes in the skin, or the neurological manifestations of chorea (St Vitus' Dance) which mercifully almost never coincided with polyarthritis, or least obvious of all 'growing pains' with slight or no fever, pains in muscles or joints with nothing to see and much debility. Any of the three was likely to be complicated or followed by valve disease. If the patient with acute rheumatism developed pericarditis the accompanying pericardial effusion could be life-threatening unless relieved by aspiration.

Hume's interest in cardiology was evident at once and he made studies of cardiac dysrhythmias especially in diphtheria, then very common. He used the Mackenzie ink polygraph, a much less informative instrument than the electrocardiograph which followed, but a good bit more convenient than the Marey polygraph with smoked drum which Mackenzie himself had first used for his studies in general practice in Burnley. Hume's publication 'A case in which a high speed of the auricles was not accompanied by a high speed of the ventricles' described a condition later labelled atrial flutter. In 1912 he persuaded the Governing body to purchase one of the new Einthoven galvanometers for taking electrocardiograms. It cost £250, a price which hardly changed for the next 40 years.

The first electrocardiogram was of his house physician Charles H Robson, taken on a falling photographic glass plate and, as can be seen in the illustration, was of excellent quality and normal. Sir John Charles, then a medical student, remembered the occasion, a 'Saturday morning and rather

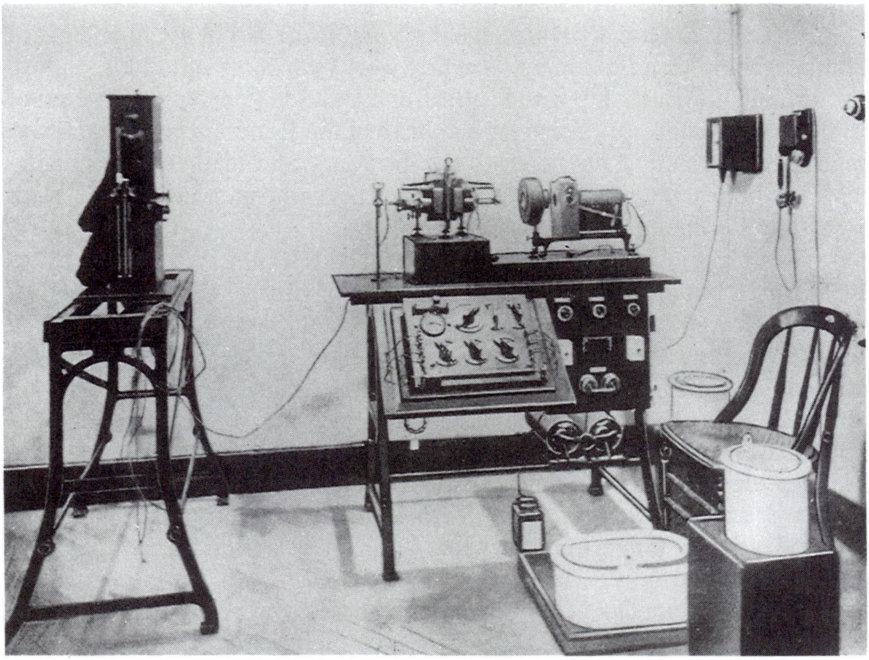

Figure 2. The 1912 Cambridge electrocardiograph at the Royal Victoria Infirmary. This was still in the Cardiology Department, though not in use, in 1947.

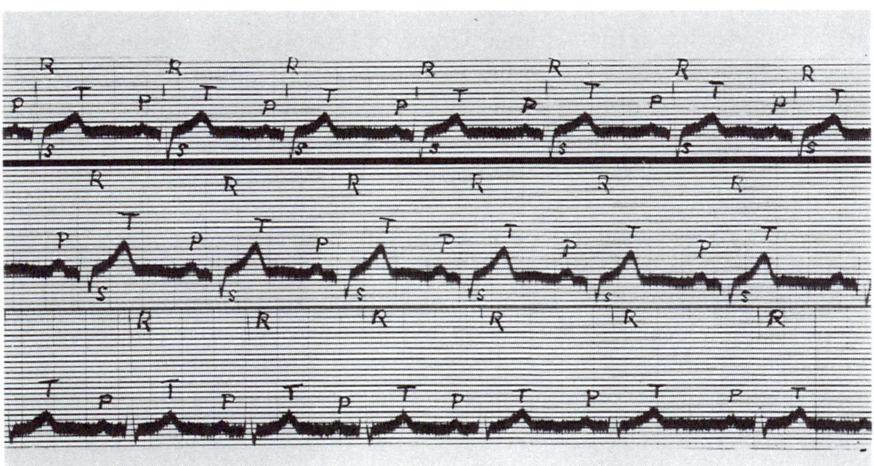

Figure 3. The first ECG taken in Newcastle by Hume.

wet'. The next record was of a case of heart block. Hume wrote a small pamphlet about the instrument[3] and had soon established links with Sir Thomas Lewis at University College, London, Professor William Ritchie in Edinburgh and other pioneers. The first world war interrupted his studies, but through his friendship with Sir Bertrand Dawson (later Lord Dawson of Penn), whose house-physician he had been at the London Hospital, he was appointed Consulting Physician to the 1st Army and made records of the cardiac abnormalities in the cases of spirochaetal jaundice which were occurring in some of the troops in the trenches.

When the war was over he returned to the RVI and developed cardiology further, but always within the framework of general medicine of which all his working life he remained a superb practitioner. Two wards in the hospital, wards 9 and 15, were linked up by electric wire and telephone, so that patients in their beds could have their ECGs recorded, by now on celluloid, by the machine in the basement. It was an admirable system, but would have worked a little better if the excellent technician in the basement had not earned his nickname 'Deafie' Thompson. Hume also acquired another instrument for his private practice and his secretary, Dillingham, his wife and other members of his own family became experts at developing and printing the records.

On the national front Hume had taken the lead in beginning the British Cardiac Society, shortly after the war, by writing in January 1922 to Cowan, suggesting that he wrote to those other physicians in the country known to be interested in heart disease, and proposing that they form a new organisation, the British Cardiac Club. The BCS grew out of it, and Hume was a prominent and popular member of both, hosting meetings of the Society in Newcastle in 1926 and 1953. As his friend Sir John Parkinson once said, 'The room always seemed to light up a bit when Hume walked in'.

Locally of course his reputation also grew and he achieved a particularly high standing in the National Union of Mineworkers, whose cases for compensation he often supported in the courts. It cannot have been the privilege of many cardiologists in the UK to be able to go to the house of a miner who had just died and in whose case he was interested, perform a limited post-mortem in the bedroom and be thanked by the widow as he left with the heart in his bag. He even had a technique for removing the heart via the rectum. As a teacher, not only of cardiology but it seemed of any branch of medicine, he was superb. He flouted the conventional rules of good lecturing by walking back and forth and peppering his discourse with innumerable "ers", but the lucidity of that discourse, its common sense, its avoidance of technical jargon and the vivid illustrations from his own experiences made his lectures masterpieces. What student could forget the moment when he broke off his exposition and said 'I think it is time I told you one or two gruey stories' and would then relate the case of the man lying in bed with a syphilitic aneurysm pulsating just beneath the skin of his upper chest, whilst his wife washed the floor with a cloth. Suddenly the end of an arc of blood landed on the floor beside her. With enormous presence of mind she clapped the floor-cloth on her husband's chest and staunched the flow. He was still just alive when Hume visited him next day.

Hume took up the study of cardiology when treatment was neither very interesting nor very rewarding. Salicylates would do much to relieve rheumatic symptoms but were not curative and would not prevent valvular disease. Digitalis had been introduced more than 100 years before by William Withering, who had himself worked out the principles of how it should be used, even if he did consider it had more effect on the kidneys than on the heart. Of true diuretics there were none and quinidine was not introduced until 1919; in the same year mercurial diuretics became available. The interesting and rewarding challenges were in diagnosis and in understanding the nature of disease. Sir James Mackenzie's adaptation of Marey's polygraph and his correlation of its recordings with long observations of his patients' progress in general practice had revolutionised cardiology. The electrocardiograph was however a much more informative tool and made it much easier to link the abnormalities seen *post mortem* in the heart with the rhythmic and the structural changes which had been seen in the ECG. Hume's museum classes in which he correlated the patient's symptoms and signs and ECG in life with the macro- and microscopic appearances at necropsy were, in the opinion of Professor Nattrass and doubtless of generations of other students, the most brilliant of his achievements as a teacher.

Not surprisingly, those who had the privilege of being his house-physicians and registrars were proud of the experience. Adrian Swan was one who learned a very great deal of cardiology from him and was much disappointed not to be elected to a vacancy on the staff of the RVI which arose shortly before the second world war. When Hume retired from the honorary staff of that hospital in 1939 at the prescribed age of 60, there was no immediate successor to take charge of cardiology there until Hewan Dewar was appointed assistant physician two years after the end of the war. In the meantime, however, Hume had been invited by Newcastle's Medical Officer of Health, Dr John Charles (later Chief Medical Officer to the Ministry of Health and knighted) to become physician, no longer honorary, at the Newcastle General Hospital.[4] There he was assisted by Paul Szekely, a Czechoslovak refugee from Hitler, who had worked with the French cardiologist Laubry in Paris.[5] Soon after the National Health Service was introduced in 1948 Hume, with his customary foresight, advised the Regional Health Authority to set up a Regional Cardiovascular Unit at the Newcastle General Hospital. Adrian Swan, who had returned from the war and already had a post at the NGH, was the obvious choice as head of it. It began functioning in 1951. Working with Swan were his deputy, Frederic Jackson,[6] a London Hospital graduate who developed a special interest in ischaemic heart disease, Paul Szekely whose many research papers especially on rheumatic heart disease and heart disease in pregnancy are recorded elsewhere in this account and Charles Henderson,[7] a Durham graduate, who had recently returned from the USA where with a Nuffield Fellowship he had been studying various aspects of cardiology, including in particular ballisto-cardiography. This was a technique for assessing the mechanical function of the heart by recording the successive tailward and headward movement of the whole body as the blood was pumped first to the arch of the aorta and then to the legs. Like apex cardiography which attracted his interest a few years later it never gave as much reliable information as its ingenuity had led people to expect and its vogue was short. Equally disappointing was the NGH's first strain-gauge manometer for cardiac catheter work which Henderson nursed most carefully during his air journey back from the USA. The manufacturers had supplied it already ruined by a puncture.

Nevertheless Henderson became a deft manipulator of that very valuable tool, the cardiac catheter, both at the NGH and also in the surgical unit at Shotley Bridge. He and Jackson performed most of the investigative procedures which had to precede operation on the numerous cases of rheumatic valvular and congenital heart disease which the Cardiovascular Unit attracted from all over the Northern Region. Marion Bethune's contribution in paediatric cardiology is described later.

On 11 December 1949 Hume invited five physicians and two surgeons to his home to form the Newcastle Cardiac Club.[8] The Club has continued to meet three or four times a year in the homes of its members. Hume himself last attended on 15 February 1958. Membership of this informal and stimulating Club has always been restricted to as many as could conveniently meet in a member's home.

Meanwhile in 1947 Dewar, with no previous special training in cardiology, inherited Hume's facilities and staff in the Royal Victoria Infirmary. It is difficult in these days of paid appointments in the NHS to realise how inevitably small these were. Between the wars Hume ran his male ward of 20 beds and his female of 10 with a staff of one registrar and one house-physician. His assistant physician (latterly James Spence) by tradition was limited to four male and two female beds for which the same junior staff served. The assistant physician's main commitment was to out-patients. Turn-over in the wards was not as rapid as today. A man with a major coronary thrombosis would spend a month in bed, the first week of it flat on his back, nourished through a feeding cup.

With a need to provide for his wife and five children entirely from private practice, and with a statutory obligation to the RVI of only two mornings a week, it is astonishing how much Hume accomplished. But the physical legacy to the RVI was one small room in the basement, with a screened off cubby-hole of a dark room shared by two cardiographers and the hospital photographer. With the Cambridge string galvanometer the ECG was recorded on photo-sensitised celluloid from which, after development, a photographic print was made, mounted on paper and despatched without a report to the ward. A 3-lead ECG took about 30 minutes to complete, a 12-lead one at least twice as long. Fortunately an early move to much more roomy though poorly ventilated premises, still in the basement, and the purchase of an American direct-writing ECG machine enabled a much faster service to be provided, accompanied for the first time by a report.

In 1940 in Germany, Forsmann had performed on himself the first cardiac catheterisation and Cournand in the USA in subsequent years had shown how valuable the technique could be in diagnosis. So Dewar paid a visit to London to learn from Frances Gardiner at the Royal Free Hospital how it was done. He met her at the Royal Free but had to travel with her to another hospital, clutching in the front passenger seat the 'manometer', a long glass tube which projected through the sunshine roof. Back in Newcastle he substituted an aneroid manometer from a BP machine and in 1949 performed the first cardiac catheterisation in the North. Soon with the help of Charles Warrick and later of Peter Hacking, the RVI radiologists, he was able to provide a full investigative service of cardiac catheterisation and angiocardiography.

These investigative procedures had assumed particular importance because of the development of cardiac surgery, of which an account is given separately. Because they were necessary before operation in a large proportion of cases, though not in all, and the apparatus was expensive, most of the cases in the Northern Region had to be seen by a cardiologist and admitted to the RVI, the NGH or Shotley Bridge. Accordingly the cardiologists began paying visits, mostly every one or two months, to the various general hospitals in the region to see new cases and follow-ups. These visits were at the invitation of the physicians in these hospitals with whom, as Hume had foreseen, they had formed friendships in the Newcastle Cardiac Club and the Assocation of Physicians of Region No 1 – both organisations which Hume had founded. Dewar used to visit North Tees and West Cumbria, Jackson Darlington and Hartlepool, Szekely Durham and Henderson Carlisle. The Regional Health Authority defrayed the travelling expenses.

Throughout, the units at the RVI and the NGH were to some extent in friendly rivalry, each keen to keep abreast of new developments. They were not in local competition for money, because funding of the cardiology unit at the RVI came from its Board of Governors which was financed directly from the Department of Health in London but which also had use of the hospital's endowment fund, dating from its days as a voluntary hospital. The Regional Cardiovascular Unit at the NGH was financed by the Regional Health Authority whose funds, also provided by the Department of Health, had to service the whole Region. A weekly review of the cases investigated, held in the Department of Radiology in the NGH, provided an excellent opportunity for mutual discussion and shared experience. It was particularly valuable in relation to congenital heart disease for Dr Marion Bethune (later Farmer), the first paediatric cardiologist, worked closely with both units. There was also some collaboration in research. Swan and Dewar did write a joint paper in 1952 on 'The Heart in Haemochromatosis'[9] but the latter's enthusiasm for fibrinolysis which began in 1961 with the 'Fibrinolytic Treatment of Coronary Thrombosis — a pilot study'[10] was not echoed in the CVS unit. Dewar however was honorary secretary of the Association of Physicians of Region No 1 for 27 years following its inception in 1950, and was thus able to recruit physicians from throughout the Region in a collaborative (and negative) project on steroid therapy in acute myocardial infarction[11] and in a trial of clofibrate in the treatment of ischaemic heart disease which began in 1968.[12]

The RVI and NGH cardiologists collaborated in the setting up in 1967 of the mainland's first (and rather unsuccessful) 'coronary ambulance'. This, copied directly from Pantridge's very successful and pioneering arrangement in Belfast, was a logical sequel to the discovery that 'coronary care units' could materially reduce the mortality of coronary thrombosis. They did so by placing the patient as early as possible, and for the first 2 or 3 days, in monitored beds under the care of specially trained medical and nursing staff who could recognise and treat dangerous disturbances of rhythm in the heart and prevent or treat cardiac arrests.[13]

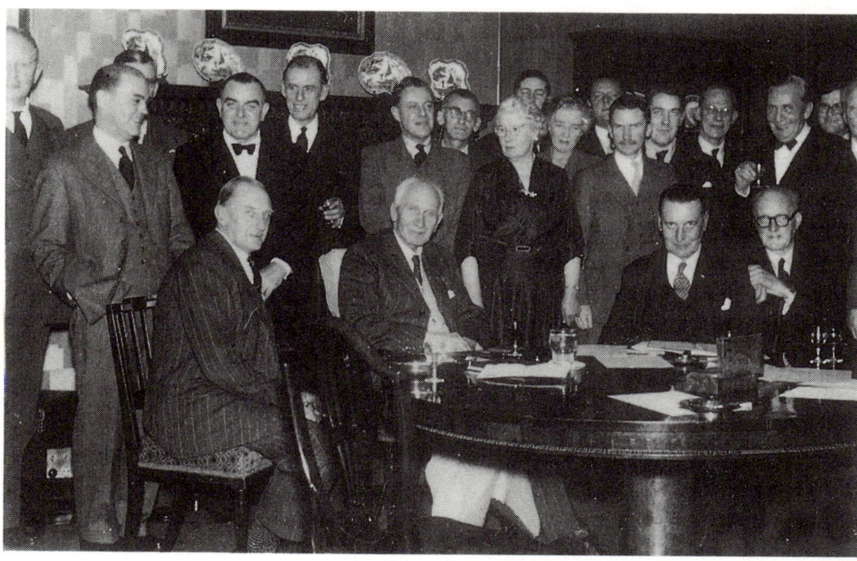

Figure 4. Hume's reunion with his former House Physicians on his 80th birthday in 1959.

The coronary ambulance, funded from patients' donations, began in December 1967 with the purchase of an old ambulance into which was put appropriate special equipment. It was stationed at the RVI and initially driven by a doctor accompanied by a nurse, most often from the CCU. The doctors were volunteers, all except one of them juniors, who at night slept in the hospital. They received no extra pay. Dewar, who generated enthusiasm by taking part, remembers one of his first 'call-outs'. The man lived in Byker, was about 70 years old and was almost unconscious with a BP of about 50 mm Hg. The ECG showed myocardial infarct and monitored over the next half hour or so his slow improvement to a BP of about 95 mm Hg. When it was then suggested to him that further recovery would be safer in the RVI his reply was firm, 'Ah'm nae gannen to that bloody place'. Nor did he, and he recovered well at home.

So 1968, the 60th year after Hume's appointment to 'that bloody place', saw Newcastle getting ready to play its part in those brilliant advances, in both medical and surgical treatment of heart disease which characterised the next two decades throughout the world.

Paediatric cardiology

In the years preceding the introduction of antibiotics, rheumatic fever and chorea were very common maladies in childhood and responsible for a high proportion of the cases of valvular heart disease which were encountered in adolescence and adult life. Toxic myocarditis was the principal cause of death when children developed diphtheria and if bacterial endocarditis complicated rheumatic or congenital heart disease it was invariably fatal. All these maladies were particularly prevalent in the North East where poverty, malnutrition and over-crowding were important contributing factors. Congenital malformations were presumably also very common and, since no surgical treatment was available, very often fatal. French physicians such as Fallot and Roger had made the clinical features of some of them recognisable and the Canadian physician Maud Abbott's atlas, published in 1936, systematised much of the knowledge available. Sir James Mackenzie (1853 – 1925), by correlating his polygraph tracings with observations of how patients fared over the years, had ensured that young people with sinus arrhythmia or a few 'extra-systoles' were not put to bed for months on end. The part played by viruses in causing heart problems was unrecognised, to begin with because viruses were unknown and later because they were thought to be unimportant.

Paediatrics as a specialty did not exist and children who needed to be in hospital for diagnosis or treatment would be cared for by consultant physicians in the children's wards of the RVI, and in the Fleming Memorial Hospital for Sick Children, or in the Infectious Diseases Hospital by general practitioners and hospital doctors. As already described, Hume took an interest in his early years in the dysrhythmias of diphtheritic myocarditis and correlated them with the pathological changes found in the heart at post mortem. He also became expert in the use of the only anti-dysrhythmia drugs available – digitalis and quinidine – and the only medicament available for active rheumatism, sodium salicylate. In the years immediately preceding the 2nd world war clinical instruction of medical students in paediatrics was in the hands of Dr James Lickley, a general practitioner erudite in anatomy and neurology and a capable and experienced if rather uninspiring teacher. Only when he retired during that war did James Spence, hitherto a general physician, take over paediatrics and establish what became a world-famous department.

After the war everything changed. The discovery of antibiotics and an enormous improvement in anaesthesia allowed surgery to be undertaken for both congenital malformations and rheumatic valvular heart disease. With universal immunisation diphtheria virtually disappeared. Both Swan's team at the NGH and presently Henderson at Shotley Bridge, and simultaneously Dewar at the RVI undertook investigation of the cases prior to surgical treatment. For some of the defects such as a patent ductus arteriosus special investigations were not needed, although occasionally insisted upon by the surgeon, but for many others they were necessary in order to assess the full severity or to exclude abnormalities such as significant valvular regurgitation or the kind of atrial septal defect which would make 'closed' surgical operations or operation under hypothermia rather than under cardiopulmonary by-pass (a later development) unsuitable.

For all of these the chief link with paediatrics was Marion Bethune. After a brilliant undergraduate career followed by experience in both cardiology and paediatrics in Edinburgh and Southampton, in 1952 she was appointed paediatric registrar to the RVI, the NGH and the Babies Hospital in Newcastle. From the outset her skill in the diagnosis and management of all forms of heart disease in children were appreciated by the cardiologists, Swan, Henderson and Dewar with whom she worked. From the latter two she learned, and rather infrequently practised, the techniques of cardiac catheterisation and angiography. The delay in her promotion to consultant status in 1966 from senior registrar (1954) was due to administrative difficulties, not lack of support by her colleagues. She got through an extraordinary amount of work in the three hospitals mentioned as well as at Shotley Bridge which was added to her remit in 1957. Yet she still found time to visit cardiological clinics at the Hammersmith Hospital and Great Ormond Street and, in 1962, similar clinics in North America. A skilled diagnostician, probably her most valued strength lay in gaining the confidence and affection of parents and children, so that they trusted her implicitly and felt after she had talked to them that they understood the technical problem as completely as was possible for a lay person. They also knew that she would be the child's doctor before, during and long after any operation.

Her liaison with other paediatric surgical centres in the UK was particularly valuable because, although the surgical unit at Shotley Bridge started operating on hearts quite early and kept abreast of new developments, it did not at first attain, especially for more difficult cases, the excellent results with low mortality which similar clinics achieved elsewhere. In the meantime a substantial proportion of the children who needed operations were sent by Marion Bethune and the cardiologists to other centres, especially in London.

Cardiac surgery

Operations on the heart developed naturally from operations on the lungs. These had their heyday between 1930 and 1950 and were mostly performed for pulmonary tuberculosis and bronchiectasis, though post-pneumonic empyema, lung abscess, 'spontaneous' pneumothorax and trauma, both civilian and military, were other indications. George Mason, a Durham graduate, specialised in thoracic surgery and in 1940 Selwyn Griffin from Liverpool joined him. Mason was keen to extend the scope of his work to the heart and shortly before the 2nd world war met Laurence O'Shaughnessy; under his stimulus Mason did some experimental work on greyhounds and then some 'cardio-omentopexies' for ischaemic heart disease. He also visited Beck in the USA, who for the same purpose was using asbestos (of all things!) to scarify the external surface of the heart and produce adhesions between it and the pericardium. The possibility of increasing blood flow through the sub-endocardium by narrowing the coronary sinus was also discussed. None of these measures was successful and perhaps fortunately the war put an end to further research on these lines.

The end of the war saw the introduction of antibiotics, improved anaesthesia and a reliable blood transfusion service; cardiac surgery became much more promising. With the help of his excellent anaesthetist Joan Millar, Mason quickly followed other surgeons in the USA and UK and in 1951 performed his first mitral valvotomy. This was a 'closed' operation, ie no artificial circulation was needed, and the procedure of enlarging the narrowed mitral valve, in the early days with the surgeon's finger, later with a cutting instrument, was performed on the beating heart through an incision in the left hemithorax and the left atrial appendage.

Other closed operations followed – ligature of a patent ductus arteriosus, the Blalock operation for Fallot's Tetralogy and pulmonary valvotomy, either for the same malady or for simple pulmonary stenosis. Within a few years hypothermia was introduced. The anaesthetised patient was placed in a bath of ice and water until body temperature fell to 30°C and this was maintained on the operating table by ice packs on the limbs. It permitted the circulation to be arrested by clamps on the great vessels whilst surgical correction of the malformation was performed. It was most suitable for the ostium secundum type of atrial septal defect. The final advance was full cardio-pulmonary by-pass, in which the patient's systemic venous blood was artifically pumped through an oxygenating device and kept warm or cooled according to requirements before being returned into the patient's arterial system. Solving the technical difficulties of this was the special responsibility of Mason's two principal anaesthetists, Joan Millar and Derek Pearson. In theory almost any operable defect, whether congenital or acquired, could be corrected, valve replacement perhaps being the most frequent.

It was sad that George Mason's own personal inadequacy as an operating surgeon and rather poor judgement resulted in the operations which he performed being less successful and more risky than those performed in other centres. He was a complex character in whom virtues and defects were blended in a confusing mixture. No-one could challenge the enthusiasm and vision which made him a pioneer of cardiac surgery in the Northern Region. He had immense drive, gave great attention to detail and could obtain selfless support from his nursing and medical staff. With a genial personality and a private income he travelled widely, made many surgical friends and invited them to visit Shotley Bridge where they inspired and charmed his medical staff. Yet he often never saw his patients before operation, and by doing ward rounds infrequently and follow-up clinics not at all, he ended by never seeing a great many of his patients except unconscious on the operating table. In the careers of his staff he had no interest and he trained them hardly at all. Though very dependent on senior assistants – first Griffin, later a senior registrar Ferguson – for help with operations, he had scant respect for them, and even when a consultant like Griffin had cases referred personally to him he had no hesitation in appropriating them for his own list. It was not surprising therefore that when in 1960 the Regional Health Authority at Swan's instigation invited Griffin, Dobson and Henry ("Paddy") Bell, an anaesthetist, to set up a separate unit for heart surgery at Seaham Hall, they leapt at the opportunity. Joan Errington provided the medical cover.

Their success was immediate and the full range of heart operations, both closed and open, was undertaken with very low mortality and the full satisfaction of the referring cardiologists who no longer needed to send their patients outside the Region.

Mason retired in 1966 and was succeeded by Ary Blesovsky, a South African surgeon, well-trained there and in the USA in both cardiology and surgery. He achieved excellent results.

Research

Research on cardiology, like everything else on the subject in Newcastle, began with Hume. Sir James Mackenzie had adapted Marey's polygraph, exchanging the smoked drum for an ink pen, and had demonstrated that, by using the instrument to distinguish between sinus arrhythmia, the different types of 'extra systoles' and atrial fibrillation, and combining the observation with many years of follow up of the patients, one could distinguish between the always harmless, the sometimes dangerous and the always sinister. Hume spent many hours in the wards of the infectious diseases hospital studying the very varied dysrhythmias which occurred in the myocarditis of diphtheria, a disease both common and dangerous in those days. He published his findings in the new journal *Heart*, of which Sir Thomas Lewis was founder and editor. One of these contributions, as already noted, was an early recognition of what subsequently was called atrial flutter. During the last world war and subsequently in civilian life he made useful contributions to medical literature on the myocarditis of spirochaetal jaundice, a dangerous malady contracted from rats in the trenches of Northern France and in the coal mines of North East England. His Bradshaw Lecture at the

Royal College of Physicians was on paroxysmal tachycardia. Between the two wars, however, the need to provide for his wife and family wholly from private practice and his many other commitments rendered it impossible for him to conduct much research himself, and the meagre staffing – one house physician and one registrar shared with the Assistant Physician – afforded little opportunity to stimulate others.

One interesting but unsuccessful piece of research was accomplished by Laurence O'Shaughnessy shortly before the 2nd world war, in the first year of which sadly he was killed. He was a Durham graduate who had passed his MB BS examination at 21 years of age and the FRCS at 23. Impressed with the extensive anastomoses which developed around the abdominal omentum in cases of cirrhosis of the liver and which conveyed into the systemic blood stream so much of what could no longer traverse the liver, he conceived the idea that the omentum, if applied to the surface of an ischaemic heart, might provide an alternative blood supply just where it was needed. Experimental work on greyhounds supported the concept and in 1938 he persuaded George Mason, who was already doing thoracic surgery, to undertake cardio-omentopexy. The patient who improved most, becoming angina-free, unkindly died later. Autopsy showed one anastomotic vessel, of the calibre of cotton thread.

The introduction of the National Health Service in 1948 gave a tremendous fillip to research. Relieved of the need to earn their living solely from private practice and with more generous staffing by juniors, consultants were able to plan and initiate research projects in which doctors in training were able to play major or minor parts. Paul Szekely, who had published his first paper on electro-cardiography within 3 years of qualifying in medicine in Prague, joined Hume in 1941 at the Newcastle General Hospital, first as house physician, later becoming registrar and consultant. Between 1941 and 1968 – the final date of this history – he published more than 40 papers. They covered a wide range of topics – cardiac involvement in spirochaetal jaundice (with Hume), cardiac pharmacology *viz* the effects on the heart of magnesium, calcium, digitalis, procaine and propanolol, cardioversion, hypothermia and pulmonary embolism. The two subjects on which his international reputation stood highest were rheumatic fever with its cardiological consequences and heart disease in pregnancy. His articles in joint authorship with his obstetrical colleague Linton Snaith on 'The Heart in Toxaemia of Pregnancy'[14] and 'The Place of Cardiac Surgery in the Management of the Pregnant Woman with Heart Disease'[15] were the forerunners of their classical text book on the subject *Heart Disease and Pregnancy*,[16] which was to appear in 1974. Fluent in five languages and an indefatigable attender and speaker at cardiological meetings world-wide, no cardiologist in Newcastle, until the arrival of Professor Julian, attained during those post-war years so high an international reputation.

Meanwhile at the Royal Victoria Infirmary Hewan Dewar, having co-operated with Ian Hill in a paper on effort syndrome,[17] had in 1947 been appointed as Assistant Physician, largely on the strength of some research, never published, on myasthenia gravis which he had begun in 1946. As soon as he learned the use of cardiac catheters, he and Tommy Grimson, later Consultant Physician at Chester-le-Street, arranged with George Mason to direct one into the thymic vein of a case of myasthenia gravis whose thymus Mason had been asked by Professor Nattrass to excise. The blood withdrawn was then applied to the neuromuscular preparation of a frog which Dewar and Grimson had prepared in the Medical School and conveyed by car to Shotley Bridge. No paralysing effect ensued and so ended a project which was imaginative, logical and wholly futile. However over the 20 years between 1948 and 1968 Dewar, in collaboration with numerous other gifted assistants, Griffith Owen, Lindsay Davidson, Alan Horler, Peter Stephenson, Satish Srivastava and JM Goodhart, pubished some 38 papers on anti-anginal and anti-hypertensive drug trials, cerebral blood flow in mitral stenosis and in 1961 the first of a series of papers on fibrinolysis *viz* 'Fibrinolytic treatment of coronary thrombosis – a pilot study',[18] a method of treatment which was to become important only in 1980. In this work on fibrinolysis a most important part was played by I Sudhakaran Menon, a very capable and enterprising Indian graduate. Over some four years, culminating in a Newcastle PhD, he initiated and collaborated in a series of experiments and trials. Several of his papers were concerned with the fibrinolytic activity (FA) in the venous effluent of different organs of the body. Other interesting topics were the demonstration that the clinical variations of FA and cortisol, though inverse, were unlikely to be causally related, and that the veins of the paralysed limb of a paraplegic patient display increased rather than decreased FA. This may explain why embolism from such a limb is infrequent.

Adrian Swan, an excellent clinical cardiologist and a good teacher of students, published little, his best paper probably being a perceptive account of 'Acute non-specific pericarditis'.[19] His long association with the venereal disease unit at the Newcastle General Hospital made him an expert on the cardiovascular effects of syphilis. He collaborated with Dewar in a paper on the heart in haemochromatosis.[8] Marion Bethune (later Mrs Farmer) wrote her MD thesis on patent ductus arteriosus of which she had experience of 110 cases, 70 of them submitted to operation. She also contributed a section on heart disease to Professor Court's book on *The Medical Care of Children*[20] and collaborated with Paul Szekely in a paper on 'Rheumatic fever and rheumatic heart disease – natural history and preventive aspects'.[21] Her paper in the *Newcastle Medical Journal* in 1958 on 'General care of a child with congenital heart disease' was a distillation of her great experience and sympathetic devotion.

Notes and references

1. Published in London by E and C Dilly, 1774. No copy of this has been located in any Newcastle library or in the British Library or Wellcome Institute.

Andrew Wilson (1718-92), an Edinburgh graduate, was Honorary Physician to the Newcastle Infirmary 1772-75. The rest of his career was in London, where he was

'Physician to the Medical Asylum'. Also wrote *An essay on the autumnal dysentery* (London,1761), of which the 2nd edit. 1777 is in the Pybus Collection. In the library of the Literary and Philosophical Society of Newcastle-upon-Tyne there is a volume (*Tracts* 379) of miscellaneous anonymous tracts, five of them noted as being by Andrew Wilson, dated 1750-1766, on Newtonian theory, human nature and revelation.

In Wilson's *Medical researches: being an enquiry into the nature and origin of hysterics in the female constitution, and into the distinction between that disease and hypochondriac or nervous disorders....1776* (copies in BL and Wellcome) there is the 'Substance of a lecture delivered at Newcastle, 28th December, 1773, on the natural powers employed in the circulation of the blood, independent of the action of the heart'. In this Wilson proposes the reactionary theory '...not to disprove that it is by the action of the heart that the blood is thrown out into the arteries...but...that that these actions have little or no concern in supporting the progress of the blood along the finer arteries...still less....on its motion through the veins back again to the heart'. He quotes Whytt on 'perpetual oscillations of the finer vessels, squeezing the blood forward in the direction of its progress..' and concludes that the heart is not 'essentially and absolutely necessary to the circulation of our fluids'. Ed.

2. Newcastle may lay some claim to another cardiologist, Byrom Bramwell (1847-1931), who was born in Dockwray Square, North Shields, qualified in Edinburgh and, after a period in General Practice with his father in North Shields, became lecturer in medical jurisprudence at the Orchard Street medical school in 1872. In 1874 he became physician and pathologist to the Infirmary. He left Newcastle in 1879 (at the age of only 31) to become physician at the Royal Infirmary in Edinburgh. He was a brilliant teacher. Among his many published works (very many of them neurological) is a textbook of 783 pages, *Diseases of the heart and thoracic aorta* (Edinburgh: Pentland, 1884). Much of the preparatory work on this must have been done in Newcastle, but it is scarcely reflected among his numerous contributions to *Proc Northumb Durh Med Soc* in the 1870s. He returned from Edinburgh to lecture to the Society on many occasions, and his two most important books (on *Diseases of the spinal cord* and *Intracranial tumours*) were, in effect, previously printed in serial form, in the Proceedings. Ed.

   See Ashworth B. *The Bramwells of Edinburgh: A medical dynasty*. Edinburgh: Roy Coll Phys Edinb, 1986.

3. Again no copy has been traced. But see — Hume WE. Demonstration of the electrocardiograph. *Univ Durh Coll Med Gaz* 1913-4; *14*:75.
4. Appointed 1938, retired 1949.
5. Appointed house physician 1941, registrar 1942, consultant 1948.
6. Appointed 1950, retired 1977.
7. Appointed registrar 1947, consultant 1958.
8. They were W C Barnsley (Thoracic Surgeon, Shotley Bridge), Dewar, Mason, R Mowbray (Physician, Dryburn), Swan, Szekely and S Whateley Davidson (Radiologist, RVI).
9. Swan WGA, Dewar HA. The heart in haemochromatosis. *Br Heart J* 1952; *14*:117-24.
10. Dewar HA, Horler AR, Cassells-Smith AJ. Fibrinolytic treatment of coronary thrombosis: a pilot study. *BMJ* 1961; *2*:671-5.
11. A group of physicians in the Newcastle Region. Steroid therapy in acute myocardial infarction: A controlled trial. *Newc Med J* 1968; *30*:82-9.
12. Group of Physicians of Newcastle upon Tyne Region (Organising secretary Dewar HA) Trial of Clofibrate in the treatment of ischaemic heart disease. *BMJ* 1971; *4*:767-75.

13. The 4 bed CCU in the RVI was established in 1968 with endowment money, the much larger unit at the NGH in 1969 with a donation by Mr Lionel Jacobson.

14. Szekely P, Snaith L. The heart in toxaemia of pregnancy. *Br Heart J* 1947; *9*:128-36.

15. Szekely P, Snaith L. The place of cardiac surgery in the management of the pregnant woman with heart disease. *J Obst Gynaec* 1963; *70*:69-73.

16. Szekely P, Snaith L. *Heart disease and pregnancy*. Edinburgh: Churchill-Livingston, 1974.

17. Hill IGW, Dewar HA. Effort Syndrome. *Lancet* 1945; *2*:161-4.

18. Dewar HA, Horler AR, Cassells-Smith AJ. Fibrinolytic treatment of coronary thrombosis — a pilot study. *BMJ* 1961; *2*:671-5.

19. Swan WGA. Acute non-specific pericarditis. *Br Heart J* 1960; *22*:651-9.

20. Court SDM. *The medical care of children*. London: Oxford Univ Press, 1963.

21. Szekely P, Bethune MB. Rheumatic fever and rheumatic heart disease — natural history and preventive aspects. *Public Hlth* 1964; *78*:78-84.

Chapter 24

TYNESIDE'S SCHEMES FOR THE CONTROL OF VENEREAL DISEASE

Elspeth M Gould

Introduction

Each of the world wars produced enormous social upheaval, one consequence of which was an increased incidence of venereal disease. National and local government concerns rose with the incidence of infection, and the increased anxiety spawned initiatives designed to diagnose and treat people with infection, as well as to educate the public about venereal disease and its prevention. Comparison of the local responses during each war shows both repetition and novelty. The 1939-45 war saw the establishment of contact tracing and ante-natal blood testing services which continue to the present.

The First World War

In September 1914, the Guardians of Newcastle-upon-Tyne Parish offered 100-200 beds at their workhouse infirmary to the War Office, 'for wounded soldiers and sailors.' The proffered facilities (at what was to become the Newcastle General Hospital) were duly inspected, but the Guardians were unhappy at the prospect of their premises being used for venereal cases. It was only when 'the Military' explained the difficulty in which they were placed, being unable 'to retain these cases in Public General Hospitals where the public were freely mixing as also to receive them into private homes' that they were 'convinced that [they] were doing a real service to the Country by permitting them to have use of the Male Block'.[1]

The beds were being used as part of the 1st Northern General Hospital, along with the Armstrong College building and part of the Royal Victoria Infirmary (RVI), and it was a physician from the RVI, Lt Col Robert A Bolam, RAMC, who had charge of those beds. He had cared for the RVI's own venereal disease patients before the war, as the Honorary Physician to the Skin Department, and was well placed to take on the infected soldiers when war broke out.[2]

The Guardians' relationship with the Military never really got over the shaky start. The number of beds at the workhouse assigned to the army grew to between 400 and 500 in January 1915, over 700 by June of that year, and reached the point when the Guardians claimed compensation for the use of 1000 beds. Throughout, the correspondence of the Guardians with, and about, the Military is of a series of petty annoyances and of disputes over payments.[1]

Writing in early 1915, Dr Harold Kerr, Newcastle's Medical Officer of Health (MOH), said:

> Subsequent to mobilisation many wild rumours were current as to moral laxity among soldiers and women in the neighbourhood of troops. The

"war-baby" scandal has proved to be a myth and a libel, and it is probable that similar statements as to disease may be relegated to the same category ... Adequate arrangements have been provided for the treatment of military cases of venereal disease.

The municipality has made no arrangement for diagnosis or treatment of venereal disease. Wasserman tests are made, and salvarsan treatment administered, at the Royal Victoria Infirmary.[3]

However, since 1913, a Royal Commission had been investigating venereal disease. Indeed, Lt Col Bolam gave evidence to it of his experience of using Kharsivan (a substitute for salvarsan which, being a German product, was not easy to obtain during the war) successfully, on 2000 cases of syphilis in Newcastle.The Commission reported in 1916, and its major recommendations were embodied in the Public Health (Venereal Diseases) Regulations of the same year. Local authorities were to provide free, confidential services for the diagnosis and treatment of venereal diseases, defined by the new law as syphilis, gonorrhoea and chancroid.[4,5]

Newcastle acted in concert with the County and County Borough Authorities of Northumberland and Durham, the Durham University College of Medicine and the RVI, and the Joint Scheme for Control of Venereal Disease came into operation on 1 January 1917.[6,7]

This scheme had three strands, bacteriological diagnosis, treatment, and health education. The College of Medicine would provide microscopic examination for spirochaetes and gonococci at 3/6 per specimen, and Wasserman reactions on a sliding scale of charges from £2 2s 0d for one to 5/- each for twenty or more. Treatment would be provided in the skin clinic at the RVI (with plans to have clinics at other hospitals in the region, too) with costs for both out and in patients recharged *pro rata* to the patients' districts of residence. To encourage attendance, secrecy was to be guaranteed to patients and expenses would be paid for necessitous cases to travel to the clinic in the area of their home. Additionally, private physicians who had had appropriate training would be supplied with salvarsan free of charge to treat their own patients. Health education was to be left to each Medical Officer of Health to arrange.[7]

Alongside his responsibilities for the venereal and skin cases of the 1st Northern General Hospital, Robert Bolam had continued as Hon Physician in Charge of the Skin Department of the RVI and he reported on the increased workload caused by the clinic's change in status.

During the year 1916 1,089 cases, including 242 syphilis were registered, whilst during the present year there have been 1,760 cases of skin disease proper, 2,369 cases of venereal disease, a grand total of 4,129.

Some idea of the magnitude of the work accomplished in the Venereal Clinic may be gathered from the fact that the patients made 15,618 attendances, and that 8,632 intravenous injections of Salvarsan were administered.[8]

However, half of the patients failed to complete their course of treatment.[8]

Lt Col Bolam organised a series of Sunday morning courses of demonstrations on the diagnosis and treatment of venereal disease, augmented by practical experience during clinic sessions, so that private practitioners could qualify to treat their own patients. Almost every doctor did so within the first year.[9]

The MOH undertook a widespread publicity campaign, addressing

> lodges, clubs, societies, brotherhoods and sisterhoods, guilds, bible classes, and other social organisations .... making known the general purpose of the scheme, and the facilities provided for free diagnosis and treatment, and the clinic was soon handling more patients than the staff as first constituted could deal with.[9]

The Newcastle Branch of the National Council for Combating Venereal Diseases (NCCVD), founded nationally in 1914, was formed after a public meeting presided over by the Lord Mayor. Its first Chairman was Sir George Hare Philipson, and it cooperated with the City Council in further health education work, including the distribution of tens of thousands of pamphlets. The Lord Chamberlain's ban on it having been lifted in 1917, Eugene Brieux's play about syphilis, *Damaged Goods*, played at the Theatre Royal for a week in December.[9,10,11]

Damaged Goods was to return to the Theatre Royal in succeeding years, but the MOH had to report decreasing interest in lectures as organisations found the novelty of the subject of venereal disease wore off.[12,13,14]

The inter-war years

With the Armistice and general demobilisation, life gradually returned to normal. The Guardians regained control of the workhouse infirmary. The MOH noted a decline in the number of cases of venereal disease treated at the RVI, and Robert Bolam was knighted in the New Years honours of 1926. The NCCVD became the British Social Hygiene Council (BSHC), but their educational work nationally and locally carried on.[15,16,17]

Treatments for venereal infection required repeated attendance at the clinic over a period of time, and involved painful procedures such as urethral irrigation. The high default rate was hardly surprising, and was a constant cause of concern. There were attempts to encourage patients to return to the clinic, with some effect, but then, as now, such attempts were fraught with the problems of false names and addresses, and the fear of breaching confidentiality. Letters appear to have been used, but whether home visiting was tried, and, if it was, by whom, is not obvious from the reports. Eventually such follow-up was abandoned.[18,19]

Over the 6-year period 1927-1932, the average death rate per 100,000 people in Newcastle, from all causes, was 106% of the rate for England and Wales. For syphilis this rate was 197% of the rate for England and Wales, and for general paralysis of the insane and tabes dorsalis it was 140%. So venereal disease was contributing to Newcastle's excess mortality.[20]

The MOH, by then Dr John A Charles, opened negotiations with the RVI for the improvement of the venereal diseases services offered at that institution. There was agreement in principle that facilities should be refurbished, but both the City and the RVI were short of money. The negotiations were protracted and became deadlocked. Eventually, the Local Authorities whose residents used the RVI decided to build a new clinic at the Newcastle General Hospital (NGH). For the Local Authorities one great advantage of the move would be greater control. As the MOH of Newcastle said, they had been paying the salaries of the staff, who were not employees of the City but of the RVI. Sir Robert Bolam's position in the negotiations had been particularly ambiguous. The Local Authorities had, thus, no control over the staff they paid for: staff were not accountable to their paymasters.[21,22,23,24,25]

The new Clinic opened on 30 August 1937 with Dr A E W McLachlan as Clinical Medical Officer. It was run by a 'Joint Committee as to Venereal Disease' on which the counties of Northumberland and Durham, and the county boroughs of Newcastle and Gateshead had representation. This arrangement brought the participating Local authorities' representatives, including Dr Charles, into close involvement with the Clinic and its concerns.[26,27]

The Second World War

War again saw a rising incidence of venereal disease. Nationally the BSHC continued its educational campaign, though its style seems to have been one of moralising rather than giving clear information. Whether for this reason or some other, the BSHC ran into financial difficulties. It was bailed out with Government money, on the condition that it transfer all its assets and responsibilities to the Central Council for Health Education (CCHE). The central figures of the BSHC were to continue to act in an advisory capacity to the CCHE.[28]

The Joint Committees Clinic met the rising tide of infection with an establishment depleted by the mobilisation, as both doctors and orderlies had been reservists. The venereal orderlies, who worked exclusively with male patients, had all originally been trained in the Army. Some of the State Registered Nurses, who worked in the female clinic, also joined the forces.[29]

The Military in Newcastle again cared for its own, running a clinic at Fenham Barracks, the temporary closure of which prompted protest from the Joint Committee when the diverted patients nearly swamped their Clinic.[27]

Both nationally and locally moves were taken to control infection. There was a particular worry that troops were being incapacitated by disease and rendered unable to fight, and a notion that certain 'promiscuous' individuals were acting as sources of infection for large numbers of people. The response was Defence Regulation 33B which came into force in 1942.

Doctors were to question patients about their consorts and record their names. An individual named more than once could be compelled to have examination and treatment, failure to comply with medical instruction would lead to prosecution and, potentially, imprisonment.[28,30]

It appears that, in practice, the military clinics reported consorts more assiduously than did the civilian ones, and that very few consorts were named more than once. Prosecutions were few, but the climate was altered and the notion that the patient was not the only person who might invite his or her sexual partners for examination became current.[31]

In the mainland of the USA contact tracing for syphilis and gonorrhoea became national policy in 1937. When America entered the war and set up bases in the UK, its army brought its public health nurses with it and continued to trace the British contacts of its personnel infected over here.[32,30]

By December of 1942, Dr Edith Summerskill M P was calling for the annulment of Regulation 33B (which actually remained in force until the end of 1947), and for 'social service' follow up of contacts named by patients at civilian clinics.[33,34] *Damaged Goods* was revived and played at London's Whitehall Theatre.[35]

The CCHE took its new responsibilities seriously and convened a conference to discuss the ways of controlling venereal infection. Held on 26 February1943, the meeting may have been attended by either Dr Charles or Dr McLachlan, but it was reported in both the BMJ and the BJVD, journals which both of them would have seen. Dr Hill, chairing the meeting, said that a lot had been done to disseminate information about venereal disease, but 'Next must come the evolution of a policy and the method of promoting action.' The Minister of Health, Ernest Brown, exhorted Medical Officers of Health to include venereal diseases in their health education work, and reminded them of the films and other material which was available from the CCHE. Universal testing for syphilis in the blood of expectant mothers was advocated by Dr David Nabarro. Miss Dorothy Manchee, Chief Almoner, St Mary's Hospital, Paddington, spoke on the value of the almoner in the Venereal Disease clinic, and the contribution she could make towards alleviating the social conditions which predisposed towards the spread of infection.[36.37]

Around the same time as the CCHE meeting, Dr Charles and the Joint Committee recognised that something needed to be done. The climate was right at the Ministry of Health (the Chief Medical Officer had broadcast to the nation on the subject), and there was support from the Local Authorities. The Committee drafted a scheme for control of venereal disease on Tyneside. The Ministry agreed to it in principle, and suggested that a grant of 75% of the cost might be forthcoming to support such a pioneering enterprise. After local consultation and extensive redrafting, they invited Miss Manchee, together with Mrs Neville-Rolfe of the BSHC, to the July meeting to hear their comments on the plans.[37,27]

Initially a 6-month experiment, the 'Tyneside Scheme for the Reduction of Venereal Disease' got off the ground in October 1943. Like its predecessor, it had three strands. Another health education campaign was to take place, alongside an extension of antenatal Wasserman testing to all pregnant women and the tracing of sexual contacts of patients with syphilis and gonorrhoea.[27,38]

Commenting at a meeting in 1944, Dr McLachlan explained that:

> Up to recently the blood testing of pregnant women in Newcastle had applied only in the case of illegitimate pregnancy; in the past six months the scope had been widened to include as many expectant mothers as possible. This had led to the recognition of a certain amount of previously undetected maternal syphilis, while, in addition, a number of defaulters were brought back to the clinic for treatment.[39]

Universal antenatal blood testing was easier to implement in the urban areas but eventually spread to the whole of the Joint Committee's area. It continued to prove its worth, and the system continues to this day.[40]

Dr Charles took his health education duties seriously and set up large and small meetings to be addressed by a variety of speakers and using the CCHE's films. The clinic's doctors and the local MOHs were heavily involved, as were Sir Drummond Shiels, Dr Otto May of the BSHC, and Dr Kennedy of the CCHE, all from London. The meetings were grouped to get the most from these eminent speakers during their stay in Newcastle, and the local press were invited along to get maximum publicity.[40,34,41]

At the end of the six months the health education strand of the Tyneside Scheme was absorbed into the ordinary work of the Health Departments of the Joint Committee's area. In Newcastle, as after the Great War, interest in Venereal Disease talks gradually petered out as the novelty of the subject wore off.

Newcastle pioneers civilian contact tracing

Miss Manchee had said at the 1943 CCHE meeting that only five London clinics and one in the provinces had almoners. Since the Newcastle Clinic had Miss Maynard in post as almoner by then, it was probably that one. At Miss Manchee's suggestion, Miss Maynard moved to another clinic in the Joint Committee's area. Into her place came the Newcastle General Hospital's almoner, Miss Brown. Miss Hilda M Johns the Director of Personal Services at the Tyneside Council for Social Service was seconded as Liaison Officer, later to be called Chief Contact Tracer. She was to start up contact tracing in conjunction with health visitors seconded from the various Local Authorities.[37,27]

Dr Charles arranged for Miss Johns and two of the health visitors to visit London for consultation and instruction with the US Army's contact tracers. Just as the system was getting underway a Col Padgett from the US Army came to speak to health visitors in Newcastle.[27,40]

Miss Johns, the almoners and health visitors involved in the scheme seem to have had responsibility for both 'case holding' and 'case finding'. They aimed to prevent default from treatment as well as to bring contacts of patients for screening. The great distances over which some patients came for treatment, the possible loss of earnings, and the difficulties mothers had in finding suitable childcare, added to the nature of treatment, meant that default continued to be a major problem. The almoners carried the responsibility for case holding, as Miss Manchee had recommended. The health visitors, known in their patches to be visiting a range of clients anyway, would have aroused little suspicion when seeking contacts named by patients in the clinic. That the health visitors were equally inconspicuous when hanging about in public houses waiting for someone to walk in who might fit a description is rather less likely, however.[27,42,43]

As this was an experiment, funded centrally, periodic reports were made on the work. Miss John's major report was printed, with a forward by Sir William Jameson, Chief Medical Officer, and circulated widely. It even reached the Library of the Surgeon General's Office, National Library of Medicine, in Washington. On the strength of the results, central funding was renewed for more 6-month periods, but the rate-payers eventually took on the whole cost of the scheme.[27,44]

Social and epidemiological information was gathered by the team at the clinic and published over the following years. The emphasis on prostitution, the categorisation of patients, and the moral judgements passed on them are all alien to the staff currently working in the clinic, but some attempt was being made to understand the people behind the diagnoses.[42,43,45,46,47]

Almoners are no longer involved, but contact tracing (now more correctly called partner notification) has continued at the clinic and is applied in the case of other, non-venereal, sexually transmitted diseases, too. Newcastle is unique in the UK in having provided 50 years of uninterrupted contact tracing.[48]

Acknowledgements

For the help they have given, I would like to thank the staffs of Newcastle Central Library Local Studies Department, Tyne and Wear Archive Service, University of Newcastle Medical School Library and Newcastle General Hospital Library.

References

1. Newcastle Guardians' correspondence re military occupation. 359/522(1) Tyne and Wear Archive.
2. Bolam R A. Arseno-benzol in syphilis. *Northumb and Dur Med J* 1911; 113-117.
3. Kerr W B. *Annual report of the Medical Officer of Health for Newcastle-upon-Tyne for 1914*; 94.
4. *Royal Commission on Venereal Disease. Final Report.* 1916; 39.
5. Brockington C F. *The Health of the Community: Principles of Public Health for practitioners and students.* London: J & A Churchill, 1954.

6. Royal Victoria Infirmary. *Minutes of the House Committee*; *51* HO/RVI/2/51 Tyne and Wear Archive.
7. Kerr W B. *Annual Report of the Medical Officer of Health for Newcastle-upon-Tyne for 1916*: 18 and 73-77.
8. Royal Victoria Infirmary. *Annual Report for 1917*; 37 HO/RVI/72/99 Tyne and Wear Archive.
9. Kerr W B. *Annual Report of the Medical Officer of Health for Newcastle-upon-Tyne for 1917*; 68-69.
10. 'A pestilential scourge. Campaign for Combating a Prevalent Disease.' Meeting in Newcastle. *The Evening Chronicle*, 29 March 1917.
11. Davenport-Hines R. *Sex, Death and Punishment*. London. Collins, 1990: Chapter 5.
12. Kerr W B. *Annual Report of the Medical Officer of Health for Newcastle-upon-Tyne for 1918*; 20-21.
13. Kerr W B. *Annual Report of the Medical Officer of Health for Newcastle-upon-Tyne for 1919*; 21-23.
14. Kerr W B. *Annual Report of the Medical Officer of Health for Newcastle-upon-Tyne for 1920*; 19-21.
15. Kerr W B. *Annual Report of the Medical Officer of health for Newcastle-upon-Tyne for 1921*; 14-15.
16. Sir R A Bolam. 'Recognition of a well known Newcastle medical man.' *The Newcastle Journal*, 7 January 1926.
17. Davenport-Hines R. *op cit* note 11, chapter 6.
18. Kerr W B. *Annual Report of the Medical Officer of Health for Newcastle-upon-Tyne for 1922*; 20-21.
19. Kerr W B. *Annual Report of the Medical Officer of Health for Newcastle-upon-Tyne for 1923*; 21-22.
20. Charles J A. *Annual Report of the Medical Officer of Health for Newcastle-upon-Tyne for 1933*; 15.
21. Royal Victoria Infirmary. *Minutes of the House Committee*; *54* HO/RVI/2/54 Tyne and Wear Archive.
22. Royal Victoria Infirmary. *Minutes of the House Committee*; *55* HO/RVI/2/55 Tyne and Wear Archive.
23. Royal Victoria Infirmary. *Sub Committee Reports*; *2* HO/RVI/154/2 Tyne and Wear Archive.
24. Charles J A. *Annual Report of the Medical Officer of Health for Newcastle-upon-Tyne for 1935*; 22-23.
25. *Newcastle Council Reports 1933-34*; 862-866.
26. Charles J A. *Annual Report of the Medical Officer of Health for Newcastle-upon-Tyne for 1937*; 29-30.
27. Joint Committee as to V.D. Clinic; *1.* 589/359 Tyne and Wear Archive.
28. Davenport-Hines R. *op cit* note 11, chapter 7.
29 Charles J A. *Annual Report of the Medical Officer of Health for Newcastle-upon-Tyne for 1939*; 12-13.
30. The venereal disease contact [editorial]. *Brit J Vener Dis* 1945; *21:* 1.
31. Wailes M. The Social Aspect of the Venereal Diseases – 2: contact tracing and the prostitute. *Brit J Vener Dis* 1945; *21:* 15-17.
32. Ramstedt K, Hallhagen G, Lundin B-I, et al. Contact tracing for human immunodeficiency virus (HIV) infection. *Sex Transm Dis* 1990; *17*: 37-41.
33. Venereal Disease: Regulation 33B [Medical notes in Parliament]. *Brit Med J* 1943; *1:* 25-26.

34. Joint Committee as to V.D. Clinic; *2*. 589/360 Tyne and Wear Archive.

35. 'Damaged Goods.' *Brit J Vener Dis* 1943; *19:* 91.

36. 'Health Education and Venereal Diseases.' *Brit Med J* 1943; *1*: 290.

37. 'Health Education and Venereal Diseases.' *Brit J Vener Dis* 1943; *19*: 85-91.

38. McCracken I E. *Annual Report of the Medical Officer of Health for Newcastle-upon-Tyne for 1944*; 23-24.

39. Prevention of Congenital Syphilis. *Brit J Vener Dis* 1944; *20:* 69.

40. *Medical Officer of Health Letter Book.* 592/465 Tyne and Wear Archive.

41. 'Anti-V.D. Vigilance Society.' *The Sunday Sun* 2 Nov 1943.

42. Johns H M. The Social Aspect of the Venereal Diseases — 3: contact tracing. *Brit J Vener Dis* 1945; *21:* 17-21.

43. Johns H M. The Social Background of Venereal Disease: a report on an experiment in contact tracing and an investigation into social conditions. *Brit J Vener Dis* 1945; *21:* 26-34.

44. National Library of Medicine. *Index and Catalogue of the Library of the Surgeon General's Office*. Fifth series, vol.III. Washington 1961.

45. Macfarlane W V. Some of the medico-social aspects of venereal diseases. *Public Health* 1948; *61*: 147-149.

46. Macfarlane W V. Further observations on the medico-social aspect of venereal diseases. *Public Health* 1948; *62:* 4-8.

47. Macfarlane W V, Johns H M, Schofield C B S. The Background of Congenital Syphilis: a search for a medico-social pattern in 200 families. Newcastle-upon-Tyne: Department of Venereology, Newcastle General Hospital [undated].

48. Wigfield A S. 27 years of uninterrupted contact tracing: the Tyneside Scheme. *Brit J Vener Dis* 1972; *48*: 37-50.

Chapter 25

THE DEVELOPMENT OF UROLOGY IN THE NORTHERN REGION

R R Hall and W Keith Yeates

Despite the use of the word *urology* in the English language since 1753, urology as a separate surgical speciality has been a phenomenon of the 20th century. In the United Kingdom its emergence was tardy and lagged behind the United States of America and most European countries. Even in 1993 the full recognition and implementation of 'urology by urologists' is incomplete, for general surgeon/urologists are still to be found operating in the Northern Region as elsewhere in Britain.

One particular early nidus of developing British urology was St Peter's Hospital ('for stricture and stone') in London; in the North of England it was the Department of Prostatic Surgery, opened in 1938 at Newcastle General Hospital, that made a unique contribution. Established specifically and primarily to provide facilities for endoscopic resection of the prostate for the citizens of Newcastle upon Tyne, it did so for 13 eventful years. In 1951 a metamorphosis produced a modern specialist urology service, which, in its turn, was translocated and superseded by the current Department of Urology at Freeman Hospital. However, the history of urology in the Northern Region really began at the Infirmary.

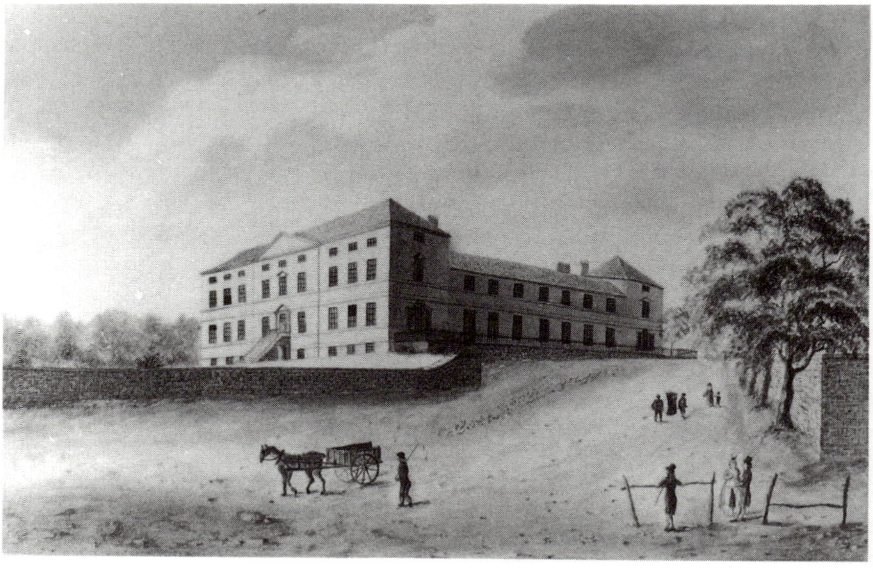

Figure 1. The Infirmary, Forth Banks 1753. Watercolour by Robert Johnson, reproduced with permission of the Laing Art Gallery, Newcastle upon Tyne (Tyne and Wear Museums).

The Infirmary

The first Infirmary in Newcastle was founded in 1751 and opened its doors on 23 May in temporary accommodation in a rented house in Gallowgate, just outside the northern city boundary. The first urological operation, the removal of a bladder stone, was recorded in the minutes of the House Committee of the 14 November 1751: 'Edward Lough age 51, the first patient cut for the stone in this infirmary, from whom a stone of 2 ounces weight was extracted, appeared before the committee and returned thanks'.[1]

The new Infirmary was built on Forth Banks overlooking the Tyne, but outside the city walls, at a cost — including bedding, linen and furniture — of £3697 7s 9¾d raised by public subscription.[2] Provision was made for 90 inpatients, but the wards soon became overcrowded as the Infirmary witnessed the growth of pre-Listerian surgery. The annual record for 1781 shows that urology accounted for 3.5% of the inpatient surgery and comprised:

Stones in the bladder	3
Fistula in perinea	3
Hydrocoele	6
Swollen testicle	1
Inflamed testicle	1
Schirrous testicle	2
Mortification of the testicle	1

In the 18th century incontinence was treated by physicians. The shorter expectation of life was naturally associated with a much lower incidence of prostatic obstruction than in later times, and retention of urine was managed by catheterisation on an outpatient basis.

The Newcastle upon Tyne School of Medicine and Surgery was founded in 1832. In 1852 the school became associated with the University of Durham under the title, 'The Newcastle upon Tyne College of Medicine in connection with the University of Durham', in 1870 becoming 'The University of Durham College of Medicine'.

The first Professor of Surgery in the College was George Yeoman Heath (1820–1892), the son of a well known ship owner. Heath joined the staff of the School of Medicine as lecturer on surgery in 1845, lecturer on anatomy 1846–47 and Surgeon to the Infirmary in 1854. In 1874 he was elected President of the College of Medicine and in 1889 became the first Professor of Surgery. He is recorded as 'always a student, well read and original thinker and blessed with a wonderful memory. He was a tall, powerful man who always dressed in rough tweeds like a country gentleman. He was unpunctual, sometimes exhibited a violent temper, was often impetuous and could be sarcastic. He was a giant from every point of view'.[3] Heath was a distinguished lithotomist and between 1854 and 1880 carried out 70 consecutive lithotomies without a death. He was able to resect a stone from the bladder in two minutes. He performed 104 lateral lithotomies before taking up lithotrity.

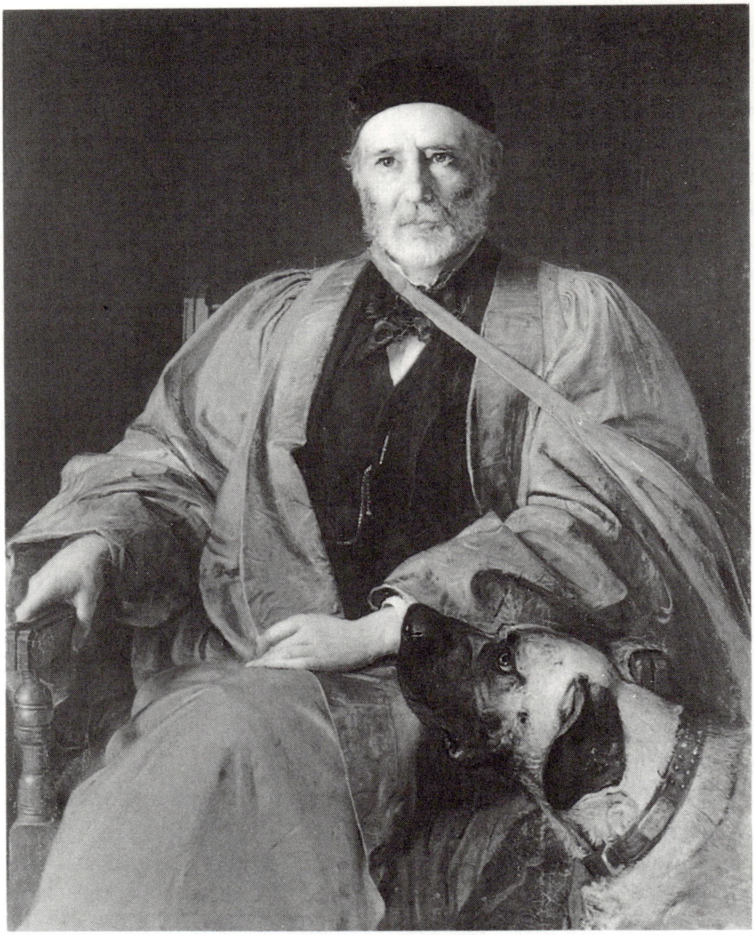

Figure 2. Professor George Yeoman Heath (1820-1892).
Oil painting by C Joy, The Medical School, University of Newcastle upon Tyne.

A friend and colleague of Heath was Dr CJ Gibb who was lecturer of surgery from 1848 and, from 1855 to 1870, an Honorary Surgeon to the Infirmary. Gibb was a popular surgeon who in private practice charged 2s 6d to rich and poor alike. His popularity is recorded in the song 'Blaydon Races':

> When we gat the wheel put on, away we went again,
> But them that had thor noses broke, they came back-owr hyem:
> Some went to the dispensary and some to Dr Gibb's,
> And some to the Infirmary to mend their thor broken ribs's.

During the first half of the 19th century, the surgeons' urological repertoire changed little; by the 1880s it included nephrotomy, perurethral lithotripsy, open removal of bladder tumour and internal urethrotomy. There is no record of attempts being made in Newcastle to relieve bladder

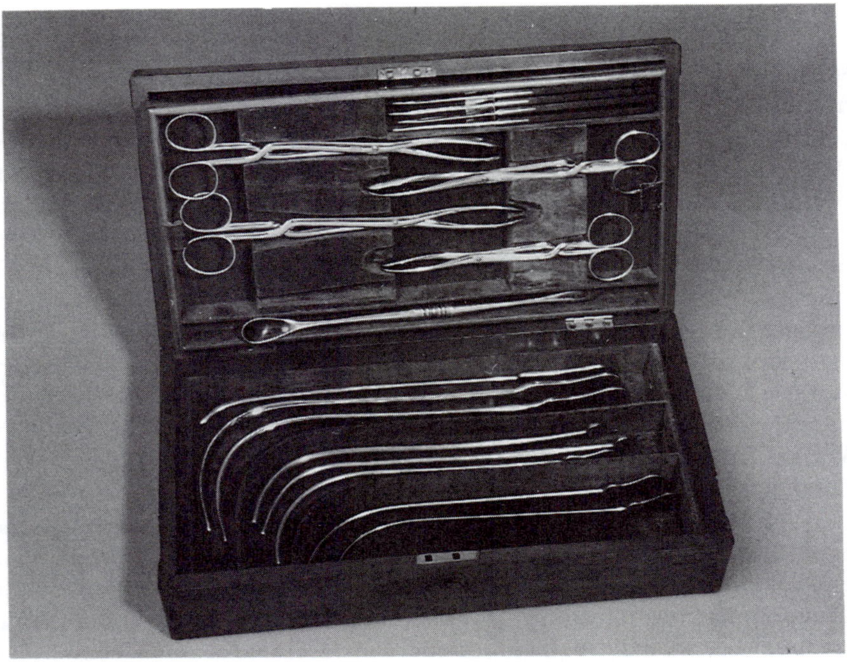

Figure 3. Lithotomy Set used by Dr CJ Gibb, (Honorary Surgeon to the Newcastle Infirmary, 1855-1870) showing metal 'sounds' to confirm the presence of a calculus in the bladder; a selection of knives, stone-grasping forceps and a curette.

outlet obstruction by blind transurethral techniques or incision or excision of small amounts of bladder neck tissue as were being attempted elsewhere. Table 1 lists the urological operations performed at the Infirmary towards the end of the 19th century.

Urological surgery in Newcastle at the end of the 19th century

	1884	1885	1887	1891
Nephrotomy	–	4	1	2
Nephorraphy	–	–	1	–
Suprapubic Lithotomy	9	4	5	6
Per-urethral lithotomy	1	5	7	2
Tapping of bladder	2	13	2	–
Tapping of hydrocoele	37	51	17	–
Perineal section	4	6	6	8
Internal urethrotomy	6	7	5	4
Median cystotomy	1	3	–	1
Removal of tumour from bladder	2	2	–	–
Amputation of penis	4	2	3	3
Amputation of testis	5	–	3	11
Circumcision	17	25	24	29
Radical cure of varicocoele	–	2	–	–

Table 1. Data from records of the Infirmary, Newcastle upon Tyne.

The first nephrectomy in Newcastle was performed in 1890 by Professor Frederick Page (Professor of Surgery 1899-1910). Page had a reputation as a skilful operator. The first 'examination of the bladder' and the first open prostatectomy (pioneered by McGill in Leeds in 1887) were done in 1898. At the turn of the century urology still accounted for only 3.5% of operations performed; in 1899, 80 out of a total of 20 283 surgical cases were urological.

The Infirmary had been enlarged in 1800 and again in 1854. But besides becoming progressively inadequate in size, 'during the east winds in the spring months it is considerably annoyed by immense clouds of smoke brought from the town and glasshouses'.[4] Also it was inconveniently near the cattle market and later was in line for the noises from the new railway station. A move had to be made. On 20 June 1900 the foundation stone of what was henceforth the Royal Victoria Infirmary was laid by HRH The Prince of Wales. The new infirmary with 560 beds received its first patient on 17 September 1906.

In 1907 Rutherford Morison, who was to become a most distinguished Professor of Surgery (1910-1921) stressed the disadvantages of blind open enucleation of prostatic enlargement: 'I do not like the ordinary operation of suprapubic prostatectomy. It is done in the dark, removes more than is essential, occasionally requires considerable force and is only accomplished by tearing all resisting tissues'.[5] He reported four successful operations performed under vision by wide exposure. However, open prostatectomy continued to be an operation associated with an undesirable degree of haemorrhage, mortality and length of hospital stay. The indications for advising its being undertaken were correspondingly strict.

Other Newcastle general surgeons with an interest in urology at the Infirmary included Grey Turner, RJ Willin, J Brumwell, J Gilmour and GY Feggetter who introduced the Stern McCarthy resectoscope to the Royal Victoria Infirmary in 1934, after working for a year at All Saints' Hospital, London.

Newcastle General Hospital

During the early 19th century the Newcastle Infirmary flourished with a growing number of patients all of whom, except surgical emergencies, had to be 'recommended' for treatment by the relatively affluent subscribers to the hospital.[6] Others, less fortunate, were accommodated in the Poor Houses. For the 'able-bodied poor' the Board of Guardians of the City built a single work-house in 1839 on the site of the present Newcastle General Hospital in Westgate Road. To care for the 'Sick, maternity cases, imbeciles..... and lame poor' a new Workhouse Hospital was built in the grounds in 1870 and was subsequently known as the Wingrove Hospital. This new hospital comprised 225 beds and was staffed by six nurses and one visiting doctor. In 1902 further wards were added including an 'Itch and venereal ward' which was later to become the Department of Prostatic Surgery. The hospital was renamed Newcastle General Hospital in 1930.

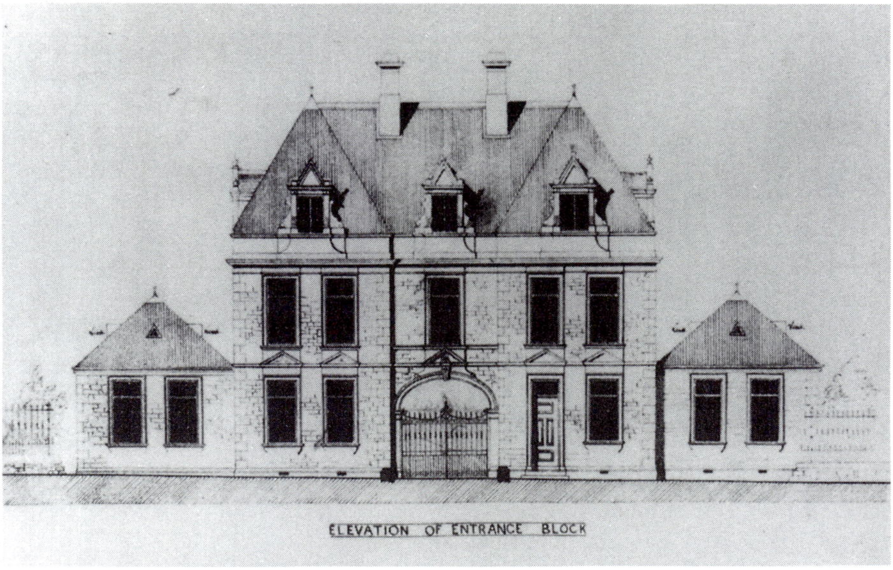

Figure 4. The Union Workhouse, Westgate Road, Newcastle upon Tyne. Front elevation of Entrance Block (1818-1839).

No surgery was performed in the Wingrove Hospital until 1922 when Morison was appointed to the staff. (His home became the Marie Curie Conrad House Hospice in 1957.) An assistant surgeon, Mr WEM Wardill, joined the staff in 1927. Wardill was a general surgeon who specialised initially in plastic surgery. In 1934 he was introduced to the early Stern McCarthy 'resecting cystoscope' by his colleague from the Infirmary Mr GY Feggetter, but showed no inclination to use it himself. However, a few years later he was to introduce the 'cold punch' resectoscope to Newcastle General Hospital instead.

By the early 1930s two quite separate techniques of perurethral resection of the prostate had developed in the United States. In one, originating and practised almost exclusively in the Mayo Clinic, the tissue was resected with a cylindrical steel knife blade – the 'cold punch'. Haemostasis was obtained by spot coagulation with a diathermy electrode. The alternative Stern McCarthy instrument resected tissue by means of a diathermy current passing through a fine wire loop. Hence the 'hot loop' resectoscope. Almost simultaneously, and for quite different reasons, the tissue-resecting ability of each instrument greatly improved. The Braasch-Bumpus cold punch, (which was a 'blind' instrument requiring rather tedious technical manipulations) was redesigned by Gershom Thompson at the Mayo Clinic, and a new diathermy circuit – the 'spark gap' – much enhanced the cutting ability of the hot loop under water.

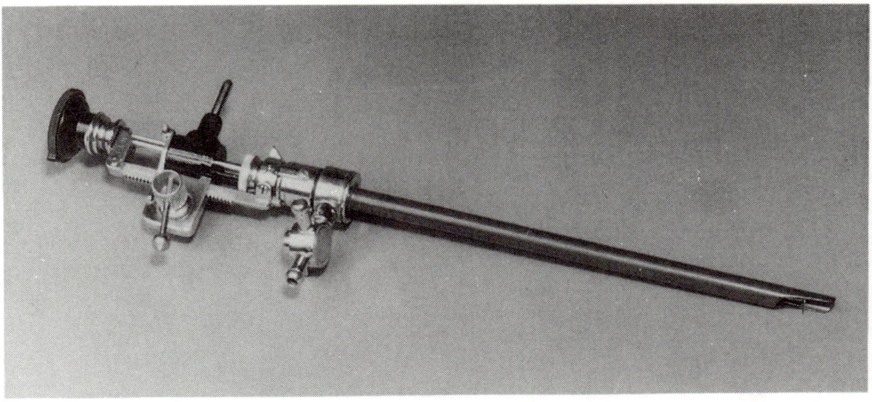

Figure 5. Stern McCarthy 'hot loop' resectoscope used at the Royal Victoria Infirmary, Newcastle, by Mr GY Feggetter.

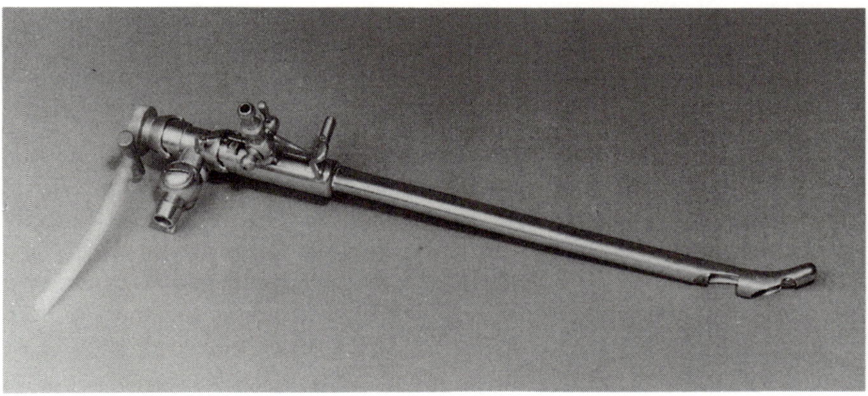

Figure 6. Gershom Thompson 'cold punch' resectoscope used in the Department of Prostatic Surgery, Newcastle General Hospital (before the addition of the 'thumb ring' by J Swinney).

As a result, by 1935, perurethral resection had become the usual procedure, in urological departments in the United States, for all except the very large prostates. The few British surgeons who were interested in replacing open prostatectomy by endoscopic prostatectomy seem to have visited the Mayo Clinic, with its cold punch technique, rather than other clinics using the hot loop. This may have been due to the inferior quality of the diathermy machines already installed in the United Kingdom, which did not have a spark gap current.

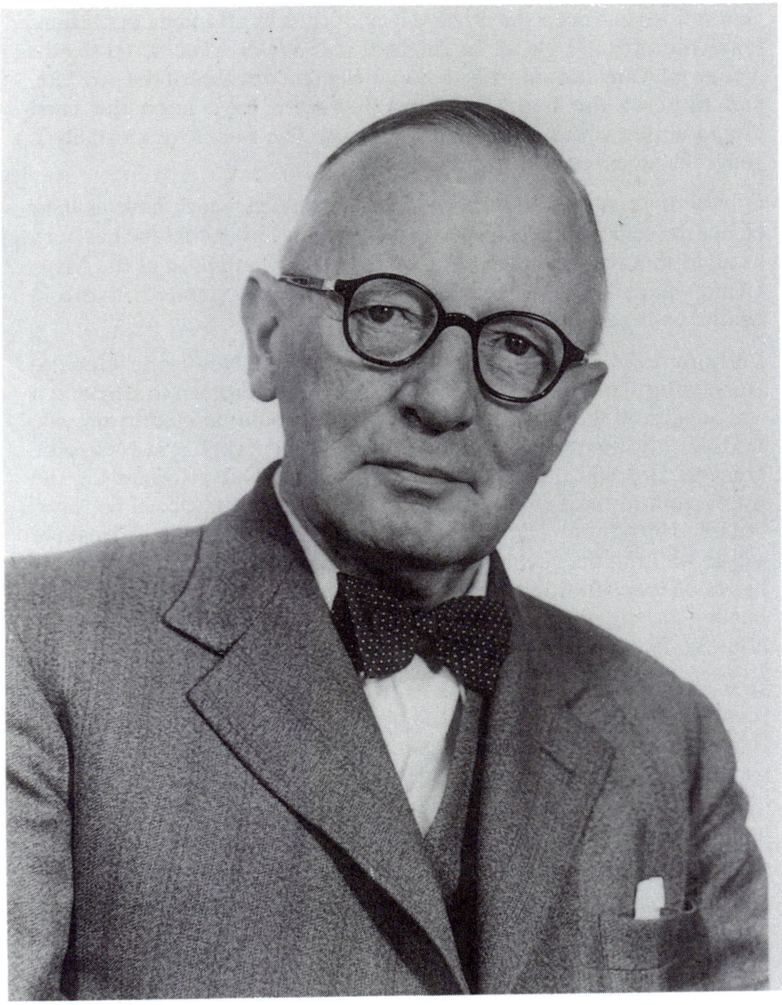

Figure 7. Mr William EM Wardill, Surgeon to the Department of Prostatic Surgery, Newcastle General Hospital (1927-1948).

In 1938 Wardill visited Gershom Thompson at the Mayo Clinic and returned with a cold punch resectoscope. Dr John Charles, Medical Officer of Health for Newcastle, later Sir John Charles, Chief Medical Officer of the Department of Health, was keen to establish specialist departments at Newcastle General Hospital and Wardill was provided with a Department of Prostatic Surgery which opened in 1938. The following extracts from the report of the Medical Officer of Health in Newcastle in 1938 describes vividly the enthusiasm with which this innovation was greeted.

> One of the most difficult questions which has perplexed surgeons for generations has been the relative lack of success attending operations upon the prostate gland. In England and Wales some 4,700 deaths among men are due annually to non-malignant diseases of the prostate, and hitherto the operation mortality rates have been the most disappointing which surgeons experience. The operative mortality is generally accepted as being about 15%.
>
> Of recent years operations have been developed, which have as their object the removal of the prostate piece meal. This technique has been brought to its highest perfection by Gershom Thompson at the Mayo Clinic, where during the year 1936, 749 cases were operated on with 11 deaths, giving a case mortality of 1.5%.
>
> Early in 1938 one of the consulting staff [of Newcastle General Hospital] spent a visit at the Mayo Clinic. On his return to England it was suggested that the Health Committee would be glad to provide facilities for the establishment of a prostatic department at Newcastle General Hospital.... A special operating suite was provided for the trans-urethral resection of the prostate with certain special features, notably a large water steriliser which can deliver a continuous stream of sterile water in the vicinity of the operating table. The adjacent wards had been specially fitted out for the easy nursing of the patients...... The nursing requirements of the average patient are relatively few because after the first 48 hours he is usually up and about.
>
> It is not too early to speak of the results of this method as revolutionary........ From the stand point of the hospital administration there are other advantages and benefits. The average number of days spent in hospital by the patient who recovered after treatment by the old method was 45. Under the new condition a patient is discharged on average after 15 days.
>
> This department is unique in Great Britain at the present time, and already the interest and keenness of those concerned in its inauguration have been well rewarded.

Over 250 transurethral prostatectomies were performed each year in the new department together with a small but growing amount of general urology; very few open prostatectomies were performed.

Wardill reported his experience with 230 cases of punch prostatectomy in the *Lancet* in 1941 and concluded:[7]

> Punch prostatectomy is the operation of choice for bladder neck obstruction, whether due to cancer, prostatic hypertrophy or median bar.... The period of confinement to bed is 1-2 days with average duration of stay in hospital about 12 days. The operation can be used in patients who are bad surgical risks, and is not contraindicated by the presence of calculi or infected urine. The safety of the operation excels that of any other method of surgical treatment available.... Punch resection is an operation carried out on the best surgical principles......... but the operative technique is difficult to acquire; in Gershom Thompson's opinion 'to put a resectoscope in the hands of a man who

is not prepared to study its use is like giving a submachine gun to a small boy who has been reading Deadwood Dick.'

On the introduction of the National Health Service, in 1948, Wardill retired. In the Department of Prostatic Surgery he was succeeded by Mr John Swinney who had previously been Assistant Surgeon to the Department and subsequently a Urologist at the Lovelace Clinic, Albuquerque, New Mexico. Swinney immediately expanded the breadth of the interest of the department as indicated by its change of title to the Department of Urology and the following year (1949) the department was established as the Regional Centre for Urological Surgery.

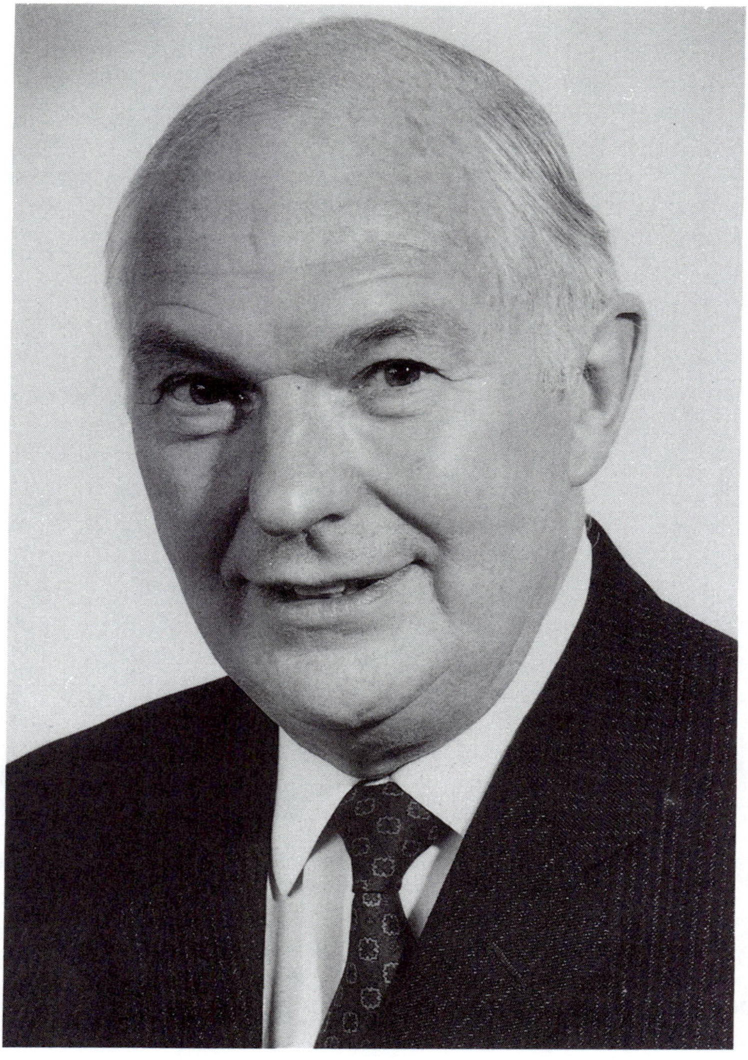

Figure 8. Professor John Swinney, Department of Urology, Newcastle General Hospital (1948-1974).

Mr WK Yeates who had been appointed Assistant Surgeon in 1947 and Senior Registrar in 1948 joined the Consultant Staff in 1951.

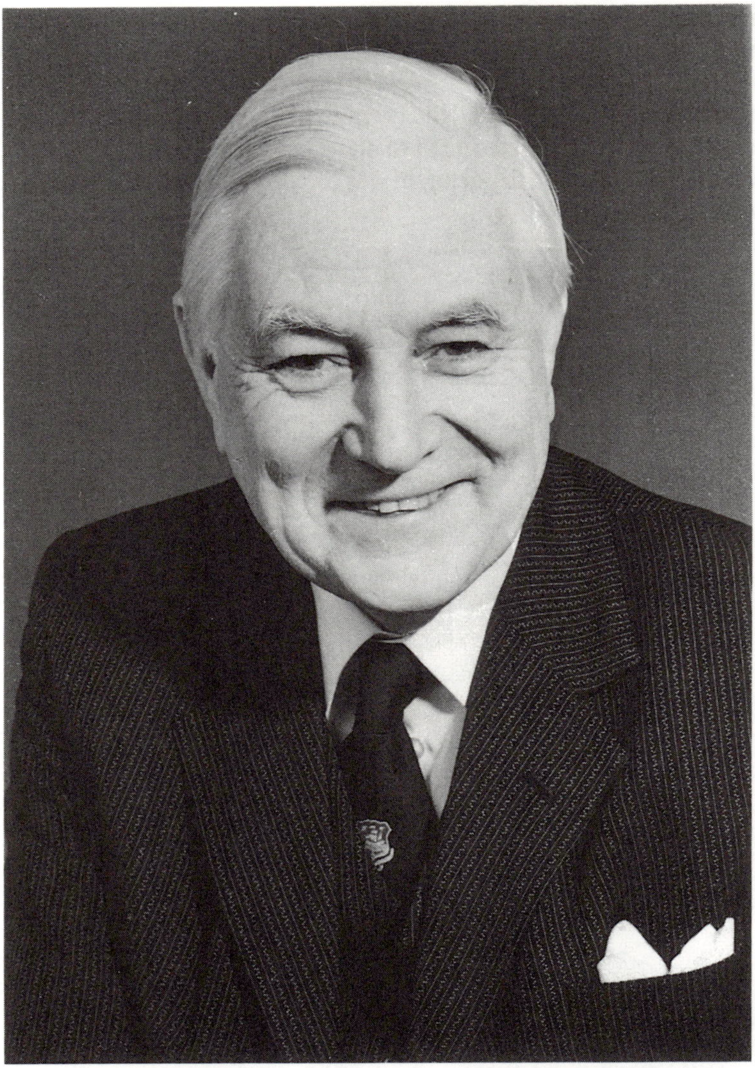

Figure 9. Mr W Keith Yeates, Consultant Urologist, Newcastle General Hospital (1951-1978) and Freeman Hospital (1978-1985).

The work of the department expanded rapidly and in 10 years the number of outpatients seen and operations performed more than trebled. The practice of punch prostatectomy was maintained and Swinney added his 'thumb ring' to the Gershom Thompson instrument. Such was the demand for specialist urology that the Department was rebuilt and enlarged on site in 1961 to provide 53 beds (43 male and 10 female), four consulting rooms, X-ray facilities, an outpatient cystoscopy suite and an inpatient operating theatre. Swinney's particular research interest was renal transplantation, which he helped to pioneer and for which he was subsequently awarded a personal Chair. The first renal transplantation in Newcastle was performed in this department in 1964.

Despite the excellence of these facilities, they were soon too small to cope with the demand for urology. A new hospital with a large urology department was being planned for Newcastle but, to bridge the gap, 26 beds and operating facilities were borrowed 15 miles away at Shotley Bridge General Hospital, County Durham, and a third consultant urologist, Mr DM Essenhigh, was appointed. Eight beds and operating theatre facilities were also provided at the Royal Victoria Infirmary where the general surgeons welcomed the aid of a specialist urologist.

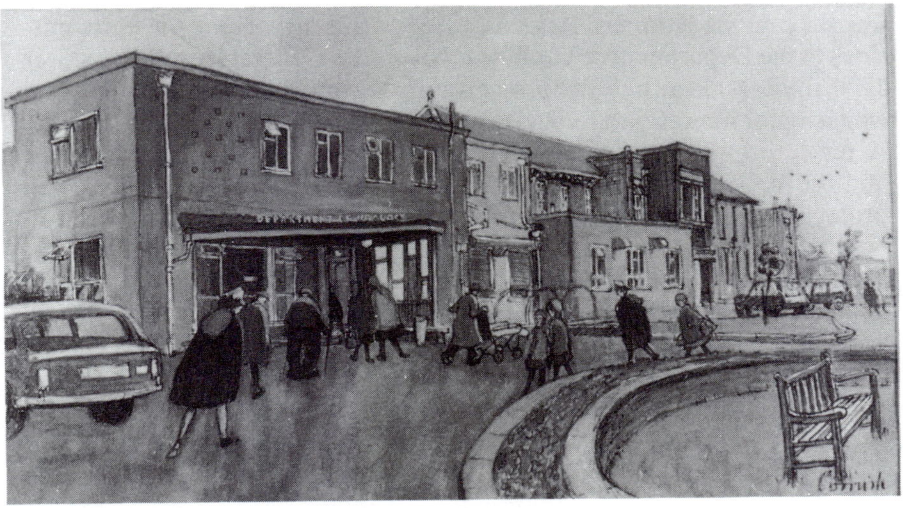

Figure 10. Department of Urology, Newcastle General Hospital. Original watercolour by Cornish, presented to Professor J Swinney on his retirement in 1974.

Professor Swinney retired in 1974 and was succeeded by Mr RR Hall. In 1978 the department was united as a single unit at the new Freeman Hospital, High Heaton, in the eastern end of the city. The consultant staff of three was augmented further by the appointment of Mr PD Ramsden in 1980. In 1985 Mr WK Yeates retired and was succeeded by MR PH Powell. At this time, endowments from the Northern Counties Kidney Research Fund and the William Leech Trust enabled the medical school to establish a new academic post at senior registrar level. It was named the Leech Green First Assistant in honour of Sir William Leech and Mr R Green, Chairman of the NCKRF. The first incumbent of this post, Mr DE Neal, was subsequently appointed Senior Lecturer and Honorary Consultant in Urology in 1990 and, in 1992, he was appointed Professor of Surgery in the Newcastle Medical School. The appointment of a urologist to the Chair of Surgery re-establishes the precedent of George Yeoman Heath after an interval of 103 years.

The present Urology Department at Freeman Hospital has 90 inpatient beds in three wards plus 11 day-case beds, two operating theatres, one outpatient cystoscopy theatre, a urodynamics suite, specialist uroradiology, andrology, a uro-oncology unit and research facilities, and it houses the Regional Lithotripsy Centre.

Development of Urology in the Northern Region outside Newcastle

A major boost in the evolution of urology in the United Kingdom was the founding of the British Association of Urological Surgeons (BAUS) in 1948 by the very few designated urologists and a group of general surgeons with particular interest in urology. Wardill was a founder member of the Association. The expansion of urology as a speciality throughout the country was slow. In the Northern Region in 1965, when the waiting list for admissions to the Department of Urology at Newcastle General Hospital was over 1000, there were still only two urologists on the staff plus one general surgeon with a major interest in urology, namely, Mr Hamilton Ross in Sunderland. At a meeting with representatives of the Northern Regional Hospital Board and the BAUS on 10 August 1965 it was proposed to appoint a second urologist in Sunderland, one in Middlesbrough, one in Carlisle and others in South Durham and Darlington in the next few years. For a number of reasons, partly financial, partly professional, these intuitive proposals were not implemented with alacrity. Nonetheless, at the present time, specialist urologists are working in Ashington (Mr JGW Feggetter), Carlisle (Mr RG Willis and Mr JA Cumming), Durham (Mr P English), Hartlepool (Mr JR Rhind), South Cleveland (Mr RS Hole, Mr JR Hindmarsh and Ms MJ Whiteway), North Tees (Mr RW Thompson), South Tyneside (Mr TG Armitage) and Sunderland (Mr C Parker and Mr RR Roy). With 16 urologists serving a population of approximately three million, the Northern Region is more than half way to the desirable proportion of about eight urologists per million. In the meantime the numerical deficiency is filled by the invaluable contributions of ten General Surgeons with a major interest in urology: in Bishop Auckland, Darlington, Durham, Gateshead, North Tyneside, Hexham, Shotley Bridge, South and West Cumbria.

Paediatric Urology

The surgical treatment of children with lesser genito-urinary disorders has been undertaken by urologists and general surgeons throughout the Region but a specialist paediatric urological service was provided for many years by Mr JES Scott at the Fleming Memorial Hospital for Sick Children, Newcastle. He was appointed in 1960 as Lecturer in the Department of Surgery, University of Durham, with a special interest in paediatric surgery.

From the late 1970s until his retirement in 1991, Scott devoted his work almost exclusively to urological surgery in neonates and children, together with the management of many of the more common nephrological disorders and childhood renal failure. Paediatric urology in Newcastle is currently undertaken by the surgical team of the Fleming Wing at the Royal Victoria Infirmary which was established following the closure of the Fleming Memorial Hospital in 1987.

Conclusion

In common with most forms of medicine, the nature and prevalence of disease afflicting the urinary and male genital systems have changed with the passing of two centuries. Men live much longer but very rarely die of 'benign' prostatic enlargement; the industrial revolution and cigarette smoking have caused many thousands of bladder cancers; the cold punch resectoscope has been made redundant by technological innovations that have made the hot loop far more versatile and much safer; sophisticated physiological measurement has revealed some, but not all, of the mysteries of bladder function. Investigatory techniques have become not only more accurate but less invasive. Bladder stones are now rare but kidney stones are much more common. Professor Heath would smile to see the computerised wonder of the 1990s lithotriptor, but might well suggest that the swiftness of the lithotomist's knife still had something to recommend it.

References

1. Minutes of the House Committee, Newcastle General Infirmary. The City Archives, Newcastle upon Tyne.
2. Mackenzie E. *A descriptive and historical account of the Town and County of Newcastle upon Tyne*. Newcastle upon Tyne: Mackenzie and Dent, 1827; II:503.
3. Turner G. *The Newcastle upon Tyne School of Medicine 1834-1934*. Newcastle upon Tyne: Andrew Reed, 1934: 169-173.
4. Mackenzie E. *op cit* note 2:II: 510.
5. Morison JR. *Surgical Contributions from 1881-1916. Vol II, Abdominal Surgery*. Bristol: John Wright, 1916:709-10.
6. Mackenzie E. *op cit* note 2:II: 510.
7. Wardill WEM. Punch Prostatectomy. *Lancet* 1941; *II*:127-29.

Chapter 26

IN MEMORIAM EDMUND ANTHONY SPRIGGS

David Gardner-Medwin

Edmund Anthony Spriggs was born on the 30 March 1918, in Banff.

His father, Dr Edmund Ivens Spriggs, had been a physician at Guy's and later St George's Hospitals but had been advised, when he developed pulmonary tuberculosis, to leave London. So he had moved north and had founded a distinguished private clinic at Duff House, a handsome mansion near Banff built by William Adam for the Duke of Fife in 1735. He and Tony's mother, Alice Watson before their marriage, had both been brought up in Foxton in Leicestershire where her father owned a farm and was the local Squire.

In 1919, when Tony was still a baby, his two elder sisters died in a drowning accident. Not long after, in the early 1920s, the Clinic moved, with the family and many of the staff, to Ruthin Castle in the Vale of Clwyd. There Tony's father, already a widely respected diagnostician and an early expert, for example, in the use of insulin for diabetes and of liver extract for pernicious anaemia, attracted many notable patients. His distinction continued to be recognised also by his peers for, in 1944, he delivered the Harveian Oration at the Royal College of Physicians, and in 1945 he was awarded the KCVO. Tony and his younger brother Arthur had memories of some of the patients. John Buchan took an interest in their plans for a hill-walking expedition; they were intimidated by Maynard Keynes but were enthralled by the Maharajah of Nawasagar and by the cricketer Duleep Singh. The Princess Victoria was also for a long time a patient at the clinic. It was at Ruthin too that Conacher, the gamekeeper from Banff, taught Tony to fish, his lifelong passion.

After prep school, at Summer Fields in Oxford, Tony went up to Winchester in 1931. There he seemed to have been an industrious and rather serious young man. But there too his love of fishing flourished, further stimulated when he heard Earl Grey of Fallodon speak about it at the College. Another school memory was of Sir Robert Hutchinson who was consulted when he developed erysipelas.

Despite his often idyllic surroundings and his devotion to his stimulating and exuberant father, Tony was not always a happy young man. His mother had died when he was 14 years old. Even after going up to New College, Oxford in 1936, he remained rather shy, burying himself in work. Soon afterwards, in 1937, he and Arthur were taken on the long sea voyage to New Zealand, together with their new stepmother, when their father was invited to give the opening address at the BMA Congress in Wellington.

He concentrated on physiology in his third year. War intervened after his first degree (BA Oxon 1939) and with other medical students Tony was housed in Worcester College during his clinical course. He qualified in 1942 and immediately went to the Postgraduate Medical School (founded only 7 years earlier) as House Officer, promptly gaining the MRCP the following year. As soon as he had registered, Tony joined the RAMC in time to prepare for the Normandy landings, sealed off from the world at Purbeck. Two months after D-Day he crossed to Normandy but his supply ship struck a mine and he spent three frustrating months based at Caen, without adequate equipment, unable to put his enthusiasm fully into practice and 'visiting cathedrals'. Then in 1945 he was posted to India, to the Coromandel Coast which he loved, but was again deeply frustrated in his work, caring for war-weary troops with war- weary nurses, all longing to be demobilised. His matron 'broke down' and had to be sent home.

It must have been a vast relief to return to England and the Hammersmith in 1947. There he spent the next three years working with P Sharpey-Schafer, Sir John McMichael (appointed Professor of Medicine the previous year) and Sheila Sherlock; there too he met Avery Jones, a lifelong friend. In Professor Aird's department he worked with EJ Holborow on the use of nebulised penicillin in the prevention of chest complications after abdominal surgery, but his main interest at that stage was in gastroenterology and it was this that he studied during his Fellowship at the Mayo Foundation in 1950-51.

Just before he left for the States he and Sheila More were married. They had known each other since they were infants together in Banff, where Sheila's father had been Sheriff, and where her family had lived in the Dower House in the grounds of Duff House. Sheila had been born in Strathpeffer and lived in Banff from 1918 to 1938 before moving to St Andrews, and it was there that they were married.

At the Mayo Clinic Tony worked with the physiologist Charles F Code and the physician Dr JA Bargen on the motility of the pelvic colon and rectum. They used a system of tandem balloons to study the bowel in ulcerative colitis, concluding that haustral activity was diminished and occasional mass movements of the colon were increased in comparison with normal subjects. The study was the subject of his DM thesis (1952) and characteristically Tony inscribed its title page with a quotation from Benjamin Franklin 'What comfort can the vortices of Descartes give to a man who has whirlwinds in his bowels?'

Tony and Sheila returned home to Ruthin Castle in 1951 and he stayed as Physician for two years. Sir Edmund had died in 1949 and for a while Tony considered whether to carry on his work at the Castle (at that stage run by Dr SW Patterson), no doubt tempted by his love of the country and the beauties of the Vale of Clwyd as well as by the family ties. But the Health Service had started just before his father had died, and Tony devoted himself to its principles. It was also clear to him that private clinics like Ruthin Castle were in decline. So he and his brother sold their shares in the concern, enabling the employees there to receive pensions, and Tony moved north with his family in 1953.

One paper published in the *BMJ* in 1954 reflected his work at Ruthin Castle – on 'Kinking, rotation and twisting of the stomach' – written in collaboration with OA Marxer, the Swiss radiographer who had worked for the Clinic since the Duff House days. Together they collected 44 cases concluding, with Tony's usual common sense, that the X-ray appearances were 'usually unimportant incidental findings, and the greatest harm they are in most cases likely to do is to interest a physician or surgeon who does not recognise this fact.' Tony presented this paper at the meeting of the Association of Physicians held in Dublin in June 1954 using a model of the stomach made for him by his wife for a graphic demonstration. It was an occasion in which he took pride and it was a longstanding disappointment to him that he was never proposed for membership of the Association. Some years later he combined his experience of the mechanical function of the stomach and bowel in an article on flatulence for the *British Journal of Clinical Practice*.

The move to the north in 1953 meant starting again in a more junior post, as Senior Registrar at the Brierton Hospital in West Hartlepool. He and Sheila, by now with a young family, lived in Sedgefield. In South East Durham he was impressed by the pioneer work of Dr JB Robinson and Dr KM Chalmers in treating patients with pulmonary tuberculosis 'with a minimum of rest and, in a large proportion of cases, at work'. In 1955, having now developed an interest in chest medicine eclipsing that in gastroenterology, he took on the isolated tuberculosis sanatorium at Barrasford in Northumberland, as Physician Superintendent, with consultant sessions as Physician to the West End Chest Clinic in Newcastle. At Barrasford he and the family lived in the Superintendent's house overlooking the North Tyne Valley. His predecessor, Dr DGR Goodwin, an enthusiast for exercise in the treatment of TB at a period when this was not the fashion, had occupied the post since 1918. At the time tuberculosis sanatoria everywhere were at the end of their useful lives and Tony knew that it was his task to preside over the closure of Barrasford and to develop from his joint appointment a new pattern of practice as a Chest Physician. In an article in 1957 for the *NAPT Bulletin* he wrote 'The modern chest physician is not a thoroughbred. He is by the tuberculosis officer out of the general physician, and the stable which bred him in 1948 – the National Health Service – must sometimes be puzzled about his proper functions and most useful future'. His provisional opinions depended 'on impressions of successful trends in the prevention of tuberculosis, and of satisfactory permanent results of treatment, and both are still statistically *sub judice*'. He strongly favoured the appointment of consultant physicians who would have a specialist interest in chest diseases, but with general responsibilities and with beds in general medical wards as well as in isolation wards. They would need access to convalescence units and these should be on the outskirts of the cities where, unlike the isolated sanatoria, they could attract staff.

His sense of history made him keenly aware that he was working at a time of rapid change in the importance of tuberculosis, and in the early 1960s he wrote three articles on rest, exercise and the institutional treatment of pulmonary tuberculosis. Characteristically the first was a detailed historical survey which began 'The best reason for reading the history of medicine is the fun of it. But it also puts into perspective the fashions of today' and, after recounting the fluctuating fashions since the time of Hippocrates and commenting on the new practice of statistical analysis of the effects of treatment, ended 'How could anyone familiar with this extraordinary story ever accept a clinical impression about treatment as final?' With Dr AA Bruce, his colleague at Barrasford, a comparative trial of rest and exercise was arranged at the Chest Clinic and the Sanatorium. They started in 1955, accepted 382 patients, retained 315 for analysis and followed them up for four years, finding no substantial difference in outcome in the two groups when they published their paper in 1964. Tony went to Amsterdam to present the work with a delightfully light touch to a meeting of the Netherlands Tuberculosis Association in 1961, commenting in his published text 'Yesterday, as I was going through Leiden, I was just able to catch a glimpse of the statue of Boerhaave; he once maintained that a tuberculosis cavity should be ripened and broken up by riding on horse-back.'

Other interests in the 1960s were the management of mucopurulent chronic bronchitis (he contributed to the British Tuberculosis Assocation multicentre trial of cephaloridine treatment); and seasonal asthma on which he did a study with Dr F Blackburn from the Department of Plant Science in Newcastle University, of air borne pollen and mould counts and the value of sensitivity testing and desensitisation of patients. This was published in 1968 in the *Newcastle Medical Journal.*

One of his major campaign interests was in the dangers of smoking. As far as I know his only publication on this subject was an unsigned little article in the Newcastle General Hospital *Nurses League Journal* (1962); but he worked tirelessly, using his influence as a doctor, as he exhorted his colleagues and friends to do, 'in our professional work and in our private lives and in any public activities which we may enjoy, to persuade people to avoid an unnecessary risk of contracting lung cancer'. Shortly after this he was one of the founders of the North of England branch of 'ASH'. He startled at least one young registrar by writing to him after he had overheard him objecting to smoking in the hospital dining room, to recruit his support for a campaign to ban smoking in the dining rooms and the sale of cigarettes by the hospital's League of Friends.

In 1959 the Barrasford Sanatorium closed and Tony was able to concentrate on his work in Newcastle. It was also the opportunity for the family to move to River House in Wylam. Since 1955 he had had a consultant post at the West End Chest Clinic in Elswick Road where he continued to work until he retired. In 1959 he became Consultant Chest Physician at Newcastle General Hospital with beds in Ward 9. Dr George Hurrell had founded the Chest Unit there in 1949, and when Hurrell retired in 1961 Tony succeeded him as the Consultant in Charge. He added a pulmonary function laboratory to the unit in the early 1960s. He also shared duties on a general medical firm, and this was more formally recognised when in 1964 he and Dr JR Lauckner (appointed Chest Physician in 1961) both became Consultant Physicians to the hospital, ending the tradition of appointing pure chest physicians.

One had only to be swept into a conversation with Tony to know that he was a good teacher. The youngest Newcastle doctors to have known him remember him as an inspiring teacher, a friendly physician and, like most people who encountered him however briefly, above all as a gentleman. He was deeply involved in the setting up of the Postgraduate Medical Centre at Newcastle General Hospital; his first moves in this direction had been to try to improve the hospital's library services and were recorded in the Hospital Medical Staff Committee's minutes from 1963. He began soon after this to twist the sometimes reluctant arms of his colleagues into pooling the resources of their departmental libraries to create a really good hospital medical library. He remained Honorary Librarian and Chairman of the Library Committee until he retired. In June 1966 the first part of the Postgraduate Centre was established with a large lecture theatre and a dining room, both reconstructed from the dining room once used by the inmates of the Wingrove Workhouse. The Library was added above it during the next two years and on 19 September 1968 the Postgraduate Medical Centre was officially opened by Professor GA Smart.

Tony did not relish administration, but he was too good at it for his colleagues to allow him to escape and in 1972 and 1973 he was a very effective Chairman of the Hospital Medical Committee. His diplomatic skills were needed in coping with one particularly difficult senior colleague and the matter was dealt with so unobtrusively that few members of the staff knew that anything had happened.

He retired in 1983. A large and entirely delightful party was held at Close House. His speech on that occasion some thought the best retirement speech they had ever heard.

Many other important themes ran through Tony's life. To an outsider his family life was transparently the greatest happiness of his very happy life. He was a member of the local parish church — St Oswins, Wylam, faithful in attendance, frank about his doubts, and active in the life of the church, even taking responsibility for cutting the churchyard hedge.

He was a countryman at heart all his life. Like his father, he loved retrievers and trained them. One of his special joys was shooting in Northumberland. My earliest memory of him was when we had just moved north from London and met Tony walking his dogs by the Tyne. 'Come beagling with us on Boxing Day' he said. We did, and afterwards went on to the first of many glorious buffet parties at his home. Later he and Sheila invited friends to regular Scottish country dance parties where the living room carpet was rolled back and we danced, enough of us for three or four sets, and were scrumptiously fed afterwards. He loved wild places, and fishing, learned as a boy on the Clywyd and the Itchen, was a passion all his life. For many years he had fishing rights in the North Tyne and he was overjoyed in the mid-1970s when the pollution of the Tyne was sufficiently controlled to allow the return of salmon to the river. Characteristically his first Tyne salmon was shared with friends at a party. The family say that Tony admitted to only one ambition – to catch a Tyne salmon, and later, when this had been achieved, to catch a big one. In his last season this too was fulfilled when he caught a 20 pound fish near Wylam. Tony's son Michael says that the only time he ever saw his father agitated was when another son, Edmund, was playing his first salmon.

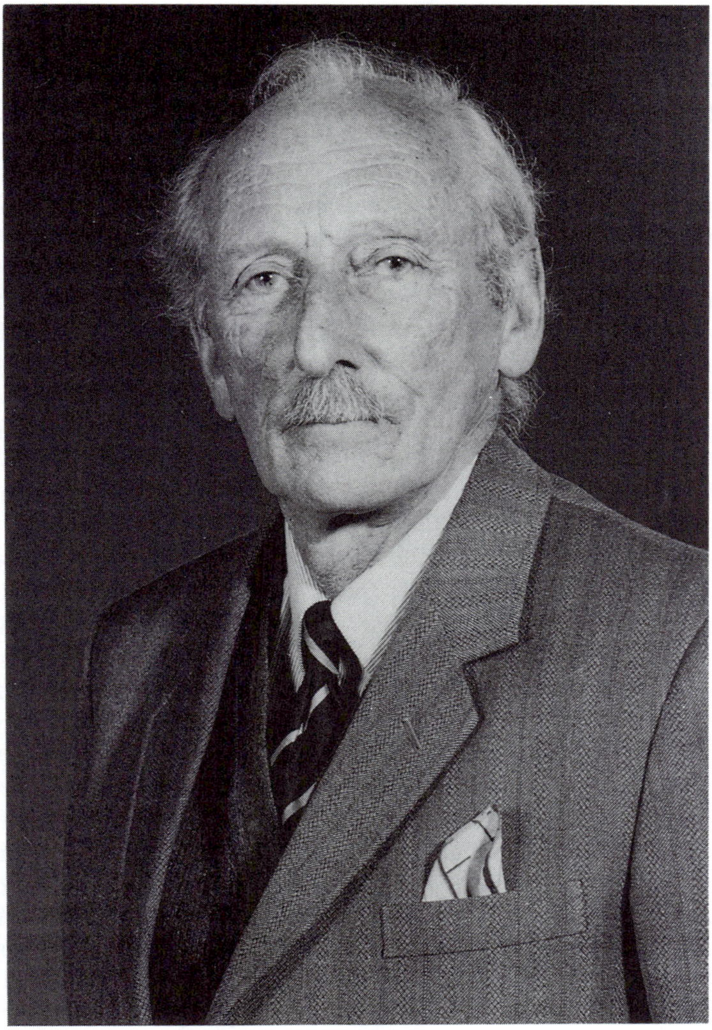

Figure 1. Tony Spriggs

When he retired Tony and Sheila took up bookbinding. Tony continued binding for the rest of his life with great care and considerable flair, though always modestly disparaging his artistic ability. An early project was to bind his father's collected offprints, and later his own, and many of the books to which he had devoted many weeks were given to his family, a special prayerbook, and a precious set of early 19th century flower paintings by one of the Lorraine family of Little Harle for his daughter Kitty. He was imperturbable in important matters but loved to show his impatience at the more pedestrian binding tasks, always with a twinkle in his eye that brought merriment to his friends in the binding class. On one occasion he had planned an elaborate and handsome gold tooled eider drake for the cover of his lovingly bound *Birds of Northumbria*. It came out beautifully, but upside down. Everyone in the class suffered agonies for him but Tony cheerfully inset a new bit of leather and just did it again.

One of Tony's most abiding joys was medical history. At Oxford his essay 'John Hunter and his approach to Pathology' won the Radcliffe Infirmary Prize in Pathology for 1941. In a footnote he wrote 'it is the preliminary to a more extended study which it is hoped to make when the present emergency is over'. The essay was later published in the *Annals of Science* (December 1942). It is a sparkling account of Hunter's place in 18th-century society, displaying an astonishing breadth of reading outside the scope of medicine, as well as the persistence he must have shown in ploughing through the works of one of the most notoriously bad writers of all the great figures in British medical history. 'Hunter's writing, though badly set out, and often difficult to follow, is not on the whole dull' was Tony's imperturbable way of putting it. Sadly 'the present emergency' was followed by other distractions and his next published contribution to medical history was not until 1960 ('Rest and exercise in pulmonary tuberculosis: a study of fashions in treatment'), and indeed he never returned to John Hunter himself though he did to one of his entourage in 'The illnesses and death of Robert Walpole' in 1982. That the 'Rest and exercise' paper was published during the planning stage of his research project at Barrasford, is a tribute to Tony's deep understanding of the importance of medical history and an object lesson to those of us who add a pinch of history as an afterthought to a paper after the work is done.

In 1975, together with Joan Emmerson and Jim Longrigg, who was already running a series of medical history seminars in the University Department of Classics, Tony founded the Pybus Club and for the next 9 years or so he and Jim ran the Club in two parts, the 'Classical wing' and the 'Hospital wing', an unconventional but entirely harmonious and successful arrangement. There had been earlier gatherings of a dining club in which Mr Dudfield Rose, Dr Robert Mowbray, Dr MHA ('Peter') Davidson, the University Librarian Dr McKenna, Miss Joan Emmerson, Professor Peter Isaacs and Dr CE Kellett had been active, largely centred on early medical books. Tony's concept was different; with a light touch he persuaded speakers to talk on a wide variety of topics, holding meetings in attractive surroundings varying from Close House to the West End Chest Clinic. He contributed papers himself: on John Hutchinson of Ryton, the first man to use spirometry in clinical practice (this was later presented in collaboration with Dr B Gandevia of Sydney, Australia and Mr PJ Bishop, librarian at the Brompton Hospital, at a meeting of the Royal Society of Medicine); on the history of spirometry; on Robert Walpole; and on Dr Hector Gavin 1815-55. Gavin was the brother of Sheila Spriggs' great grandmother. His father's manuscript biography of him was then still in the family's possession and was later presented to the Wellcome Library at Tony's suggestion. He gave an account of Gavin's life, his work for the Sanitary Movement, especially on Tyneside, during the period of devastating urban epidemics of cholera (likening the tribulations of the Movement's campaign to those of the anti-smoking campaign in which he himself was engaged at the time), and describing his assignment as Sanitary Commissioner to the Army in the Crimea and his tragic death there when a revolver he was handing to his brother went off accidentally. Most of these papers were later published in *Medical History*.

Tony was a keen supporter of the British Society of the History of Medicine and represented the Pybus Club at many of its meetings. After he retired, the hospital wing of the club became inactive for three years despite his attempts to find a successor. He was very glad when it revived in 1986, but only rather reluctantly agreed to chair the first meeting, and when pressed repeatedly to become President he always managed to disappear mysteriously. It was clear that he felt his creation should find its own feet.

One evening in November 1988, Tony made some uncharacteristic mistakes in his bookbinding. He seemed uneasy, but his conversation was as wide ranging as ever. Ten days later a scan had shown a brain tumour. He told me so when I visited him in the neurology ward, discussed with diagnostic shrewdness why he thought it was a glioma not a metastasis (he was right); announced that he had requested the opinion of a neurosurgeon who would try no unnecessary heroics; discussed which fishing pools on the North Tyne he would choose next season if his now hemiparetic leg was still troubling him; and asked me to find out for him, for a friend who had enquired, the details of the Newcastle physician George R Murray's first use of thyroid extract in treating myxoedema. Only later did the conversation seem like a summing-up. He died on the 28th December 1988.

At the memorial service in Wylam on the 6th January 1989, St Oswin's Church was crowded to the doors. Three years later a stained glass window, made by LC Evetts, was dedicated there to Tony's memory.

While he was ill, and after he died, the word that came to everyone's lips was 'gentleman', several independently quoted Chaucer's 'a verray parfit gentil knyght'. But Tony Spriggs' special quality was to combine his instinctive and unvarying courtesy with gaiety, generosity and enthusiastic interest in those he met and in everything they did, as well as in his own many interests. His patients must have loved him; his friends certainly did.

Acknowledgements

I am grateful to the Spriggs family from whom most of the information was gleaned; and to many of Tony's colleagues and friends.

EA Spriggs' bibliography

1. Spriggs EA. John Hunter and his approach to pathology. *Ann Sci* 1942; *5*:177-184.
2. Holborow EJ, Spriggs EA. Nebulised penicillin and post-operative pulmonary complications. *Lancet* 1948; *2*:688.
3. Spriggs EA. *The motility of the human pelvic colon and rectum in health and in certain abnormal conditions*. Thesis for the degree of DM at the University of Oxford 1952.
4. Spriggs EA and Marxer AO. Kinking, rotation, and twisting of the stomach with special reference to cascade stomach and chronic gastric volvulus. *Brit Med J* 1954; *2*:325-30.
5. Spriggs EA, Code CD, Bargen JA, Curtiss RK, Hightower NC. Motility of the pelvic colon and rectum of normal persons and patients with ulcerative colitis. *Gastroenterology* 1957; *19*:480-491.
6. Spriggs EA. The Modern Chest Physician: a series of articles contributed by invitation. What is his future? *Nat Assoc Pulm Tuberculosis Bull* 1957; *20*:66-7.
7. Spriggs EA. Flatulence. *Brit J Clin Prac* 1959; *13*:795-801.
8. Spriggs EA. Rest and exercise in pulmonary tuberculosis: a study of fashions in treatment. *Tubercle* 1960; *41*:455-62.
9. Spriggs EA. Rest and exercise in pulmonary tuberculosis. *Proc Tuberculosis Res Council* 1961; *48*:3-10.
10. Anon (Spriggs EA). Smoking and lung cancer. *Newcastle General Hospital Nurses' League Journal* 1962; (No vol nos):26-29.
11. Brace AA and Spriggs EA. Bed rest and institutional treatment in pulmonary tuberculosis. *Amer Rev Resp Dis* 1964; *90*:183-193.
12. Citron KM, Emerson PA, Joyce CRB, May JR, Selkon JB, Sommer AR and Spriggs EA. Cephaloridine compared with penicillin and streptomycin in exacerbations of chronic mucopurulent bronchitis: Report to the Research Committee of the British Tuberculosis Association. *Lancet* 1968; *2*:592-594.
13. Blackburn F, Spriggs EA. Seasonal asthma in Newcastle upon Tyne. *Newcastle Med J* 1968; *30*:197- 203.
14. Spriggs EA, Gandevia B and Bishop PJ. John Hutchinson (1811-1861), inventor of the spirometer. *Proc Roy Soc Med* 1976; *69*:450 (abstract).
15. Spriggs EA. John Hutchinson, inventor of the spirometer – his North Country background, life in London and scientific achievements. *Med Hist* 1977; *21*:357-364.
16. Spriggs EA. The history of spirometry. *Brit J Dis Chest* 1978; 72:165-180.
17. [Spriggs EA]. The revenge of Freeman Hospital. Anonymous contribution to the 'In England Now' column. *Lancet* 1979; *1*:1134.
18. Spriggs EA. The illnesses and death of Robert Walpole. *Med Hist* 1982; *26*:421-428.
19. [Spriggs EA]. Clinical encounter: Death on the train. Anonymous contribution *Brit Med J* 1983; *286*:1727.
20. Spriggs EA. Hector Gavin, MD, FRCSE (1815-1855) – his life, his work for the sanitary movement and his accidental death in the Crimea. *Med Hist* 1984; *28*:283-292.

INDEX

Books! 'tis a dull and endless strife:
Come, hear the woodland linnet,
How sweet his music! on my life
There's more of wisdom in it.
And hark! how blithe the throstle sings!
He too is no mean preacher:
Come forth into the light of things,
Let Nature be your Teacher.

William Wordsworth
Lyrical Ballads, 1798